theclinics.com

CLINICS IN PERINATOLOGY

Infectious Diseases in Pregnancy

GUEST EDITORS
Lisa M. Hollier, MD, MPH
George D. Wendel, Jr, MD

September 2005 • Volume 32 • Number 3

SAUNDERS
An Imprint of Elsevier, Inc.
PHILADELPHIA LONDON TORONTO MONTREAL SYDNEY TOKYO

W.B. SAUNDERS COMPANY
A Division of Elsevier Inc.

Elsevier, Inc., 1600 John F. Kennedy Blvd., Suite 1800, Philadelphia, PA 19103-2899

http://www.theclinics.com

CLINICS IN PERINATOLOGY **Volume 32, Number 3**
September 2005 **ISSN 0095-5108**
Editor: Carin Davis **ISBN 1-4160-2756-4**

Reprints. For copies of 100 or more, of articles in this publication, please contact the Commercial Reprints Department, Elsevier Inc., 360 Park Avenue South, New York, New York 10010-1710. Tel. (212) 633-3813, Fax: (212) 462-1935, e-mail: reprints@elsevier.com.

Clinics in Perinatology (ISSN 0095-5108) is published quarterly by Elsevier, Inc., Corporate and editorial offices: Elsevier, Inc., 1600 John F. Kennedy Blvd., Suite 1800, Philadelphia, PA 19103-2899. Accounting and circulation offices: 6277 Sea Harbor Drive, Orlando, FL 32887-4800. Periodicals postage paid at Orlando, FL 32862, and additional mailing offices. Subscription prices are $155.00 per year (US individuals), $237.00 per year (US institutions), $183.00 per year (Canadian individuals), $293.00 per year (Canadian institutions), $215.00 per year (foreign individuals), $293.00 per year (foreign institutions), $78.00 per year (US students), and $108.00 per year (foreign students). Foreign air speed delivery is included in all Clinics subscription prices. All prices are subject to change without notice. POSTMASTER: Send address changes to *Clinics in Perinatology*, W.B. Saunders Company, Periodicals Fulfillment, Orlando, FL 32887-4800. **Customer Service: 1-800-654-2452 (US). From outside of the US, call 1-407-345-4000.** E-mail: hhspcs@harcourt.com.

Clinics in Perinatology is also published in Spanish by McGraw-Hill Interamericana Editores S.A., P.O. Box 5-237, 06500 Mexico D.F., Mexico.

Clinics in Perinatology is covered in *Index Medicus, Current Contents, Excerpta Medica, BIOSIS,* and *ISI/BIOMED.*

Printed in the United States of America.

GUEST EDITORS

LISA M. HOLLIER, MD, MPH, Assistant Professor, Division of Maternal-Fetal Medicine, Department of Obstetrics, Gynecology, and Reproductive Sciences, University of Texas Houston Medical School, Lyndon B. Johnson General Hospital, Houston, Texas

GEORGE D. WENDEL, Jr, MD, Professor, Department of Obstetrics and Gynecology, University of Texas Southwestern Medical School, Dallas, Texas

CONTRIBUTORS

JAMES M. ALEXANDER, MD, Associate Professor, Department of Obstetrics and Gynecology, University of Texas Southwestern Medical Center at Dallas, Dallas, Texas

KIM A. BOGGESS, MD, Assistant Professor, Department of Obstetrics and Gynecology, Division of Maternal Fetal Medicine, University of North Carolina School of Medicine, Chapel Hill, North Carolina

JENNIFER F. CULHANE, PhD, The Department of Obstetrics and Gynecology, Drexel University College of Medicine, Philadelphia, Pennsylvania

JANE E. ELLIS, MD, PhD, Maternal-Fetal Medicine Fellow, Department of Gynecology and Obstetrics, Emory University School of Medicine, Atlanta, Georgia

SEBASTIAN FARO, MD, PhD, Clinical Professor, Department of Obstetrics, Gynecology, and Reproductive Sciences, The University of Texas Houston Health Sciences Center, Houston, Texas

ROBERT L. GOLDENBERG, MD, Center for Obstetric Research, Department of Obstetrics and Gynecology, Division of Maternal-Fetal Medicine, University of Alabama at Birmingham, Birmingham, Alabama

HEIDI GRISSOM, MD, RPh, Resident, Department of Obstetrics, Gynecology, and Reproductive Sciences, University of Texas Houston Medical School, Lyndon B. Johnson General Hospital, Houston, Texas

JAMES HILL, MD, Chief of Obstetrics, Department of Obstetrics and Gynecology, Department of the Army, Womack Army Medical Center, Fort Bragg, North Carolina

LISA M. HOLLIER, MD, MPH, Assistant Professor, Division of Maternal-Fetal Medicine, Department of Obstetrics, Gynecology, and Reproductive Sciences, University of Texas Houston Medical School, Lyndon B. Johnson General Hospital, Houston, Texas

DENISE J. JAMIESON, MD, MPH, Medical Officer, Division of Reproductive Health, National Center for Chronic Disease Prevention and Health Promotion, Centers for Disease Control and Prevention; Clinical Associate Professor, Department of Gynecology and Obstetrics, Emory University School of Medicine, Atlanta, Georgia

DANIEL B. JERNIGAN, MD, MPH, Medical Officer, National Center for Infectious Diseases, Centers for Disease Control and Prevention, Atlanta, Georgia

DEREK C. JOHNSON, BA, The Department of Obstetrics and Gynecology, Drexel University College of Medicine, Philadelphia, Pennsylvania

VANESSA R. LAIBL, MD, Postdoctoral Fellow, Division of Maternal-Fetal Medicine, Department of Obstetrics and Gynecology, University of Texas Southwestern Medical Center at Dallas, Dallas, Texas

JOAN M. MASTROBATTISTA, MD, Associate Professor, Division of Maternal-Fetal Medicine, Department of Obstetrics, Gynecology, and Reproductive Sciences, University of Texas Health Science Center at Houston, Houston, Texas

POOJA MITTAL, MD, Clinical Fellow, Division of Maternal-Fetal Medicine, Department of Obstetrics-Gynecology, Hutzel Women's Hospital, Wayne State University, Detroit, Michigan

JOSE G. MONTOYA, MD, Associate Professor of Medicine, Department of Medicine, Division of Infectious Diseases and Geographic Medicine, Stanford University School of Medicine, Stanford; Department of Immunology and Infectious Diseases, Research Institute, Palo Alto Medical Foundation, Palo Alto, California

EDWARD R. NEWTON, MD, Professor; Chair of Obstetrics and Gynecology, Brody School of Medicine, East Carolina University, Greenville, North Carolina

JASON A. PATES, MD, Postdoctoral Fellow, Division of Maternal-Fetal Medicine, Department of Obstetrics & Gynecology, University of Texas Southwestern Medical Center at Dallas, Dallas, Texas

MILDRED M. RAMIREZ, MD, Associate Professor, Division of Maternal-Fetal Medicine, Department of Obstetrics, Gynecology, and Reproductive Sciences, University of Texas Health Science Center at Houston, Houston, Texas

SCOTT ROBERTS, MD, Associate Professor, Division of Maternal-Fetal Medicine, Department of Obstetrics and Gynecology, University of Texas Southwestern Medical Center, Dallas, Texas

FERNANDO ROSSO, MD, Visiting Scholar, Department of Medicine, Division of Infectious Diseases and Geographic Medicine, Stanford University School of Medicine, Stanford, California; Department of Immunology and Infectious Diseases, Research Institute, Palo Alto Medical Foundation, Palo Alto, California; Fundación Clínica Valle del Lili, Cali, Colombia

STEPHANIE SCHRAG, D Phil, Epidemiologist, Division of Bacterial and Mycotic Diseases, National Center for Infectious Diseases, Centers for Disease Control and Prevention, Atlanta, Georgia

ANNE SCHUCHAT, MD, Acting Director, National Center for Infectious Diseases, Centers for Disease Control and Prevention, Atlanta, Georgia

JEANNE S. SHEFFIELD, MD, Assistant Professor, Division of Maternal-Fetal Medicine, Department of Obstetrics and Gynecology, University of Texas Southwestern Medical Center at Dallas, Dallas, Texas

TRACEE A TREADWELL, DVM, MPH, Medical Epidemiologist, National Center for Infectious Diseases, Centers for Disease Control and Prevention, Atlanta, Georgia

DIANE M. TWICKLER, MD, Professor, Departments of Radiology and Obstetrics & Gynecology, University of Texas Southwestern Medical Center at Dallas, Dallas, Texas

DEBORAH A. WING, MD, Associate Professor and Director, Division of Maternal-Fetal Medicine, Department of Obstetrics-Gynecology, University of California, Irvine Medical Center, Orange, California

KIMBERLY WORKOWSKI, MD, FACP, Associate Professor of Medicine, Division of Infectious Diseases, Emory University; Guidelines Unit, Epidemiology and Surveillance Branch, Division of STD Prevention, Centers for Disease Control and Prevention, Atlanta, Georgia

MARK H. YUDIN, MD, MSc, Assistant Professor, Department of Obstetrics and Gynecology, St. Michael's Hospital, University of Toronto, Toronto, Ontario, Canada

CONTENTS

GOAL STATEMENT

The goal of *Clinics in Perinatology* is to keep practicing neonatologists and maternal-fetal medicine specialists up to date with current clinical practice in perinatology by providing timely articles reviewing the state of the art in patient care.

ACCREDITATION

The *Clinics in Perinatology* is planned and implemented in accordance with the Essential Areas and Policies of the Accreditation Council for Continuing Medical Education (ACCME) through the joint sponsorship of the University of Virginia School of Medicine and Elsevier. The University of Virginia School of Medicine is accredited by the ACCME to provide continuing medical education for physicians.

The University of Virginia School of Medicine designates this educational activity for a maximum of 60 category 1 credits per year, 15 category 1 credits per issue, toward the AMA Physician's Recognition Award. Each physician should claim only those credits that he/she actually spent in the activity.

Category 1 credit can be earned by reading the text material, taking the CME examination online at http://www.theclinics.com/home/cme, and completing the evaluation. After taking the test, you will be required to review any and all incorrect answers. Following completion of the test and evaluation, your credit will be awarded and you may print your certificate.

FACULTY DISCLOSURE

Disclosure of faculty financial affiliations:

As a provider accredited by the Accreditation Council for Continuing Medical Education (ACCME), the Office of Continuing Medical Education of the University of Virginia School of Medicine must ensure balance, independence, objectivity, and scientific rigor in all its individually sponsored or jointly sponsored educational activities. All authors/editors participating in a sponsored activity are expected to disclose to the readers any significant financial interest or other relationship (1) with the manufacturer(s) of any commercial product(s) and/or provider(s) of commercial services discussed in an educational presentation and (2) with any commercial supporters of the activity (significant financial interest or other relationship can include such things as grants or research support, employee, consultant, stock holder, member of speakers bureau, etc.) The intent of this disclosure is not to prevent authors/editors with a significant financial or other relationship from writing an article, but rather to provide readers with information on which they can make their own judgments. It remains for the readers to determine whether the author's/editor's interest or relationships may influence the article with regard to exposition or conclusion.

The authors/editors listed below have identified no professional or financial affiliations related to their article:

James M. Alexander, MD; Kim A. Boggess, MD; Jennifer F. Culhane, PhD; Carin Davis, Acquisitions Editor; Jane E. Ellis, MD, PhD; Sebastian Faro, MD, PhD; Robert L. Goldenberg, MD; Heidi A. Grissom, MD; James B. Hill, MD; Lisa M. Hollier, MD, MPH; Denise J. Jamieson, MD, MPH; Daniel B. Jernigan, MD, MPH; Derek C. Johnson, BA; Vanessa R. Laibl, MD; Joan M. Mastrobattista, MD; Pooja Mittal, MD; Jose G. Montoya, MD; Eward R. Newton, MD; Jason A. Pates, MD, CPT, MC, USA; Mildred M. Ramirez, MD; Scott Roberts, MD, MS; Fernando Rosso, MD; Stephanie Schrag, PhD; Anne Schuchat, MD; Jeanne S. Sheffield, MD; Tracess A. Treadwell, DVM, MPH; Diane M. Twickler, MD; George D. Wendel, Jr., MD; Deborah A. Wing, MD; Kimberly Workowski, MD, FACP; and, Mark H. Yudin, MD, MSc, FRCSC.

Disclosure of Discussion of non-FDA approved uses for pharmaceutical products and/or medical devices: The University of Virginia School of Medicine, as an ACCME provider, requires that all faculty presenters identify and disclose any "off label" uses for pharmaceutical and medical device products. The University of Virginia School of Medicine recommends that each physician fully review all the available data on new products or procedures prior to instituting them with patients.

All authors who provided disclosures will not be discussing any off-label uses except:
Lisa M. Hollier, MD, MPH and Heidi A. Grissom, MD will discuss the use of acyclovir, valacyclovir, famcyclovir for the prevention of HSV recurrence at delivery.
Jose G. Montoya, MD and Fernando Rosso, MD Spiramycin is a drug approved in Europe to attempt to prevent congenital transmission of T. gondii. The drug is not approved by the FDA but it can be recommended by our laboratory (Toxoplasma Serology Laboratory at Palo Alto Medical Foundation Research Institute) and can be obtained in the United States through the FDA.
Scott Roberts, MD, MS will discuss the reports of prophylaxis trials with valacyclovir and famcyclovir.

TO ENROLL

To enroll in the *Clinics in Perinatology* Continuing Medical Education program, , call customer service at 1-800-654-2452 or visit us online at www.theclinics.com/home/cme. The CME program is available to subscribers for an additional fee of $165.00

FORTHCOMING ISSUES

December 2005

Cardiovascular Disease of the Fetus and Neonate
Gil Wernovsky, MD, Stuart Berger, MD, and
S. David Rubenstein, MD, *Guest Editors*

March 2006

The Science Behind Neonatal Resuscitation
Jeffrey Perlman, MB, *Guest Editor*

June 2006

Cerebral Functional Monitoring
Robert White, MD, and
Alan Spitzer, MD, *Guest Editors*

RECENT ISSUES

June 2005

Multiple Gestations
Keith A. Eddleman, MD, and
Joanne Stone, MD, *Guest Editors*

March 2005

Risk Management in Neonatal-Perinatal Medicine
Marcus C. Hermansen, MD, *Guest Editor*

December 2004

Management of High-Risk Pregnancy
Baha M. Sibai, MD, *Guest Editor*

CLINICS IN PERINATOLOGY

Clin Perinatol 32 (2005) xv–xvii

Preface

Infectious Diseases in Pregnancy

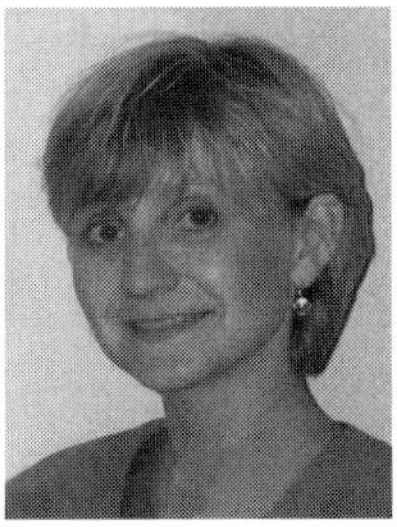

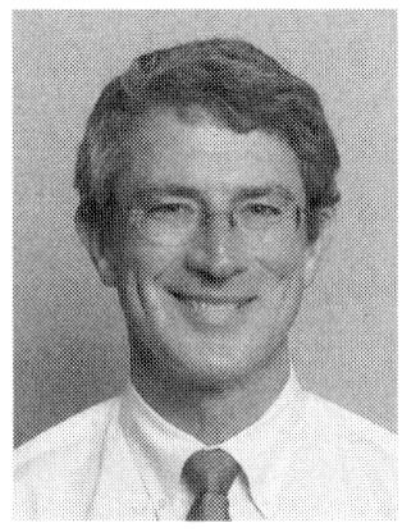

Lisa M. Hollier, MD, MPH George D. Wendel, Jr, MD
Guest Editors

Infectious diseases are important causes of both morbidity and mortality worldwide. Women and infants bear a significant proportion of disease morbidity because of complications associated with pregnancy. Sexually transmitted infections like gonorrhea and chlamydia can cause infertility or ectopic pregnancy. Many infections have been associated with preterm birth. Infections with viruses such as cytomegalovirus and varicella can cause structural fetal abnormalities. These and other perinatally acquired infections can lead to neonatal blindness or stillbirth. When considered as a group, infections are one of the most common complications of pregnancy. The economic and social burdens of these diseases among women are staggering and worthy of significant attention.

This issue of the *Clinics in Perinatology* presents the unique aspects of selected infectious diseases that cause important complications of pregnancy. Dr. Goldenberg and colleagues open the issue with an excellent discussion of the impact of infectious diseases on specific pregnancy outcomes. Preterm birth remains one of the most important problems in obstetrics and gynecology today. Evidence continues to emerge implicating infection as a major etiologic factor, particularly in the earliest of these births. Dr. Boggess presents the latest research in this exciting field. The current evidence supporting interventions for preterm labor and preterm premature rupture of the membranes is reviewed by Dr. Newton, who provides important practical clinical information. This section is

doi:10.1016/j.clp.2005.07.001 *perinatology.theclinics.com*

rounded out by Drs. Schrag and Schuchat who present an excellent review of interventions to prevent neonatal sepsis. They address strategies for the prevention of group B streptococcal disease and developing concerns about antimicrobial resistance.

Articles in the next section review management of specific infections during pregnancy. Bacterial vaginosis is a common alteration in the vaginal flora and is increasingly recognized as an important contributor to preterm birth. Dr. Yudin presents an update regarding the optimal strategies for diagnosis, screening, and management of this complication. Drs. Hollier and Workowski review the management of STDs during pregnancy and highlight new changes in the Centers of Disease Control and Prevention Guidelines for the Treatment of Sexually Transmitted Diseases. Herpes simplex virus infections affect approximately one fifth of the United States population, but many infected individuals remain undiagnosed. Drs. Hill and Roberts review new diagnostic techniques and their application for pregnant patients. They also discuss the latest research regarding management of the patient with a history of genital infection and the prevention of neonatal herpes. Drs. Hollier and Grissom address the latest research regarding prenatal diagnosis of cytomegalovirus infections and also review complications associated with Epstein-Barr virus and varicella zoster virus infections. Practical management tips and algorithms are included. A clinically oriented guide for the diagnosis and management of pregnancies with possible and confirmed infection with human parvovirus B19 is provided by Drs. Ramirez and Mastrobattista. Dr. Montoya is one of the leading experts in the United States in the diagnosis and management of pregnancies complicated by *Toxoplasma gondii* infection. He and Dr. Rosso provide a well-organized plan for maternal and fetal testing and subsequent intervention. They present new information to help the clinician in the difficult situation of deciding which pregnancies are truly at risk for fetal toxoplasmosis.

Drs. Laibl and Sheffield review two important infections with pulmonary manifestations: influenza and tuberculosis. They review important changes in the recommendations for influenza vaccination during pregnancy and discuss appropriate therapeutic interventions. Strategies for evaluation of the asymptomatic patient with tuberculosis exposure and infection are reviewed, as are new recommendations for treatment of women with active disease. Urinary tract infections contribute to preterm birth and may contribute to adverse neurologic outcomes. Optimal management for the pregnant patient with urinary tract infections is presented by Drs. Mittal and Wing. Led by Dr. Jamieson, experts from the Centers for Disease Control and Prevention review important emerging infections including West Nile virus and severe acute respiratory syndrome (SARS).

This issue would not be complete without a discussion of current research involving the association between epidural analgesia and fever during labor. Dr. Alexander presents an excellent discussion of this common occurrence. Drs. Pate and Twickler provide an outstanding overview of radiologic modalities and appropriate use in patients with infections. They emphasize the importance of system-wide protocols for evaluating pregnant women with imaging resources to minimize confusion and streamline care. The issue concludes with an up-to-date guide for antimicrobial use in the prevention and treatment of postoperative pelvic infections written by Dr. Faro.

We would like to thank the contributors for sharing their expertise and experience and providing the readers with timely updates on research and practical clinical information. The authors are all busy physicians or researchers who worked extra hours into already busy schedules to prepare these outstanding articles. We would like to especially thank the editorial staff at Elsevier, particularly Carin Davis for her expert input and for her patience as she guided this project to completion.

Lisa M. Hollier, MD, MPH
Department of Obstetrics, Gynecology, and Reproductive Services
University of Texas Houston Medical School
Lyndon B. Johnson General Hospital
5656 Kelley Street
Houston, TX 77026, USA
E-mail address: lisa.m.hollier@uth.tmc.edu

George D. Wendel, Jr, MD
Department of Obstetrics and Gynecology
University of Texas Southwestern Medical School
5323 Harry Hines Boulevard
Dallas, TX 75390-9032, USA
E-mail address: george.wendel@utsouthwestern.edu

ELSEVIER
SAUNDERS

Clin Perinatol 32 (2005) 523–559

CLINICS IN
PERINATOLOGY

Maternal Infection and Adverse Fetal and Neonatal Outcomes

Robert L. Goldenberg, MD[a,*], Jennifer F. Culhane, PhD[b], Derek C. Johnson, BA[b]

[a]*Center for Obstetric Research, Department of Obstetrics and Gynecology, Division of Maternal-Fetal Medicine, University of Alabama at Birmingham, 1500 6th Avenue South, Birmingham, AL 35233, USA*
[b]*Department of Obstetrics and Gynecology, Drexel University College of Medicine, 245 North 15th Street, MS#495, 17th Floor, Philadelphia, PA 19102, USA*

The relationship between pregnancy outcome and maternal colonization with a wide variety of bacterial, fungal, protozoan, and viral organisms has been studied for many years [1,2]. The more classic sexually transmitted diseases, including syphilis, gonorrhea, herpes, trichomonas and *Chlamydia*, are almost always transmitted between adults as a result of sexual contact. The majority of human immunodeficiency virus (HIV) infections in women of reproductive age are also transmitted sexually; however, there are other maternal infections that are not easily classifiable. Group B streptococcus, hepatitis B virus, cytomegalovirus, and the organisms associated with bacterial vaginosis, such as the mycoplasmas, *Gardnerella vaginalis*, *Bacteroides*, and *Mobiluncus* species, are all found more commonly in sexually active women than non–sexually active women, but their mode of transmission is often not apparent. Other maternal infections that are associated with adverse pregnancy outcomes, including malaria, parvovirus, rubella, and listeria, are not generally transmitted sexually.

In this article, the authors define a number of adverse pregnancy outcomes, and then explore the evidence that various types of maternal infections are responsible for these outcomes, which include stillbirth and neonatal death; congenital anomalies; short-term neonatal morbidity such as intraventricular hemorrhage (IVH), respiratory distress syndrome (RDS), and necrotizing entrocolitis (NEC); long-term morbidity, including cerebral palsy and mental

* Corresponding author.
E-mail address: rlg@uab.edu (R.L. Goldenberg).

0095-5108/05/$ – see front matter
doi:10.1016/j.clp.2005.04.006 ***perinatology.theclinics.com***

retardation; and preterm birth and fetal growth restriction. Before we address specific adverse pregnancy outcomes, however, it should be noted that several sexually transmitted diseases, such as gonorrhea and chlamydia, have been associated with a failure to achieve pregnancy, predominantly through fallopian tube damage. Additionally, fallopian tube damage secondary to chlamydia and gonorrhea infection is the leading cause of ectopic pregnancy, which complicates close to 100,000 pregnancies in the United States each year [3].

Measurement of pregnancy outcome

The specific definitions of the most important adverse pregnancy outcomes collected through the vital statistics reports are as follows: in most states, abortion is defined as a pregnancy which terminates or is terminated before 20 weeks' gestational age, whereas a stillbirth is usually defined as a fetus born at 20 weeks' gestational age or more having no heartbeat or respiratory effort. A liveborn infant is generally defined as an infant born at any gestational age having a heartbeat or respiratory effort. Death of a liveborn infant can occur in the neonatal period (in the first 28 days of life) or in the post neonatal period (between 28 days and 1 year of age). An infant death is defined as the death of a liveborn baby that occurs before 1 year of age, both neonatal and post-neonatal deaths. Perinatal mortality is frequently defined as the sum of fetal and neonatal deaths, although other definitions are used. Preterm birth is defined as a birth occurring before 37 weeks of gestation, and a growth-restricted infant is defined as one born at less than the 10th percentile birth weight for a specific gestational age. There are many definitions of long-term morbidity, but those children who have structural anomalies, blindness, deafness, cerebral palsy, or mental retardation are frequently defined as handicapped.

Routes of transmission

Adverse pregnancy outcomes associated with maternal infections can occur because of direct infections of the fetus or neonate, or because of infections that cause early delivery without directly involving the fetus. For those organisms that attack the fetus directly, the transmission may occur within the uterus via transplacental or ascending infection, or in the intrapartum period secondary to fetal contact with infected genital secretions or maternal blood. Postpartum transmission occurs through breast-feeding or other types of maternal contact.

Diagnosing intrauterine infection

In general, organisms causing intrauterine infections enter the uterus through the placenta or ascend from the vagina into the uterus through the cervix.

Organisms can be found in the space between the decidua and the membranes, within the membranes, in the amniotic fluid, or within the placenta or fetus. Over time, evidence has accumulated in support of the causal role of intrauterine infection in various adverse pregnancy outcomes. As a result, growing attention has been focused on the optimal criteria for diagnosing intrauterine infection. Obviously, finding organisms in one of the above locations, before possible contamination from the vagina after membrane rupture, conclusively proves colonization (but not necessarily an adverse outcome associated with that colonization); however, many of the early studies, and in fact many studies reported recently, do not use a positive culture or even a positive polymerase chain reaction (PCR) for bacterial or viral DNA as the standard for diagnosing intrauterine infection. Instead, histologic chorioamnionitis or white cell infiltration into the chorion and amnion is often used as the criterion for diagnosing an intrauterine infection. Furthermore, in recent years there have been many investigations in which various markers of intrauterine infection—including elevations in various cytokines such as interleukin(IL)-6, IL-1β, and IL-8, increases in some of the matrix metalloproteinases, and the presence of white cells in the amniotic fluid—have been used as surrogate markers for an intrauterine infection [4–9]. Although finding bacteria in the amniotic fluid or in the membranes must be considered the most important indicator of any intrauterine bacterial infection, in women in preterm labor, the correlations between bacteria in the membranes, histologic chorioamnionitis, and elevated cytokines are all reasonably strong [5].

Types of intrauterine infection

As stated above, infections within the uterus may be located: (1) in the space between the decidua and the membranes, (2) within the membranes themselves, (3) in the amniotic fluid, or (4) within the placenta or fetus. Studies suggest that infection is most commonly found adjacent to or within the membranes. Importantly, of the women who have infection in the membranes, only half also have bacteria in the amniotic fluid [10]. A far smaller percentage also have a fetal infection. This pattern suggests that most intrauterine infections move from the membranes to the amniotic fluid and then to the fetus.

Recent studies demonstrate that there are a wide array of clinical presentations associated with intrauterine bacterial infections. Some women who have an intrauterine bacterial infection develop clinical signs of a systemic infection, including fever, uterine tenderness, and an elevated white cell response. These women are labeled as having clinical chorioamnionitis; however, it is now clear that many women can have an intrauterine infection without having these clinical symptoms. For example, several studies suggest that only 5% to 10% of the women who have histologic chorioamnionitis or women who have organisms in the membranes have clinical chorioamnionitis [11]. Therefore, many investigators studying this issue now believe that intrauterine infection rarely presents as clinical chorioamnionitis. Instead, uterine contractions or preterm labor, or preterm rupture of the membranes, appear to be far more common presentations of intrauterine infection. Furthermore, it is likely that many women who have an intrauterine infection will have no signs or symptoms at all.

Early pregnancy loss

The incidence of first trimester spontaneous abortion is highly dependent upon how one defines pregnancy. Using the standard obstetric definition, which includes a missed period and a positive urinary pregnancy test between 4 weeks and 6 weeks after the last menstrual period, approximately 15% to 20% of all pregnancies end in spontaneous miscarriage. The etiology of these miscarriages is generally secondary to maldevelopment of the ovum and associated chromosomal abnormalities. It is very rare to spontaneously abort a normally developing fetus during the first trimester. In fact, most of the pathologic material from spontaneous abortions fails to demonstrate any fetal tissue whatsoever. In some reports, maternal infections such as syphilis, rubella, and HIV have been associated with early spontaneous abortion; however, there is little evidence that these infections play an important role in first trimester spontaneous abortion [12].

Second trimester abortions (ie, those that occur between the 13th and 20th week of pregnancy) differ substantially from first trimester abortions in that a fetus is nearly always present. Spontaneous second trimester abortions occur in approximately 1% to 2% of all pregnancies. Although the etiology of these losses is often less clear than that of those occurring at other times, second trimester losses certainly include anomalous fetuses, some having chromosomal abnormalities, and those losses which occur secondary to uterine malformations, incompetent cervix and leiomyomata [12]. Most of the spontaneous second trimester losses, however, occur in the face of a normal uterus and a normally developed fetus. In these cases, there is either "spontaneous" labor or rupture of membranes leading to delivery, or a fetal death that ultimately leads to delivery. Obstetric complications such as twin pregnancy, placental abruption, the presence of maternal anticardiolipin antibodies, or the lupus anticoagulant and fetal growth retardation are also associated with spontaneous pregnancy losses between 12 to 20 weeks' gestation; however, the relative importance of these etiologies is not well quantified. Because the etiology of so many of the second trimester losses is not clear, and a majority of them are associated with spontaneous labor and ruptured membranes, there is ample room to hypothesize that intrauterine infection, which has been implicated in both of these pregnancy complications, may also be an important etiologic component of spontaneous second trimester losses. Indeed, chorioamnionitis has frequently been described, and there are numerous case reports of amniotic fluid infection that have occurred during this gestational age period. Additionally, isolation of microorganisms from pregnancy products has been reported to be more common in women who have spontaneous midtrimester pregnancy loss when compared with women who have induced abortions [13,14]. Furthermore, several treatment trials have shown a reduction in second trimester abortions with antibiotics.

Stillbirth

A stillbirth is one of the most common adverse outcomes of pregnancy. In the United States, a stillbirth occurs in nearly 1% (or 7 per 1000) of all births, and in the year 2000, there were nearly 27,000 of these events [15,16]. The fetal death rates are approximately twice as high in African American women compared with white women. Stillbirth occurs far more frequently in developing countries than in developed countries, with rates as high as 100/1000 reported in some areas. Worldwide, nearly 4 million stillbirths occur in developing countries yearly [17]. In many countries, and especially the most developed ones, over the last several decades there has been a significant reduction in stillbirths. For example, from 1970 to 1998 the stillbirth rate in the United States fell from 14.0 to 6.7 per 1000 births [16]. Much of this decrease has occurred in term or near-term stillbirths, and is mostly due to improvements in medical care [18,19]. With these changes, stillbirths now account for about half of all perinatal mortality and more than a third of all mortality from 20 weeks' gestation to 1 year of age.

Because of the reduction in term stillbirths in the United States over the last several decades, most stillbirths now occur in the preterm gestational ages. In a US multicenter study [18], approximately half of the stillbirths occurred before 28 weeks gestational age, and another third of the stillbirths occurred between 28 weeks and 37 weeks. In this study, and in a number of others, the etiology of many of the stillbirths was not clear; however, many of the early gestational age fetuses died in conjunction with spontaneous preterm labor or rupture of the membranes. Placental histologic changes consistent with chorioamnionitis are found frequently in association with these early stillbirths, and these mothers are also more likely to develop postpartum endometritis. Therefore, there is substantial reason to believe that intrauterine infection may contribute to the etiology of many stillbirths, either as an initiator of preterm labor, as an initiator of ruptured membranes, or as an initiator of fetal death that ultimately results in the birth of a stillborn infant.

In developed countries, 10% to 25% of all stillbirths appear to be caused by a maternal/fetal infection, whereas in developing countries, which often have far higher stillbirth rates, the relative contribution of infection may be even greater [19–21]. The authors have recently reviewed the relationship between various types of maternal infections and stillbirth [22]. In that review, we found that this relationship was strongly influenced by gestational age. The earlier the stillbirth, the more likely it will be related to an infection. For example, in one study [23], 19% of fetal deaths at less than 28 weeks were associated with an infection, whereas only 2% of term stillbirths were infection-related.

For a number of reasons, the relationship between maternal infection and stillbirth is often not very clear [21]. First, it is often difficult to know exactly why a specific fetus died. For example, an autopsy of the fetus and histologic study of the placenta may have findings suggestive of both infectious and hypoxic etiologies. Second, simply finding histologic evidence of infection or specific types of organisms in the placenta or on the fetus does not prove causation, nor does finding serologic evidence of infection prove causation. Neither does the presence of organisms in internal fetal tissues, although this finding clearly increases suspicion of an infectious etiology. Third, infection may cause a stillbirth that initially may not appear to be related to infection at all. The stillbirths associated with rubella-induced congenital anomalies, or with the nonimmune hydrops caused by parvovirus, were not originally seen as infection-related. Finally, organisms that now are quite clearly associated with stillbirth, such as parvovirus and *Ureaplasma urealyticum*, are hard to identify, and are often not sought in studies of infectious etiologies of stillbirths [10].

Conceptually, infection may result in fetal death through many different pathways [19–23]. First, a maternal infection may lead to a systemic illness whereby the mother is severely ill. Perhaps because of the high maternal fever, maternal respiratory distress, or other systemic reactions to the illness, the fetus may die, although the organisms are never transmitted to the placenta or fetus. The increased fetal mortality associated with influenza epidemics or maternal polio is likely due to this phenomenon [24,25]. Second, the placenta may be directly infected without spread of the organisms to the fetus. In these situations, reduced blood flow to the fetus may result in stillbirth. The stillbirths associated with maternal malaria infection are likely due to placental damage [26]. Third, the fetus may be directly infected through the placenta or membranes, with the infectious organisms damaging a vital fetal organ such as the lungs, liver, heart, or brain. Examples of this type of infection include the fetal pneumonia associated with *Eschericia coli* or group B streptococcal chorioamnionitis, or systemic infections with viruses such as coxsackie A or B [27–29].

If an infection occurs very early in gestation, the fetus may not die, but may develop a congenital anomaly, with a fetal death occurring later secondary to the anomaly. Rubella infection has been associated with stillbirths via this mechanism [30,31]. And lastly, an infection in the uterus or anywhere else in the mother's body may precipitate preterm labor. Some of these fetuses, often deemed to be too small to be salvageable by cesarean section, cannot tolerate labor and are born dead. *U urealyticum* is an organism that may precipitate early preterm labor by infecting the fetal membranes without causing a fetal infection. A urinary tract infection with *E coli* is an example of a non–genital tract infection that might precipitate early preterm labor. Periodontal infections are also associated with preterm labor, but the mechanism by which periodontal disease is associated with preterm birth has not yet been elucidated [32].

Ascending bacterial infection, both before and after membrane rupture, with organisms such as *E coli*, group B streptococci, and *U urealyticum* is usually the most common infectious cause of stillbirth; however, in areas where syphilis is very prevalent, up to half of all stillbirths may be caused by this infection alone. Malaria may be an important cause of stillbirth in women infected for the first time in pregnancy. The two most important viral causes of stillbirth are parvovirus and coxsackie virus, although a number of other viral infections appear to be causal. *Toxoplasma gondii*, leptospirosis, *Listeria monocytogenes*, and the organisms that cause leptospirosis, Q fever, and Lyme disease have all been implicated as etiologic for stillbirth. Table 1, from our review, updated to reflect a few new reports, describes each of the organisms that to date have been studied in relationship to stillbirth [22].

Neonatal death

Neonatal deaths are defined as those that occur within the first 28 days of life. In most Western countries, these deaths occur at a rate of between 3 and 7 per 1000 live births. In general, about 70% of these deaths are associated with a preterm birth, and 25% are associated with a major congenital anomaly, with the remainder due to asphyxia, sepsis, meconium aspiration, birth trauma, and more rare conditions such as immune or nonimmune hydrops. Infection as a specific cause of neonatal death occurs predominantly in preterm infants, and is often part of the picture that includes RDS, IVH, and NEC. Because of the multiple system failures, it is often difficult to define a single cause of death in these cases, but infection frequently plays a role.

In developed countries, group B-streptococcus is one of the most common organisms implicated in systemic neonatal infection, but many other organisms, mostly gram-negative, including those that normally colonize the vagina (*E coli, Klebsiella*) and those that are acquired in the nursery (often staphylococcus), have also been implicated in sepsis related neonatal deaths [33,34]. In many developing countries, neonatal group B streptococcal infections are rare and the contribution of gram-negative organisms to neonatal sepsis is proportionately greater. Many of these neonatal infections appear to be contracted in utero before delivery. For the most part, these organisms enter the fetus by way of the amniotic fluid, infecting the lungs, causing a fetal or neonatal pneumonia. Both group B streptococous and the gram-negative organisms cause meningitis as well. Finally, infections such as syphilis and some virus infections such as cytomegalovirus (CMV), varicella, echovirus, coxsackievirus, measles, and herpes simplex are clearly causal for neonatal death, as are other transplacentally transmitted infections such as listerosis and even occasionally tuberculosis. In any case, based on these reports, the authors estimate that in the United States and other developed countries, less than 10% of neonatal mortality is due to neonatal sepsis, pneumonia, and meningitis, with a much smaller portion of the mortality attributable to other infections. In lesser developed countries, the neonatal mortality rates are considerably higher and the contribution of infection considerably greater. For example, in Pakistan it is estimated that half of the neonatal mortality, or as many as 30 per 1000 live births, is infection related [35]. Overall, the World Health Organization (WHO) estimates that of the nearly 5,000,000 neonatal

Table 1
Maternal infections and stillbirths

Organism	Maternal disease	Comment
Spirochetes		
T pallidum	Syphilis	Major cause of SB when maternal prevalence is high
B burgdorferi	Lyme disease	Confirmed, but not a common cause of SB
B recurrentis	Tick-borne Relapsing fever	Of unknown importance as a cause of SB
Leptospira interrogans	Leptospirosis	Confirmed, but not a common cause of SB
Protozoa		
T brucei	Trypanosomiasis	Not a certain cause of SB
T cruzi	Chagas disease	Confirmed as a cause of SB in South America but of unknown importance
P falciparum *P vivax*	Malaria	Likely an important cause of SB in newly endemic areas or in newly infected women
T gondii	Toxoplasmosis	Confirmed, but not a common cause of SB
C burnetti	Q fever	Confirmed as a cause of SB but of unknown importance
Viruses		
Parvovirus (B-19)	Erythema infectiosum	Confirmed as a cause of SB and likely the most common viral etiologic agent
Coxsackie A & B	Various presentations	Confirmed as causes of SB and may be an important contributor
Echovirus	Various presentations	Confirmed as a cause of SB but of unknown importance
Enterovirus	Various presentations	Confirmed as a cause of SB but of unknown importance
Polio virus	Polio	Historically a cause of SB but since routine vaccination no longer seen in developed countries
Varicella-zoster	Chickenpox	Confirmed, but not a common cause of SB
Rubella	German measles	Confirmed, but no longer a cause of SB in developed countries
Mumps	Parotitis	Possibly historically, but no longer a cause of SB in developed countries
Rubeola	Measles	Possibly a cause of SB historically
Cytomegalovirus	Generally asymptomatic in adults	Rarely if ever a cause of SB
SARS virus	Respiratory illness	Case reports
Variola	smallpox	Historically a cause of SB but no longer seen
Lymphocytic choriomeningitis virus	Lymphocytic choriomeningitis	Not confirmed as a cause of SB and of unknown importance
HIV	AIDS	Associated with SB, but not likely causative

(continued on next page)

Table 1 (*continued*)

Organism	Maternal disease	Comment
Bacteria		
Escherichia coli	Generally asymptomatic	Confirmed and probably the most common organism associated with SB
Group B streptococcus	Generally asymptomatic	Confirmed as a common cause of SB
Klebsiella	Generally asymptomatic	Confirmed as a common cause of SB
Enterococcus	Generally asymptomatic	Confirmed
Ureaplasma urealyticum	Generally asymptomatic	Confirmed
Mycoplasma hominus	Generally asymptomatic	Confirmed
Bacteroidaceae	Generally asymptomatic	Confirmed
Listeria monocytogenes	Listerosis	Confirmed, generally transmitted transplacentally
Other bacteria including brucellosis, clostridia, agrobacterium radiobacter, salmonella, pseudomonas, etc.		Suggested by case reports
Chlamydia trachomatis	Pelvic infection	Suggested by case reports
Neiserria gonorrhoeae	Pelvic infection	Suggested by case reports
Mycobacterium tuberculosis	Tuberculosis	Confirmed by case reports, but rare in developed countries
Fungi		
Candida albicans	Thrush, vaginitis	Confirmed as a cause of SB by case reports

Data from Goldenberg RL, Thompson C. The infectious origins of stillbirth. Am J Obstet Gynecol 2003;189:863.

deaths that occur each year worldwide, up to 40%, or 2,000,000 deaths per year, are due to infection [36]. Of these, 800,000 deaths, mostly in developing countries, occur due to acute respiratory infections.

Post-neonatal deaths

In developed countries, post-neonatal deaths occur in approximately three infants per 1000 live births. Sudden infant death syndrome is the most common etiology, and congenital anomalies, accidents, and infection account for most of the other deaths. The most common infectious-related causes of post-neonatal mortality include meningitis, pneumonia, and diarrhea. Although deaths from these causes are rare in middle class women in western countries, they are more frequently seen in rural areas and among the poor. In underdeveloped countries, infection may cause up to several hundred infant deaths per thousand live births. Nearly all the infectious causes of neonatal mortality cause postneonatal deaths as well.

Long-term disability

In addition to mortality, there has been a wide range of permanent structural and neurological morbidity associated with maternally transmitted infectious diseases. These include: (1) structural congenital anomalies with a defect in one or more organs; (2) structural or functional damage to the brain resulting in decreased cognitive ability, mental retardation, or both; and (3) a motor disorder such as a diminution of fine or gross motor skills, or an increase in spasticity or athetosis such as that associated with cerebral palsy. These morbidities, in addition to blindness, deafness, and hydrocephalus, have all been associated with infectious diseases [1].

Cerebral palsy

Cerebral palsy is found in about 2 infants per 1000, but is far more common in preterm infants. For example, among the lowest gestational age infants who survive (23 and 24 weeks), between 25% and 50% end up having cerebral palsy. Perhaps the most commonly used definition of cerebral palsy is that of Nelson and Ellenberg [37], who defined cerebral palsy as "a chronic disability characterized by aberrant control of movement or posture appearing early in life and not the result of recognized progressive disease." Cerebral palsy is associated with damage to the upper motor neurons within the brain, and most cases present as excessive muscular tonus, spasticity with increased stretch reflexes, and hyperactive tendon reflexes. The authors also emphasize that cerebral palsy is a neuromuscular condition only, and does not imply alterations in cognitive function. Although children who have cerebral palsy are statistically more likely to have low intelligence quotients (IQs), mental retardation, or various types of seizure disorders, many children who have cerebral palsy have normal intelligence and are free of other types of neurologic disability [38].

Many bacterial and viral infections of the fetus, infant, and young child have been associated with cerebral palsy, although quantification is difficult [39]. For example, Stanley [40] notes that a fairly large number of cases of cerebral palsy associated with congenital rubella syndrome were described before the initiation of the rubella vaccination program, but this relationship rarely occurs in the United States today. Congenital infection with *Toxoplasma gondii* and CMV can also cause cerebral palsy. Older literature suggests that infection of the infant with measles, mumps, varicella, and rubella was once reported as a common cause of central nervous system (CNS) injury leading to cerebral palsy. Since the development of vaccines for many of the common childhood diseases, however, it appears that a viral etiology for postpartum acquired cerebral palsy is rare. Nelson [41] agrees, stating that although numeric documentation is lacking, judging from medical writing in the 19th century when infectious diseases were more frequent and less effectively treated, infection-related cerebral palsy was more common than it is now in developed countries. Because of these reductions, it appears that CMV has become the most common viral infection associated with a cerebral palsy-like syndrome [39]. In addition to the infections described, herpes virus infection as well as meningococcal, pneumococcal, and group B streptococcal infections of the neonate also may manifest later in life as a cerebral palsy-like syndrome.

More important numerically, many studies now link chorioamnionitis to the development of cerebral palsy [42–44]. Nelson and Ellenberg [37], using data from the Collaborative Perinatal Project, showed that in low–birth weight infants, chorioamnionitis was associated with a tripling of the risk of cerebral palsy from 12 per 1000 to 39 per 1000 live births. Among term infants in that study, chorioamnionitis increased the risk of cerebral palsy from 3 per 1000 to 8 per 1000 live births. In a more recent study, Grether and colleagues [45] examined prenatal and perinatal factors related to cerebral palsy in very low–birth weight (VLBW) California infants. In this study, chorioamnionitis was associated with a fourfold increased risk of cerebral palsy. Even more recently, term infants who have evidence of chorioamnionitis had a significantly greater risk of cerebral palsy [46]. Murphy and coworkers [47], investigating the relationship of various antenatal and intrapartum risk factors to cerebral palsy in infants born at less than 32 weeks' gestational age, showed that in such infants, chorioamnionitis increased the risk of cerebral palsy from 3% in controls to 17% in infected infants.

In a number of other studies, intrauterine infection has preceded neonatal IVH, a precursor of cerebral palsy. For example, Groome and colleagues [48], using data from the March of Dimes multicenter study, showed that clinical chorioamnionitis was associated with a twofold to threefold increased risk of IVH. Damman and Leviton [49,50] have also explored the relationship between maternal intrauterine infection and evidence of brain damage in the preterm newborn. They revealed an association between intrauterine infection in the mother and both IVH and white matter damage in the newborn. In a study of more than 1000 preterm infants, intrauterine infection was associated with a doubling of the infant's risk for having IVH, periventricular leukomalacia (PVL), and ventriculomegaly. Additional data from the National Institute of Child Health and Human Development Neonatal Research Network [51,52] confirm that both early-onset and late-onset sepsis in VLBW newborns is associated with an increased incidence of IVH.

Bejar and coworkers [53] found that chorioamnionitis was present in more than half of the preterm infants who developed white matter echolucencies within 3 days after birth. Leviton [54] notes that the histologic abnormalities of white matter have been associated with sepsis in the baby and with gynecologic and urinary tract infection in the mother. Mays and colleagues [55] report that acute maternal appendicitis is associated with IVH and PVL, even when the gestational age at birth is controlled for. Therefore, even extrauterine intra-abdominal infections appear to be able to initiate the cascade of events linking infection, labor, and neonatal brain injury [56]. Hansen and coworkers [57] studied the correlation between placental pathology and IVH in preterm infants. Placental characteristics of inflammation, including umbilical vasculitis, chorionic vasculitis, and inflammation of the subchorion, chorion, and amnion, were associated with an increased risk of IVH. Grafe [58], Salafia and colleagues [59], and others confirmed the relationship between both periventricular hemorrhage and leukomalacia and cerebral palsy and placental membrane and umbilical cord evidence of inflammation and associated thrombosis [60,61].

In a further attempt to understand this phenomenon, Kuban and Leviton [62] studied echolucent images in periventricular white matter in relationship to maternal uterine infection. The odds ratio for development of an echolucency was highest for infants whose placentas had vasculitis of the chorionic plate or umbilical cord (odds ratio = 9.8). Zupan and coworkers [63], in a study of risk factors for PVL, found a strong link between intrauterine infection and the development of PVL, and that this relationship was increased in the face of premature rupture of membranes and infection. They also suggest that most of the PVL originates before birth, that susceptibility to the condition closely depends on the developmental age, and that the major etiologic components of white matter lesions in infants born late in the second trimester relate to the presence of an intrauterine infection. Perlman and colleagues [64] noted that cystic PVL, which occurred in 3% of infants weighing less than 1500 g, was associated with two clinical indicators: prolonged rupture of membranes and chorioamnionitis. The odds ratio for cerebral palsy after prolonged rupture of membranes was 6.6, and the odds ratio for cerebral palsy with chorioamnionitis was 6.8.

In recent years, much evidence has emerged suggesting that various cytokines mediate the relationship between cerebral palsy and intrauterine infection, IVH, and PVL. Certainly various cytokines, such as IL-6, IL-1, tumor necrosis factor (TNF) alpha, and others, are elevated in the amniotic fluid of pregnant women who have chorioamnionitis. Andrews and coworkers [13] have emphasized that amniotic fluid cytokines are elevated even with infection confined to the amniotic membranes. Adinolfi [65] was among the first to propose that cytokines produced in relationship to maternal infection were harmful to the developing brain of the unborn infants. Figueroa and colleagues [66] showed that elevated amniotic fluid IL-6 predicted neonatal PVL and IVH. Yoon and coworkers [67], Kashlan and colleagues [68], and others showed that elevated IL-6 levels in the umbilical cord were also related to the subsequent development of periventricular echodensities and echolucencies. Recent papers document the association between elevated umbilical cord blood cytokine levels and cerebral palsy [69,70]. From these data, there seems little question that intrauterine infection, a clear predictor of preterm delivery [14], is also a predictor of white matter lesions, IVH, and ultimately cerebral palsy. If, as has been proposed [71], 70% to 80% of VLBW births are associated with an intrauterine infection, the high rate of cerebral palsy in these infants may well be related to this intrauterine infection.

Mental retardation

Mental retardation, usually defined by an IQ cutoff less than 70 or 75, is another outcome measure of great importance, but one whose prevalence in the population is difficult to determine with certainty. Prevalence is undoubtedly influenced by definition, timing of testing, and many other factors as well, but in most populations about 3% of all infants and children receive this diagnosis. Babies born prematurely and babies born following intrauterine growth retardation are all at greater risk for the development of mental retardation regardless of the definition [72,73]; however, most babies who have these diagnoses will eventually have IQs within the normal range. For example, on average, infants who survive weighing less than 1000 g at birth, have an average IQ about 10 points below appropriate controls. As with cerebral palsy, intrauterine infection is thought to play a role in this reduction in IQ. What is clear, however, is that the socioeconomic status and educational background of the parents greatly influence the ultimate rate of mental retardation in the population. Although perinatal infections that attack the fetus, such as group B streptococcus, herpes simplex virus, CMV, syphilis, and toxoplasmosis all are demonstrated causes of mental retardation, infection-initiated preterm birth, which will be described in detail, appears to be a more important cause of mental retardation from the overall public health perspective [74,75].

Psychiatric disease/schizophrenia

A variety of psychiatric and developmental disorders, and especially schizophrenia, have been associated with various maternal infections. Prenatal influenza has been the most studied [76–78]. Interestingly, several recent studies have shown that increased levels of amniotic fluid cytokines during the second trimester of pregnancy may contribute to a greater risk in offspring developing schizophrenia [79]. Those relationships that are positive are at best associations, with no proven causality. Relationships between pre- and perinatal infections with childhood autism have also been studied, and as with schizophrenia, the data supporting the relationship are mixed. Further research is necessary to confirm or refute each of these relationships.

Congenital anomalies

Structural anomalies of the fetus occur in about 3% of all births. Among the most serious, and those that contribute to the most long-term morbidity and mortality, are neural tube defects, urinary tract anomalies, and cardiac defects. Overall, about 20% of stillbirths and neonatal deaths are caused by an anomaly, as is a portion of mental retardation. Although maternal virus infections clearly can cause structural anomalies, only a very small percentage of all anomalies are likely to be viral related. For example, rubella infections, especially those occurring in the first trimester, as well as varicella infections, are associated with a wide variety of anomalies. Because of routine vaccinations to prevent rubella and other viral infections, however, these anomalies are rarely seen today in developed countries. Coxsackieviruses B3 and B4 have been associated with congenital heart disease [80]. Maternal parvovirus infection, especially in the second trimester, has been associated with a fetal nonimmune hydrops, sometimes leading to fetal death. Whether it is appropriate to consider these cases as congenital anomalies is not clear. In addition, there are isolated case reports of CNS anomalies associated with parvovirus infection, but this relationship has not been confirmed epidemiologically.

Growth retardation

Fetal growth retardation is generally defined as a birthweight less than the 10th percentile birthweight for gestational age; however, the standards used to define the 10th percentile birthweight for gestational age are highly variable and often do not apply to the population being evaluated [81]. Also, because the gestational age measures used for defining the standard are so variable, it is difficult to compare rates of growth retardation from one time period to another, or from one study to another. Growth retardation has many etiologies, including low maternal height, low maternal weight, smoking, preeclampsia, congenital anomalies, and intrauterine infection. With changes in obstetric recommendations about maternal weight gain over the last several decades, it appears that the rate of growth retardation is decreasing.

Nearly all infections of the mother and fetus have been associated with growth retardation, but it is unknown whether maternally transmitted infections other than those that infect the fetus or placenta early and directly, such as rubella, toxoplasmosis, CMV, syphilis, and malaria, actually cause growth retardation. Assuming they do, the mechanism may lie in fetal cell death caused by direct infection or by changes in placental or fetal blood flow. Maternal malaria, for example, which often attacks the placenta and seems to inhibit gas and nutrient exchange, is associated with a two- or threefold increase in fetal growth restriction [26]. The impact of syphilis is similar, and in general, in developing countries, a wide variety of maternal infections are very likely responsible for a large proportion of the growth retarded infants. Because growth retardation in developed countries often appears to be associated with below average maternal size, poor nutritional status, various adverse health behaviors and hypertension, however, it is unclear what portion of the growth retardation in developed countries can be explained by an infectious etiology.

Preterm birth

Preterm birth is the most significant problem confronting obstetricians in industrial countries today. Preterm births, defined as those occurring at less than 37 weeks' gestational age, are associated with approximately 75% of the perinatal mortality and as much as 50% of the long-term neurologic handicap [82]. In the last 20 years, the preterm rate in the United States has risen from approximately 9.5% to 12% [83]. Although we have made tremendous strides in keeping preterm infants alive, we have been less successful in reducing the long-term handicap rates among the survivors [84,85]. Much of the mortality and the long-term handicap associated with prematurity occurs in the smallest or earliest gestational age newborns. For example, it is estimated that 60% of the neonatal mortality and much of the long-term handicap accrue to infants born weighing less than 1000 g and less than 28 weeks' gestational age. Many of these early preterm births occur secondary to an intrauterine infection [86]. This section explores the relationship between infection and preterm birth.

The relationship between genital tract infection and preterm birth has been appreciated by some physicians for more than half a century. For example, in 1950 Knox and Hoerner [87] noted that "infection in the female reproductive tract can cause premature rupture of the membranes and induce premature labor." In their series, they noted that the membranes in all premature cases showed evidence of infection. Perhaps the most influential paper on infection and preterm birth was written in 1977 by Bobitt and Ledger [88]. In this study, they performed amniocenteses in 10 women in preterm labor with intact membranes. Seven of the women had bacterial colony counts higher than 1000 per mL, with anaerobic organisms predominating. These authors posited that bacteria can penetrate the fetal membranes and contaminate the amniotic fluid, and suggested that in patients in premature labor, the role of unrecognized amnionitis should be reevaluated. Elder and colleagues [89] approached the issue of infection and preterm birth somewhat differently. Believing that bacterial infection was causal for preterm birth, in 1971 they treated 279 "non-bacteriuric women" with a 6-week course of 1 g of tetracycline daily beginning at less than 32 weeks' gestational age, and compared the outcomes to women treated with a placebo. In the tetracycline-treated group there were statistically fewer preterm births.

Because of the more frequent use of amniocentesis, we now have ample data relating amniotic fluid infection to preterm labor. Beginning with Bobitt and Ledger's study [88] and extending to the present, there have now been a large number of studies in which women presenting with preterm labor and intact membranes have had an amniocentesis performed and the amniotic fluid cultured [90–94]. The percent of positive cultures in these studies has varied widely, ranging from no positive cultures in several small studies to as high as 50% in others. In a review of the studies performed before 1992, 100 of 863 or 12% of amniotic fluid cultures were positive. Knowing what we know now, the reason for the relatively low culture rates are quite apparent. First, many of these studies did not focus on early preterm infants, and we know that the percent of positive cultures are gestational age-related, with the proportion of positive cultures increasing with decreasing gestational age [86]. Second, few of these studies cultured for *Ureaplasma* or *Mycoplasma* or other hard-to-grow anaerobes. We now know that the most common organisms found in the uterus are *Ureaplasma* and *Mycoplasma*. We also know that in the presence of an intrauterine infection, the amniotic fluid will be positive on only half the occasions when organisms are present in the membranes [10]. For each of these reasons and possibly others, the rates of positive amnionic fluid cultures in women in preterm labor are lower than the actual rate of intrauterine infection.

Relationship to gestational age

A concept developed more than 20 years ago, but more widely held today, is that the relationship of intrauterine infection and preterm labor is not consistent across all preterm gestational ages. In 1979, Russell [95], using histologic chorioamnionitis as a marker of infection, showed that virtually all births at 21 to 24 weeks were associated with an intrauterine infection, compared with only about 10% of the preterm births at 33 to 36 weeks. Mueller-Heubach and colleagues [96] and Chellam and Rushton [97] reported similar findings, which were also confirmed by Andrews and coworkers [5] in Alabama. Therefore, there is no question that the earliest preterm births are strongly associated with histologic chorioamnionitis.

Rather than evaluating histologic chorioamnionitis as the marker of intrauterine infection, in 1992, Watts and coworkers [98] studied amniotic fluid cultures in women in labor who had intact membranes. They showed that at 23 and 24 weeks' gestation, more than 60% of the women in preterm labor had organisms in the amniotic fluid. That number fell to less than 20% for women in labor at 33 to 34 weeks. To further investigate this issue, Hauth and colleagues in Alabama [99] cultured the chorioamnions of over 600 women having a cesarean section who had intact membranes. In this study, after delivery the placental membranes were opened and cultures were taken from the space between the chorion and amnion. This study design precluded vaginal or ascending infection following membrane rupture contamination of the membranes, because membranes were not delivered through the vagina and the membranes were intact at the time of delivery. The study authors found that in women in spontaneous labor delivering a less than 1000-g infant, 83% had chorioamnion cultures that were positive, whereas those delivering a more than 2500-g infant had a 20% positive culture rate [99]. For those women not in labor, undergoing an indicated cesarean section, and delivering a less than 1000-g infant, only about 10% of the cultures were positive. The researchers therefore believe that based on histology and culture results, 80% or more of women in early preterm labor, destined to deliver a less than 1000-g infant, will have organisms in the membranes before membrane rupture. They believe this association is likely to be causal for preterm birth.

Chronicity

There is also ample evidence suggesting that intrauterine infections are often chronic. As evidence, intrauterine infections have been documented weeks or even months before a preterm birth [100–102]. For example, in Alabama, at the time of routine genetic amniocentesis at 16 to 18 weeks, it was occasionally noted that the amniotic fluid was cloudy [100–102]. For this reason, fluids were sent for routine bacterial culture, and cultures for *Ureaplasma* and *Mycoplasma* were often performed. Occasionally the cultures were positive. In nearly all cases in which the amniotic fluid was found to be infected with *Ureaplasma*, the women were initially asymptomatic; however, many of these women went on to deliver spontaneously at 24 to 28 weeks' gestation without clinical chorioamnionitis. The placentas, however, were nearly always positive for histologic chorioamnionitis. Similarly, using PCR techniques for the diagnosis of *Ureaplasma* infection in amniotic fluid, it has been demonstrated that women who are PCR-positive are substantially more likely to experience spontaneous preterm labor later in the second trimester [103]. More recently, using IL-6 as a marker of infection, it has been observed in several series that women undergoing routine genetic amniocentesis at 16 to 18 weeks and who are found to have high amniotic fluid IL-6 levels frequently deliver at less than 32 weeks [104–106].

Organisms

Between 50 and 100 different organisms have been associated with intrauterine infections before the rupture of membranes [93,94]. What is interesting about these infections is that certain common vaginal organisms, such as group B streptococcus and *E coli*, are rarely found in the uterus before rupture of membranes. Furthermore, gonorrhea or *Chlamydia* are hardly ever found inside the uterus before membrane rupture. On the other hand, a number of other organisms, such as *Ureaplasma*, *Mycoplasma, Gardenerella*, *Mobiluncus*, *Peptostreptococcus*, and *Bacteroides*, are quite commonly found in the uterus before membrane rupture. Why some organisms invade the uterus before membrane rupture and others do not is not clear. Galask and colleagues [107] showed that neither *Chlamydia* nor gonorrhea bind to the fetal membranes, and offered the failure to attach as an explanation for their lack of entrance into the uterus before membrane rupture. What is clear about the organisms generally found in the uterus before delivery is that they generally are of low virulence. It may be that this low virulence accounts for both the chronicity described above and the fact that most of the intrauterine infections do not cause a clinical chorioamnionitis.

Mechanisms

The mechanisms by which an intrauterine bacterial infection precipitates preterm labor are relatively clear. Placing either living organisms or bacterial endotoxin into an animal's uterus under experimental conditions precipitates preterm labor in a fashion similar to that which occurs in humans with naturally acquired organisms [108]. In both cases, the intrauterine infection elicits an immune response that includes an increasing production of a wide variety of cytokines, prostaglandins, and metalloproteinases [4,5,86]. These analytes are capable of causing contractions, cervical softening, and membrane rupture, which together ultimately result in spontaneous preterm birth.

Origin of the organisms

Conceptually, there are at least several pathways by which bacteria can enter the uterus. For example, if the mother has a bacteremia or viremia, organisms can enter the uterus hematogenously through the placenta. Although it is believed that hematogenous spread through the placenta is rare, it almost certainly does occur. As evidence, fetuses have been infected by a wide variety of organisms during maternal septicemia, including those causing *Listeria* and tularemia. These organisms appear to reach the fetus through the maternal circulation [22]. Dental organisms such as *Capnocytophaga* and various fusiform organisms are also most likely to enter the uterus through the placenta [109,110]. Theoretically, bacteria can enter the uterus through the fallopian tubes; however, the abdominal cavity is usually sterile. Organisms have been introduced inadvertently into the amniotic cavity at the time of amniocentesis, but this route of infection seems quite rare. Finally, and most commonly, it appears that bacteria from the vagina can ascend into the uterus through the cervix. The organisms most commonly found in the uterus are those typically found in the vagina, of which *Ureaplasma* is the most common. It is therefore widely believed that the organisms responsible for most early preterm birth are vaginal organisms that ascend directly from the vagina through the cervix into the uterus.

Timing of ascent

It is widely held that organisms from the vagina ascend into the uterus during the pregnancy, traversing the space between the membranes and the decidua. The bacteria then take up residence in the membranes, and in about 50% of the cases enter the amniotic fluid. In a much smaller percentage of the cases, the fetus is infected as well. An alternate hypothesis is that the organisms that ultimately cause histologic chorioamnionitis actually reside in the uterus before the pregnancy. Korn and colleagues [111] observed in 1995 that nonpregnant women who had bacterial vaginosis were nearly ten times more likely to have bacterial vaginosis-associated organisms residing in the uterus than were women who did not have bacterial vaginosis. These women were far more likely to have an associated chronic plasma cell endometritis. Andrews and coworkers [112] also observed a large number of bacterial vaginosis related organisms in the uterus in healthy nonpregnant women. These data suggest that there are women who have their endometrium colonized with bacteria before pregnancy. These women are, for the most part, asymptomatic, and would probably remain so until pregnant, because these colonizations do not seem to cause much in the way of symptoms, do not hinder conception to any large degree, and have little impact on the pregnancy until the second trimester. It has been hypothesized by the authors' group [71,86] that once the membranes become tightly applied to the decidua, essentially forming an abscess, only then do these colonizations become symptomatic. With the adherence of the membranes to the decidua at about 20 weeks' gestation, the inflammatory process accelerates, ultimately leading to a preterm birth, which usually occurs before 28 or 30 weeks' gestational age.

Bacterial vaginosis and preterm birth

Bacterial vaginosis (BV) is a vaginal syndrome associated with an alteration of the normal vaginal flora, rather than an infection specific to any one microorganism. BV is diagnosed clinically by the Amsel criteria, which include: (1) the presence of clue cells, (2) a pH higher than 4.5, (3) a profuse whitish discharge, and (4) a fishy odor when that discharge is treated with potassium hydroxide (KOH) [113]. For research purposes, bacterial vaginosis is often defined by the Nugent criteria, whereby air-dried vaginal smears are Gram-stained, and are scored based on the number of lactobacillus (which tend to be low), and the presence of organisms that look like *Mobiluncus* and *Bacteroides*, which tend to be high [114]. A score of 7 to 10 has traditionally been used to diagnose BV; however, a recent study [115] suggests that only the very highest scores (ie, 9 and 10) may be associated with preterm birth.

Nevertheless, BV diagnosed by a score of 7 to 10 has been associated with a one and a half- to threefold increased risk of preterm birth in more than 20 studies [116–118]. Therefore, there is more evidence for this association than for most epidemiologic associations reported in the literature. Interestingly, black women are considerably more likely to have BV than white women [119]. Though not explained by different rates of sexual intercourse or feminine hygiene practices, this two- to threefold difference may explain part of the racial differences in spontaneous preterm birth [120]. In fact, nearly 50% of the excess preterm births and preterm-associated mortality in black versus white infants may be explained by the increase in vaginal and intrauterine infections. Importantly, from a mechanistic point of view, women who have large quantities of these bacteria in the vagina appear more likely to have the same bacteria in the uterus associated with histologic chorioamnionitis. Gravett and colleagues [91], Silver and coworkers [121], Watts and colleagues [98], Hillier and colleagues [122], Krohn and coworkers [123], and others have all shown that there is an association linking BV and subsequent amnionitis, often with similar organisms. The mechanism by which BV is associated with amnionitis and preterm birth is uncertain, but it likely is the result of ascension of the vaginal organisms into the uterus either before, or early in, the pregnancy.

Sexually transmitted diseases and preterm birth

One of the difficult questions to answer related to genital tract infections with gonorrhea, chlamydia, trichomonas, group B streptococcus, and other organisms is whether they are causally associated with preterm birth. With virtually each of these organisms, a range of associations has been reported, varying from none to a strong relationship with preterm birth. In total, it appears that spontaneous preterm birth (defined as a birth following labor or rupture of the membranes) occurs more frequently in women who have and infection than in those who do not; however, even though gonorrhea, chlamydial infection, and other sexually transmitted diseases are usually found more frequently in women who have a spontaneous preterm birth, these women often have other risk factors as well. Furthermore, most studies claiming an association between various infections and preterm birth have not considered many of these confounding variables. As an example, gonorrhea has been associated with spontaneous preterm birth in a number of studies [124]. Almost none of these adjusted for most risk factors and especially for the presence of BV [125]. Therefore, although it is likely that maternal gonorrhea infection is associated with an independent two- or threefold risk for spontaneous preterm birth, this conclusion is not certain. As opposed to the organisms associated with BV, the gonococcus is rarely found in the amniotic fluid or the fetal membranes in women who give birth prematurely. Syphilis is widely reported to be associated with a twofold increased risk of preterm birth, and this relationship is relatively consistent in most studies [126].

Chlamydial infection has been associated with prematurity in some studies but not in others, with the majority of the studies showing no increased risk [118,127]. Sweet and coworkers [128], however, reported that women who had *Chlamydia trachomatis* infection and IgM antibodies were more likely to have a spontaneous preterm birth compared with women who have chlamydia infection and IgG, but not IgM, antibodies. In the Preterm Prediction Study [129], women tested for *Chlamydia trachomatis* at 24 weeks' gestation had about twice as many preterm births associated with the presence of this organism as did uninfected women; however, after adjusting for other risk factors, this association was no longer significant, contributing to the continuing uncertainty about whether chlamydia infection plays a causative role in preterm birth. Many of the other sexually transmitted diseases, such as HIV, hepatitis B, and genital herpes simplex virus, have been associated with an increased risk for spontaneous preterm birth in some, but not most, studies. In general, the evidence for a causative link between maternal infection with these organisms and spontaneous preterm birth is poor [75].

Non–genital tract infections and preterm birth

Several non–genital tract infections seem to be related to, and are probably causal for, preterm birth. The first of these is urinary tract infection. In a meta-analysis of the existing literature by Romero and colleagues [164], urinary tract infection was clearly associated with preterm birth, and antibiotic treatment of urinary tract infection did result in a reduction of preterm birth. Maternal pneumonias and other systemic infections such as appendicitis also appear to increase the risk of preterm birth. Recently, research efforts have focused on exploring the relationship between maternal periodontal disease and subsequent preterm birth [110,130]. This association has now been confirmed at several study sites. Importantly, recent evidence suggests that treatment of the periodontal disease with deep cleaning, as opposed to the use of antibiotics, may reduce the associated preterm birth [131].

Viral infections and preterm birth

In comparison with bacterial infections, the evidence that viral infections are causal for preterm birth is quite sparse; however, in cases of viral infection when the mother has a severe systemic illness, such as varicella pneumonia or polio, a preterm delivery may occur [22,23]. Recent reports suggest that a maternal infection with the severe acute respiratory syndrome (SARS) virus can result in preterm birth as well [132]. In the absence of major systemic disease, the evidence for a relationship between maternal viral infection and preterm delivery is based mostly on case reports. For example, a number of fetuses that had an intrauterine CMV infection have been noted to deliver preterm, although the denominator for such observations is unknown. In the several studies in which asymptomatic women undergoing genetic amniocentesis were evaluated for intra-amniotic viral infection using PCR techniques, a number of different viral DNAs were identified in the amniotic fluid, but their presence was not related to subsequent preterm birth [133]. Therefore, it seems unlikely that maternal viral infection plays an important role in preterm birth. Because of the limited information available, however, further study of this potential relationship is in order.

Maternal infections and the types of adverse pregnancy outcomes

Based on the authors' review of the literature, Table 2 [76,134–136] presents a summary of the types of adverse perinatal outcomes that have been associated with specific maternal infections.

Many of the infants infected with a specific organism during fetal life or during delivery and who manifest disease, do so in the neonatal period. These include most of the infants infected with herpes simplex virus, syphilis, and gonorrhea; however, for many others, the disease will not become apparent for months or years later. For example, although the ophthalmologic damage caused by *Neisseria gonorrhoeae* and *C trachomatis* becomes apparent within several days or weeks after birth, the pneumonia associated with chlamydia infection may occur months after delivery [137,138]. The deafness associated with neonatal cytomegalovirus is often not apparent until later in childhood, and the

Table 2
Adverse reproductive outcomes associated with maternal infection

Maternal colonization/ organism	Infertility	Abortion	Congenital anomalies	Stillbirth	IUGR
Bacterial vaginosis	−	−	−	−	−
Chlamydia	+	−	−	−	−
Coxsackievirus	−	−	±	+	−
Cytomegalovirus	−	−	−	−	+
Echovirus	−	−	−	±	−
Gonorrhoea	+	−	−	−	−
Group B streptococcus	−	−	−	+	−
Hepatitis B	−	−	−	−	−
Hepatitis C	−	−	−	−	−
Herpes simplex	−	−	−	−	−
HIV	−	−	−	−	±
HPV	−	−	−	−	−
Influenza	−	+	−	±	−
Listeria	−	+	−	+	+
Lyme borreliosis	−	−	−	+	+
Malaria	−	+	−	+	+
Measles	−	−	−	−	+
Mumps	+	±	−	±	−
Parvovirus	−	+	−	+	−
Rubella	−	±	+	+	+
SARS	−	+	−	+	±
Syphilis	−	+	+	+	+
Toxoplasmosis	−	+	−	+	+
Trichomonas	−	−	−	−	−
Tuberculosis	−	−	−	±	−
Varicella	−	−	+	±	+

−, Occurs rarely if at all; +, established relationship; ±, may occur, uncommon.
Data from Refs. [75,134–136].

neurological sequelae of fetal or neonatal infections with toxoplasmosis, CMV, rubella, herpes virus, Group B streptococcus and syphilis are often not apparent until later as well [40,139]. The most important outcome in HIV-infected neonates, childhood acquired immunodeficiency syndrome (AIDS), does not usually appear until after infancy. The chronic hepatitis resulting from perinatal infection with the hepatitis B virus is usually not symptomatic in the neonatal period, and the late sequelae of perinatal hepatitis B infection, including cirrhosis and hepatocellular carcinoma, generally occur decades later [140,141]. Congenital infection with the human papilloma virus has been implicated in laryngeal papillomas and several childhood cancers [142,143].

Prevalence and the timing of transmission

There are many definitions of "prenatal," "perinatal," and "intrapartum" in use today. In the following discussion, prenatal refers to the period between

Preterm birth	Neonatal death	Postnatal disease	Long-term disability		
			Deafness	Eye disease	Neurologic
+	−	−	−	−	−
+	−	+	−	+	−
−	−	−	−	−	±
+	+	+	+	+	+
−	+	−	−	−	−
+	−	−	−	+	−
−	+	+	−	−	+
−	−	+	−	−	−
−	−	+	−	−	−
−	+	+	−	+	+
±	−	+	−	−	±
−	−	+	−	−	−
+	−	−	−	−	−
+	+	+	−	−	+
±	−	−	−	−	±
±	−	−	−	−	−
+	+	+	−	−	−
−	−	−	−	−	−
−	−	−	−	−	−
−	+	+	+	+	+
±	−	−	−	−	−
+	+	+	+	−	+
−	−	−	−	+	+
+	−	−	−	−	−
−	+	+	−	−	−
+	+	+	−	+	+

conception and the events leading to delivery, perinatal refers to the time between the onset of labor or rupture of membranes and approximately 1 month after delivery, and intrapartum refers to the period between the onset of labor and delivery. The numerical values used for infection and transmission rates and the percentage of infected infants who had various sequelae used in the following tables are based on a wide variety of sources with widely discrepant estimates [76,134]. These differences may reflect differences in study design, laboratory methodology, or population differences (race and socioeconomic status or size of study population), or case definition.

Table 3 describes the maternal prevalence of a number of infections, as well as the timing of transmission and the percent of neonates infected when the mother is colonized. For example, syphilis, hepatitis B, and HIV infections are currently found in approximately 0.10% to 0.2% of pregnant women in the United States [144,145]. Gonorrhea infections are found in about 1% of all pregnant women, and trichomonas and chlamydia in about 5% [146–148]. Maternal colonization with herpes simplex virus, and bacterial vaginosis is found in approximately 20%

Table 3
Perinatal transmission of major human pathogens

Maternal infection/ organism	Approximate maternal prevalence (%)	Usual timing of transmission		Neonates infected/ colonized (%) when mother colonized and not treated
		Prenatal	Intrapartum	
Bacterial vaginosis	20.0	−	−	0
Chlamydia	5.0	−	+	50.0
Coxsackievirus	1.0	+	−	±
Cytomegalovirus	33.0[a]	+	+	3.0
Echovirus	Variable	−	+	±
Gonorrhoea	1.0	−	+	50.0
Group B streptococcus	20.0	±	+	50.0
Hepatitis B	0.2	−	+	30.0
Hepatitis C	2.0	−	+	8
Herpes simplex	20.0[a]	±	+	0.2
HIV	0.2	+	+	25.0
HPV	5.0	−	+	5.0
Influenza	Variable	+	−	±
Listeria	Rare	+	−	±
Lyme borreliosis	0.1	+	−	±
Malaria	Variable	+	−	4.0
Measles (rubeola)	Rare	+	−	±
Mumps	Rare	+	−	±
Parvovirus	1.0	+	−	20.0
Rubella	Rare	+	−	50.0
Syphilis	0.12	+	±	40.0
Toxoplasmosis	1.0	+	−	30.0
Trichomonas	5.0	−	−	0
Tuberculosis	Rare	+	−	±
Varicella	Rare	+	−	2.0

+, Established relationship; ±, may occur, uncommon; −, occurs rarely if at all.
[a] By serology.
Data from Refs. [75,134–136].

of pregnant women. Cytomegalovirus infection is estimated to be present in about one third of all pregnant women [149,150].

Infants are virtually never infected with *Trichomonas.* Manifestation of bacterial vaginosis in the infant is unknown; however, neonatal infections with *U urealyticum*, *Mycoplasma hominis*, various bacterioides spp, *Gardnerella* or other bacterial vaginosis-related organisms have been reported, although rarely [151]. Congenital syphilis is usually transmitted after the first trimester, but can be transmitted at any time during the pregnancy or at delivery. *N gonorrhoeae, C trachomatis,* and the hepatitis B virus rarely infect the fetus in the prenatal period and are almost never found in the uterus before rupture of the membranes [1,74,124,152–154]. Instead, the fetus generally acquires these organisms as it passes through the birth canal. Fetal infections with herpes simplex virus rarely occur before the rupture of the membranes [155,156]. Instead, the vast majority of transmissions occur after the rupture of the membranes or in the intrapartum period. Transmission rates to the fetus vary depending on whether the infection is primary or recurrent. Neonatal HIV infection may be acquired prenatally, but studies of second trimester abortuses suggest that early in utero infection is rare. Using a mathematical model, Rouzioux and colleagues [157] estimated that one third of the transmissions occur in the last 2 weeks of pregnancy and two thirds occur in the intrapartum period. Women who have an HIV infection and whose membranes rupture more than 4 hours before delivery or who are delivered vaginally are, in most studies, more likely to transmit this infection to their neonates [158–160].

If the mother is infected, variable percents of the exposed infants, depending upon the disease, become colonized (see Table 3). Without treatment, these rates of transmission range from 0.2% for herpes simplex, to 3% for cytomegalovirus, and up to 25% to 40% for syphilis, hepatitis B virus, and HIV [161]. If routine ophthalmic prophylaxis is not used, approximately 30% to 50% of the infants [52] of infected mothers acquire gonorrhea or chlamydia ophthalmic infections.

Transmission of organisms to the fetus and newborn

Because the influence of maternally transmitted organisms on adverse outcomes of pregnancy are generally presented in individual papers, it may be instructive to compare their impact. For a subset of maternal infections that are associated with fetal infection, Table 4 indicates not only the maternal and infant prevalences in the 4 million births per year in the United States, but also the approximate number of mothers and infants who have an infection. Also displayed in this table is the approximate number of infants each year in the United States who have specific types of sequelae associated with direct fetal or infant infection. The potential excess in preterm births attributable to various infections and the sequelae associated with those preterm births are discussed later. When translated into the total US population, this means that there are approximately 4000 to 8000 pregnant women per year who have syphilis, hepatitis B, or HIV; about 40,000 pregnant women per year infected with gonorrhea; about 80,000 pregnant women who have *Trichomonas*; perhaps 200,000 pregnant women who have chlamydia; and approximately 800,000 pregnant women per year who have herpes simplex virus or BV. It is estimated that approximately 1.3 million pregnant women are infected/colonized with CMV. Again, these numbers are our best estimates for infection for the entire population of pregnant women who give birth in the United States each year. Subpopulations of women who have markedly higher and lower prevalences have been described. For both herpes simplex virus and cytomegalovirus, it is assumed that previous infection, as defined serologically, is associated with persistent infection.

Table 4
The estimated impact of direct fetal and neonatal infection with various infections on adverse outcomes of pregnancy each year in the 4,000,000 United States births

Maternal infection/ organism	Approximate maternal prevalence (%)	Mothers infected/ colonized (no.)	With current treatment in the United States, of infected mothers, % and no. of infants colonized		Adverse outcomes of fetal neonatal infection/colonized			
			%	No.	Neonatal disease without sequelae	Perinatal death	Neurologic sequelae	New onset post-neonatal illness and death
Bacterial vaginosis	20.0	800,000	0	0	0	0	0	0
Chlamydia[a]	5.0	200,000	50.0	100,000	20,000[b]	0	0	0
Cytomegalovirus	33.0	1,300,000	3.0	40,000	±	300	2000	5000[c]
Gonorrhea[a]	1.0	40,000	50.0	20,000	±	±	±	0
Group B streptococcus[d]	20.0	800,000	12.5	100,000	1200	150	150	—
Hepatitis B[e]	0.2	8000	10.0	800	0	0	0	300
Herpes simplex	20.0	800,000	0.15	1200	400	400	400	0
HIV[f]	0.2	8000	1.0	80	0	0	0	80
Rubella	Rare	—	—	—	0	0	0	0
Syphilis	0.12	4800	40.0	1920	720	720	600	0
Trichomonas	5.0	200,000	0	0	0	0	0	0

±, Occurs, but rarely.
[a] Assumes prophylaxis for eye disease.
[b] Mild pneumonia.
[c] Hearing loss.
[d] Assuming current screening and treatment programs reduce transmission by 75% and that 1.5% of colonized infants develop sepsis.
[e] Assuming current screening and treatment programs reduce transmission by 70%.
[f] Assuming current screening and treatment programs reduce transmission to 1%.
Data from Refs. [75,135,136].

Adverse outcomes associated with perinatal transmission

The next several columns in Table 4 show potential outcomes associated with fetal and perinatal infection with each of the organisms. These are estimates of outcomes achieved in the United States with current medical practices. From the existing literature, it is estimated that of the 1920 infants infected with syphilis at the time of birth, approximately 600 will be stillborn or will die as neonates, and about 600 will have long-term neurological or other sequelae. Approximately 720 of these 1920 infants will live and not have apparent long-term sequelae. With gonorrhea, assuming no ophthalmologic disease because of prophylaxis, there will be few major sequelae in the infant from neonatal infection. Of the 100,000 infants infected with chlamydia at birth, again assuming no long-term ophthalmologic sequelae because of prophylaxis, it is estimated that there will be approximately 20,000 cases of chlamydial pneumonia, nearly all of which will regress spontaneously or respond to antibiotics and not result in long-term sequelae or death [135]. Without immunoprophylaxis, of the 12,000 infants infected with hepatitis B virus at birth, approximately 4000 will ultimately develop cirrhosis or hepatocellular carcinoma [140,162]. These numbers should be substantially reduced with routine neonatal hepatitis B immunoglobulin prophylaxis and vaccination, and although the numbers are unknown, the authors estimate that about 300 will develop cirrhosis or hepatocellular carcinoma sometimes in their lives. Of the 1200 infants infected at birth with herpes simplex virus, an estimated 400 will die during the perinatal period, approximately 400 will have neurological sequelae, and 400 will have neonatal disease but no long-term sequelae. Of the 40,000 infants infected with CMV, approximately 7% will have signs of disease in the neonatal period. Of these 2800 infants, some 300 will die, whereas 2000 more will have major neurological sequelae. Newell [163] estimates that as much as 7% of all cases of cerebral palsy are due to CMV infections. Later in life, an additional 5000 infants will have significant hearing loss associated with the CMV infection [147]. As stated above, it is estimated that with maternal and infant prophylaxis, fewer than 100 infants per year in the United States will be infected with HIV. It is assumed that even with treatment, each of these infants will ultimately manifest AIDS and die of the disease.

Adverse outcomes associated with infection-related preterm birth

As discussed above, it is not absolutely clear whether maternal infections such as gonorrhea, syphilis, chlamydial infection, Group B streptococcal infection, or trichomoniasis result in preterm birth. The data supporting the association of BV with spontaneous preterm birth are more solid. Although the relationships are uncertain, based on the authors' assessment of the literature, we assumed that gonorrhea is associated with a threefold increase in the preterm birth rate, and that syphilis and chlamydial infection are associated with a twofold increase in pre-

Table 5
The estimated impact of various infections on adverse outcomes of pregnancy[a] through their effect on preterm birth

Maternal infection/ organism	Approximate maternal prevalence (%)	Mothers infected (no.)	Estimated increase in preterm birth[b] (×)	Estimated excess preterm birth[c] (no.)	Adverse outcomes linked to preterm birth[d]	
					Perinatal death (no.)	Neurologic sequelae (no.)
Bacterial vaginosis	20.0	800,000	2×	80,000	4000	4000
Chlamydia	5.0	200,000	2×	20,000	1000	1000
Cytomegalovirus	33.0	1,300,000	[e]	—	—	—
Gonorrhea	1.0	40,000	3×	8000	400	400
Group B streptococcus	20	80,000	[e]	—	—	—
Hepatitis B	1.0	40,000	[e]	—	—	—
Herpes simplex	20.0	800,000	[e]	—	—	—
HIV	0.2	8000	[e]	—	—	—
Rubella	0	0	[e]	—	—	—
Syphilis	0.12	4800	2×	480	24	24
Trichomonas	2.0	80,000	1.3	2400	120	120

[a] Assuming 4,000,000 births per year.
[b] Based on best available data in untreated women.
[c] Assuming a baseline preterm rate of 10%.
[d] Assuming 5% deaths and 5% neurologic sequelae.
[e] Insufficient evidence for a causative relationship.

Data from Refs. [75,135].

term birth. Bacterial vaginosis is associated with a twofold increase and trichomonas with a 1.3-fold increase. From these numbers and the rates of maternal infection, assuming a 10% rate of prematurity in the general population, the excess number of preterm births per year in the United States associated with maternal infection with each organism can be calculated (Table 5). As an example, if 40,000 pregnant women in the Unites States are infected per year with gonorrhea, and if these women have a 30% instead of a 10% rate of spontaneous preterm birth, maternal gonorrhea infection may be associated with an estimated 8000 excess preterm births. Of the 4800 women who have syphilis, assuming a twofold increase in preterm birth, approximately 480 excess preterm births due to syphilis may occur in the United States each year. Assuming a twofold increase in preterm birth, with 200,000 mothers having chlamydial infection each year, as many as 20,000 excess preterm births may be associated with maternal chlamydial infection. Applying this same logic to maternal BV infections and assuming a twofold increase in preterm birth associated with BV, of the 800,000 women who have BV, an excess of 80,000 preterm births may occur.

The last two columns in Table 4 show the estimated number of perinatal deaths and infants who have major neurological handicaps associated with maternal infections and preterm birth, if it is assumed that 5% of the preterm infants die and 5% are neurologically handicapped with such conditions as blindness, hydrocephalus, mental retardation, or cerebral palsy. If these assumptions are correct, prematurity secondary to maternal gonococcal infections may be responsible for approximately 400 perinatal deaths and 400 children experiencing long-term neurological sequelae. Through its influence on preterm birth, syphilis would be responsible for an additional 16 perinatal deaths and for 16 children who have long-term neurological sequelae. Through its impact on preterm birth, chlamydial infection might account for as many as 1000 excess perinatal deaths and 1000 children who have long-term disability. Maternal BV, because of its high prevalence in the population and an associated twofold increase in preterm birth, may be responsible for approximately 80,000 excess preterm births, 4000 perinatal deaths, and 4000 children who have long-term neurological sequelae. The authors emphasize that most of these adverse outcomes associated with preterm birth occur without apparent fetal or neonatal infection.

Summary

Fetal or neonatal infections with the agents of sexually transmitted diseases—syphilis, herpes simplex virus, and HIV —ay have a devastating effect, including either death or long-term neurological disability. In the United States, associated with each of these infections, between 1000 and 2500 infants per year die or are severely damaged. In contrast to these relatively rare outcomes, approximately 400,000 infants are born prematurely each year, and of these, more than 20,000 die in the fetal or the neonatal period, and another 20,000 have neurological sequelae. If the projected effect on preterm birth by BV and the other organisms proposed here is correct, as many as 100,000 preterm births and 5000 or more of the deaths, as well as a similar number of the major disabilities, may be associated with maternal infections. Because some studies suggest that some of the preterm births associated with BV and intrauterine infection may be prevented, it seems that the greatest potential for reducing adverse outcomes of pregnancy associated with maternal infection lies in preventing or treating BV and intrauterine infection-associated preterm births.

References

[1] Alberman E, Stanley F. Guidelines to the epidemiological approach. In: Stanley F, Alberman E, editors. Clinics in developmental medicine no. 87; the epidemiology of the cerebral palsies. Lavenham, United Kingdom: Spastics International Medical Publications; 1984. p. 172–83.

[2] Wendel PJ, Wendel Jr GD. Sexually transmitted diseases in pregnancy. Semin Perinatol 1993; 17:443–51.

[3] Goldner TE, Lawson HW, Xia Z, et al. Surveillance for ectopic pregnancy—United States, 1970–1989. MMWR CDC Surveill Summ 1993;42(6):73–85.

[4] Romero R, Brody DT, Oyarzun E, et al. Infection and labor. III. Interleukin-1: a signal for the onset of parturition. Am J Obstet Gynecol 1989;160:1117–23.

[5] Andrews WW, Hauth JC, Goldenberg RL, et al. Amniotic fluid interleukin-6: correlation with upper genital tract microbial colonization and gestational age in women delivered following spontaneous labor versus indicated delivery. Am J Obstet Gynecol 1995;173:606–12.

[6] Arntzen KJ, Kjolledsal AM, Halgunset J, et al. TNF, IL-1, IL-6, IL-8 and soluble TNG receptors in relation to chorioamnionitis and premature labor. J Perinat Med 1998;26:17–26.

[7] Steinborn A, Kuhnert M, Halberstadt E. Immunmodulating cytokines induce term and preterm parturition. J Perinat Med 1996;24:381–90.

[8] Maeda K, Matsuzaki N, Fuke S, et al. Value of the maternal interleukin 6 level for determination of histologic chorioamnionitis in preterm delivery. Gynecol Obstet Invest 1997;43: 225–31.

[9] Saito S, Kasahara T, Kato Y, et al. Elevation of amniotic fluid interleukin 6 (IL-6), IL-8 and granulocyte colony stimulating factor (G-CSF) in term and preterm parturition. Cytokine 1993; 5:81–8.

[10] Cassell G, Andrews W, Hauth J, et al. Isolation of microorganisms from the chorioamnion is twice that from amniotic fluid at cesarean delivery in women with intact membranes. Am J Obstet Gynecol 1993;168:424.

[11] Guzick DS, Winn K. The association of chorioamnionitis with preterm delivery. Obstet Gynecol 1985;65:11–6.

[12] Speroff L, Glass RH, Kase NG. Clinical gynecologic endocrinology and infertility. 6th edition. Baltimore (MD): Williams & Wilkins; 1999.

[13] Andrews WW, Goldenberg RL, Hauth JC. Preterm labor: emerging role of genital tract infections. Infect Agents Dis 1995;4:196–211.

[14] Gibbs RS, Romero MD, Hillier SL, et al. A review of premature birth and subclinical infection. Am J Obstet Gynecol 1992;166:1515–28.

[15] Hsieh HL, Lee KS, Khoshnood B, et al. Fetal death rate in the United States, 1979–1990: trend and racial disparity. Obstet Gynecol 1997;89:33–9.

[16] Martin JA, Hoyert DL. The national fetal death file. Semin Perinatol 2002;26:3–11.

[17] Bale JR, Stoll BJ, Lucas AO, editors. Improving birth outcomes. Reducing fetal mortality. Washington (DC): The National Academies Press; 2003.

[18] Copper RL, Goldenberg RL, Dubard MB, et al. Risk factors for fetal death in white, black, and Hispanic women. Collaborative Group on Preterm Birth Prevention. Obstet Gynecol 1994; 84:490–5.
[19] Winbo I, Serenius F, Dahlquist G, et al. Maternal risk factors for cause-specific stillbirth and neonatal death. Acta Obstet Gynecol Scand 2001;80:235–44.
[20] Benirschke K, Robb J. Infectious causes of fetal death. Clin Obstet Gynecol 1987;30:284–94.
[21] Gibbs RS. The origins of stillbirth: infectious diseases. Semin Perinatol 2002;26:75–8.
[22] Goldenberg RL, Thompson C. The infectious origins of stillbirth. Am J Obstet Gynecol 2003; 189:861–73.
[23] Herschel M, Hsieh H, Mittendorf R, et al. Fetal death in a population of black women. Am J Prev Med 1995;11:185–9.
[24] Hardy JMB, Azarowicz EN, Mannini A, et al. The effect of Asian influenza on the outcome of pregnancy. Baltimore 1957–1958. Am J Public Health 1961;51:1182–8.
[25] Horn P. Poliomyelitis in pregnancy. A twenty-year report from Los Angeles County, California. Obstet Gynecol 1955;6:121–37.
[26] Steketee RW, Wirima JJ, Slutsker L, et al. The problem of malaria and malaria control in pregnancy in sub-Saharan Africa. Am J Trop Med Hyg 1996;55:2–7.
[27] Naeye RL, Tafari N, Judge D, et al. Amniotic fluid infections in an African city. J Pediatr 1977; 90(6):965–70.
[28] Bernirschke K, Clifford SH. Intrauterine bacterial infection of the newborn infant. J Pediatr 1959;54:11–8.
[29] Blanc W. Pathways of fetal and early neonatal infection. J Pediatr 1961;59:473–96.
[30] Cooper LZ, Alford CA. Rubella. In: Remington JS, Klein JO, editors. Infectious diseases of the fetus and newborn infant. Philadelphia: Saunders; 2001. p. 347–88.
[31] Martin D, Schoub B. Rubella infection in pregnancy. In: Newell ML, McIntyre J, editors. Congenital and perinatal infections. Cambridge, United Kingdom: Cambridge University Press; 2000. p. 83–95.
[32] Jeffcoat MK, Geurs NC, Reddy MS, et al. Current evidence regarding periodontal disease as a risk factor in preterm birth. Ann Periodontol 2001;6(1):183–8.
[33] Schuchat A, Oxtoby M, Cochi S, et al. Population-based risk factors for neonatal group B streptococcal disease: results of a cohort study in metropolitan Atlanta. J Infect Dis 1990;162: 672–7.
[34] Rouse DJ, Goldenberg RL, Cliver SP, et al. Strategies for the prevention of early-onset neonatal group B streptococcal sepsis, a decision analysis. Obstet Gynecol 1994;83:483–94.
[35] Bhutta ZA, Yusuf K. Early-onset neonatal sepsis in Pakistan: a case control study of risk factors in a birth cohort. Am J Perinatol 1997;14:577–81.
[36] Stoll BJ. Neonatal infections: a global perspective. In: Remington JS, Klein JO, editors. Infectious diseases of the fetus and newborn infant. Philadelphia: Saunders; 2001. p. 139–68.
[37] Nelson KB, Ellenberg JH. Epidemiology of cerebral palsy. Adv Neurol 1978;19:421–35.
[38] Nelson KB, Ellenberg JH. Intrapartum events and cerebral palsy. In: Kubli F, Patel N, Schmidt W, et al, editors. Perinatal events and brain damage in surviving children. Heidelberg (Germany): Springer-Verlag; 1988. p. 139–48.
[39] Fowler KB, Stagno S, Pass RF, et al. The outcome of congenital cytomegalovirus infection in relation to maternal antibody status. N Engl J Med 1992;326:663–7.
[40] Stanley F. Social and biological determinants of the cerebral palsies. In: Stanely F, Alberman E, editors. Clinics in developmental medicine no. 87; the epidemiology of the cerebral palsies. Lavenham, Suffolk: Spastics International Medical Publications, Great Britain, Lavenham Press Ltd.; 1984. p. 69–86.
[41] Nelson KB. Epidemiology of cerebral palsy. In: Levene MI, Lilford RJ, Bennett MJ, et al, editors. Fetal and neonatal neurology and neurosurgery. New York: Churchill Livingstone; 1995. p. 681–8.
[42] Dammann O, Leviton A. Role of the fetus in perinatal infection and neonatal brain damage. Curr Opin Pediatr 2000;12(2):99–104.

[43] Yoon BH, Romero R, Park JS, et al. The relationship among inflammatory lesions of the umbilical cord (funisitis), umbilical cord plasma interleukin 6 concentration, amniotic fluid infection, and neonatal sepsis. Am J Obstet Gynecol 2000;183(5):1124–9.
[44] Wu YW, Colford Jr JM. Chorioamnionitis as a risk factor for cerebral palsy: a meta-analysis. JAMA 2000;284:1417–24.
[45] Grether JK, Nelson KB, Emery III ES, et al. Prenatal and perinatal factors and cerebral palsy in very low birth weight infants. J Pediatr 1996;128:407–14.
[46] Grether JK, Nelson KB. Maternal infection and cerebral palsy in infants of normal birth weight. JAMA 1997;278:207–11.
[47] Murphy DJ, Sellers S, MacKenzie IZ, et al. Case-control study of antenatal and intrapartum risk factors for cerebral palsy in very preterm singleton babies. Lancet 1995;346:1449–54.
[48] Groome LJ, Goldenberg RL, Cliver SP, et al. Neonatal periventricular-intraventricular hemorrhage after maternal β-sympathomimetic tocolysis. Am J Obstet Gynecol 1992;167: 873–9.
[49] Dammann O, Leviton A. Maternal intrauterine infection, cytokines, and brain damage in the preterm newborn. Pediatr Res 1996;42:1–8.
[50] Dammann O, Leviton A. The role of perinatal brain damage in developmental disabilities: an epidemiologic perspective. Ment Retard Dev Disabil Res Rev 1997;3:13–21.
[51] Stoll BJ, Gordon T, Korones SB, et al. Early-onset sepsis in very low birth weight neonates: a report from the National Institute of Child Health and Human Development Neonatal Research Network. J Pediatr 1995;129:72–80.
[52] Stoll BJ, Gordon T, Korones SB, et al. Late-onset sepsis in very low birth weight neonates: a report from the National Institute of Child Health and Human Development Neonatal Research Network. J Pediatr 1996;129:63–71.
[53] Bejar R, Wozniak P, Allard M, et al. Antenatal origin of neurologic damage in newborn infants. I. Preterm infants. Am J Obstet Gynecol 1988;159:357–63.
[54] Leviton A. Preterm birth and cerebral palsy: is tumor necrosis factor the missing link? Dev Med Child Neurol 1993;35:549.
[55] Mays J, Verma U, Klein S, et al. Acute appendicitis in pregnancy and the occurrence of major intraventricular hemorrhage and periventricular leukomalacia. Obstet Gynecol 1995;86: 650–2.
[56] Dammann O, Leviton A. Infection remote from the brain, neonatal white matter damage, and cerebral palsy in the preterm infant. Semin Pediatr Neurol 1998;5:190–201.
[57] Hansen AR, Collins MH, Genest D. Very low birth weight infant's placenta and its relation to pregnancy and fetal characteristics. Pediatr Dev Pathol 2000;3:419–30.
[58] Grafe MR. The correlation of prenatal brain damage with placental pathology. J Neuropathol Exp Neurol 1994;53:407–15.
[59] Salafia CM, Minior VK, Rosenkrantz TS, et al. Maternal, placental, and neonatal associations with early germinal matrix/intraventricular hemorrhage in infants born before 23 weeks' gestation. Am J Perinatol 1995;12:429–36.
[60] Kraus FT. Cerebral palsy and thrombi in placental vessels of the fetus: insights from litigation. Hum Pathol 1997;28:246–8.
[61] Redline RW, O'Riordan MA. Placental lesions associated with cerebral palsy and neurologic impairment following term birth. Arch Pathol Lab Med 2000;124:1785–91.
[62] Kuban KCK, Leviton A. Cerebral palsy. N Engl J Med 1994;330:188–95.
[63] Zupan V, Gonzalez P, Lacaze-Masmonteil T, et al. Periventricular leukomalacia: risk factors revisited. Dev Med Child Neurol 1996;38:1061–7.
[64] Perlman JM, Risser R, Broyles RS. Bilateral cystic periventricular leukomalacia in the premature infant: associated risk factors. Pediatrics 1996;97:822–7.
[65] Adinolfi M. Infectious diseases in pregnancy, cytokines and neurological impairment: a hypothesis. Dev Med Child Neurol 1993;35:549–53.
[66] Martinez E, Figueroa R, Garry D, et al. Elevated amniotic fluid interleukin-6 as a predictor of neonatal periventricular leukomalacia and intraventricular hemorrhage. J Matern Fetal Invest 1998;8:101–7.

[67] Yoon BH, Romero R, Kim CJ, et al. High expression of interleukin-6, interleukin-1β, and tumor necrosis factor-α in periventricular leukomalacia [abstract]. Am J Obstet Gynecol 1996; 174:399.
[68] Kashlan F, Smulian J, Vintzileos A, et al. Umbilical vein interleukin-6 (IL-6) levels and intracranial events in very low birth weight infants. Pediatr Res 1997;41:158A.
[69] Yoon BH, Romero R, Park JS, et al. Fetal exposure to an intra-amniotic inflammation and the development of cerebral palsy at the age of three years. Am J Obstet Gynecol 2000;182: 675–81.
[70] Duggan PJ, Maalouf EF, Watts TL, et al. Intrauterine T-cell activation and increased proinflammatory cytokine concentrations in preterm infants with cerebral lesions. Lancet 2001;358(9294):1699–700.
[71] Goldenberg RL, Andrews WW. Intrauterine infection and why preterm prevention programs have failed. Am J Public Health 1996;86:781–3.
[72] Goldenberg RL, DuBard MB, Cliver SP, et al. Pregnancy outcome and intelligence at age five years. Am J Obstet Gynecol 1996;175:1511–5.
[73] Allen M. Developmental outcome and followup of the small for gestational age infant. Semin Perinatol 1984;8:123–56.
[74] Henderson JL, Weiner CP. Congenital infection. Curr Opin Obstet Gynecol 1995;7:130–4.
[75] Goldenberg RL, Andrews WW, Yuan AC, et al. Sexually transmitted diseases and adverse outcomes of pregnancy. Clin Perinatol 1997;24:23–41.
[76] Brown AS, Begg MD, Gravenstein S, et al. Serologic evidence of prenatal influenza in the etiology of schizophrenia. Arch Gen Psychiatry 2004;61:774–80.
[77] Brown AS, Susser ES. In utero infection and adult schizophrenia. Ment Retard Dev Disabil Res Rev 2002;8:51–7.
[78] Buka SL, Fan AP. Association of prenatal and perinatal complications with subsequent bipolar disorder and schizophrenia. Schizophr Res 1999;39:113–9 [discussion: 160–1].
[79] Buka SL, Tsuang MT, Torrey EF, et al. Maternal cytokine levels during pregnancy and adult psychosis. Brain Behav Immun 2001;15:411–20.
[80] Klein RM, Jiang H, Du M, et al. Detection of enteroviral RNA (poliovirus types 1 and 3) in endomyocardial biopsies from patients with ventricular tachycardia and survivors of sudden cardiac death. Scand J Infect Dis 2002;34:746–52.
[81] Goldenberg RL, Cutter GR, Hoffman H, et al. Intrauterine growth retardation: standards for diagnosis. Am J Obstet Gynecol 1989;161:271–7.
[82] McCormick MC. The contribution of low birth weight to infant mortality and childhood morbidity. N Engl J Med 1985;312:82–90.
[83] Goldenberg RL, Rouse DJ. The prevention of premature birth. N Engl J Med 1998;339:313–20.
[84] Hack M, Fanaroff AA. Outcomes of children of extremely low birth weight and gestational age in the 1990's. Early Hum Dev 1999;53:193–218.
[85] Lorenz JM, Wooliever DE, Jetton JR, et al. A quantitative review of mortality and developmental disability in extremely premature newborns. Arch Pediatr Adolesc Med 1998;152: 425–35.
[86] Goldenberg RL, Hauth JC, Andrews WW. Intrauterine infection and preterm delivery. N Engl J Med 2000;342:1500–7.
[87] Knox Jr IC, Hoerner JK. The role of infection in premature rupture of the membranes. Am J Obstet Gynecol 1950;59:190–4.
[88] Bobitt JR, Ledger WJ. Unrecognized amnionitis and prematurity: a preliminary report. J Reprod Med 1977;19:8–12.
[89] Elder HA, Santamarina BAG, Smith S, et al. The natural history of asymptomatic bacteriuria during pregnancy: the effect of tetracycline on the clinical course and the outcome of pregnancy. Am J Obstet Gynecol 1971;111:441–61.
[90] Bobiitt JR, Hayslip CC, Damato JD. Amniotic fluid infection as determined by transabdominal amniocentesis in patients with intact membranes with premature labor. Am J Obstet Gynecol 1981;140:947–52.

[91] Gravett MG, Hummel D, Eschenbach DA, et al. Preterm labor associated with subclinical amniotic fluid infection and with subclinical bacterial vaginosis. Obstet Gynecol 1986;67: 229–37.
[92] Harger JH, Meyer MP, Amortegui A, et al. Low incidence of positive amniotic fluid cultures in preterm labor at 27–32 weeks in the absence of clinical evidence of chorioamnionitis. Obstet Gynecol 1991;77:228–34.
[93] Romero R, Sirtori M, Oyarzun E, et al. Infection and labor. V. Prevalence, microbiology, and clinical significance of intraamniotic infection in women with preterm labor and intact membranes. Am J Obstet Gynecol 1989;161:817–24.
[94] Gibbs RS, Romero R, Hillier SL, et al. A review of premature birth and subclinical infection. Am J Obstet Gynecol 1992;166:1515–28.
[95] Russell P. Inflammatory lesions of the human placenta. I. Clinical significance of acute chorioamnionitis. Diagn Gynecol Obstet 1979;1:127–37.
[96] Mueller-Heubach E, Rubinstein DN, Schwarz SS. Histologic chorioamnionitis and preterm delivery in different patient populations. Obstet Gynecol 1990;75:622–6.
[97] Chellam VG, Rushton DI. Chorioamnionitis and funiculitis in the placentas of births weighing less than 2.5 kg. Br J Obstet Gynaecol 1985;92:808–14.
[98] Watts DH, Krohn MA, Hillier SL, et al. The association of occult amniotic fluid infection with gestational age and neonatal outcome among women in preterm labor. Obstet Gynecol 1992;79:351–7.
[99] Hauth JC, Andrews WW, Goldenberg RL. Infection-related risk factors predictive of spontaneous labor and birth. Prenat Neonatal Med 1998;3:86–90.
[100] Cassell GH, Davis RO, Waites KB, et al. Isolation of *Mycoplasma hominis* and *Ureaplasma urealyticum* from amniotic fluid at 16–20 weeks of gestation: potential effect on outcome of pregnancy. Sex Transm Dis 1983;10(Suppl 4):294–302.
[101] Cassell G. Ureaplasma Infection. In: Hitchcock PJ, MacKay HT, Wasserheit JN, et al, editors. Sexually transmitted diseases and adverse outcomes of pregnancy. Washington (DC): ASM Press; 1999. p. 175–93.
[102] Horowitz S, Mazor M, Romero R, et al. Infection of the amniotic cavity with *Ureaplasma urealyticum* in the midtrimester of pregnancy. J Reprod Med 1995;40(5):375–9.
[103] Gray DJ, Robinson HB, Malone J, et al. Adverse outcome in pregnancy following amniotic fluid isolation of *Ureaplasma urealyticum*. Prenat Diagn 1992;12:111–7.
[104] Ghidini A, Jenkins CB, Spong CY, et al. Elevated amniotic fluid interleukin-6 levels during the early second trimester are associated with greater risk of subsequent preterm delivery. Am J Reprod Immunol 1997;37:227–31.
[105] Wenstrom KD, Andrews WW, Hauth JC, et al. Elevated second trimester amniotic fluid interleukin-6 levels predict preterm delivery. Am J Obstet Gynecol 1998;178:546–50.
[106] Wenstrom KD, Andrews WW, Tsuneobu T, et al. Elevated amniotic fluid interleukin-6 levels at genetic amniocentesis predict subsequent pregnancy loss. Am J Obstet Gynecol 1996;175: 830–3.
[107] Galask RP, Varner MW, Petzold R, et al. Bacterial attachment to the chorioamniotic membranes. Am J Obstet Gynecol 1984;148:915–28.
[108] Gravett MG, Witkin SS, Haluska GJ, et al. An experimental model for intramniotic infection and preterm labor in rhesus monkeys. Am J Obstet Gynecol 1994;171:1660–7.
[109] Dixon NG, Ebright D, Defrancesco MA, et al. Orogenital contact: a cause of chorioamnionitis? Obstet Gynecol 1994;84:654–5.
[110] Jeffcoat MK, Geurs NC, Reddy MS, et al. Periodontal infection and preterm birth: results of a prospective study. J Am Dent Assoc 2001;132:875–80.
[111] Korn AP, Bolan G, Padian N, et al. Plasma cell endometritis in women with symptomatic bacterial vaginosis. Obstet Gynecol 1995;85:387–90.
[112] Andrews WW, Hauth JC, Cliver S, et al. Endometrial microbial colonization and plasma cell endometritis following spontaneous or indicated preterm vs. term birth [abstract]. Am J Obstet Gynecol 2000;182:S53.

[113] Amstel R, Totten PA, Speigel CA, et al. Nonspecific vaginitis: diagnostic criteria and microbial and epidemiologic associations. Am J Med 1983;74:14–22.
[114] Nugent RP, Krohn MA, Hillier SL. Reliability of diagnosing bacterial vaginosis is improved by a standardized method of gram stain interpretation. J Clin Microbiol 1991;29:297–301.
[115] Hauth JC, MacPherson C, Carey C, et al. Early pregnancy threshold vaginal pH and gram stain scores predictive of subsequent preterm birth in asymptomatic women. Am J Obstet Gynecol 2003;188:831–5.
[116] Meis PJ, Goldenberg RL, Mercer B, et al. The preterm prediction study: significance of vaginal infections. National Institute of Child Health and Human Development Maternal-Fetal Medicine Units Network. Am J Obstet Gynecol 1995;173(4):1231–5.
[117] Hillier SL, Nugent RP, Eschenbach DA, et al for the Vaginal Infections and Prematurity Study Group. Association between bacterial vaginosis and preterm delivery of a low-birth-weight infant. N Engl J Med 1995;333:1737–42.
[118] Martius J, Krohn MA, Hillier SL, et al. Relationships of vaginal lactobacillus species, cervical *Chlamydia trachomatis*, and bacterial vaginosis to preterm birth. Obstet Gynecol 1988;71: 89–95.
[119] Goldenberg RL, Klebanoff MA, Nugent R, et al. Bacterial colonization of the vagina during pregnancy in four ethnic groups. Am J Obstet Gynecol 1996;175:1317–24.
[120] Fiscella K. Racial disparities in preterm births: the role of urogenital infections. Public Health Rep 1996;111:104–13.
[121] Silver HM, Sperling RS, St. Clair PJ, et al. Evidence relating bacterial vaginosis to intra-amniotic infection. Am J Obstet Gynecol 1989;161:808–12.
[122] Hillier SL, Krohn MA, Cassen E, et al. The role of bacterial vaginosis and vaginal bacteria in amniotic fluid infection in women in preterm labor with intact fetal membranes. Clin Infect Dis 1994;20(Suppl 2):S276–8.
[123] Krohn MA, Hillier SL, Nugent RP, et al. The genital flora of women with intraamniotic infection. Vaginal infection and prematurity study group. J Inf Dis 1995;171:1475–80.
[124] Elliott B, Brunham RC, Laga M, et al. Maternal gonococcal infection as a preventable factor for low birth weight. J Infect Dis 1990;161:531–6.
[125] Donders GG, Desmyter J, De Wet DH, et al. The association of gonorrhea and syphilis with premature birth and low birth weight. Genitourin Med 1993;69:98–101.
[126] Ingall D, Sanchez PJ, Musher DM. Syphilis. In: Remington JS, Klein JO, editors. Infectious diseases of the fetus and newborn infant. 4th edition. Philadelphia: W.B. Saunders; 1995. p. 529–64.
[127] Martin DH, Koutsky L, Eschenbach DA, et al. Prematurity and perinatal mortality in pregnancies complicated by maternal *Chlamydia trachomatis* infections. JAMA 1982;247:1585–8.
[128] Sweet RL, Landers DL, Walker C, et al. *Chlamydia trachomatis* infection and pregnancy outcome. Am J Obstet Gynecol 1987;156:824–33.
[129] Andrews WW, and the MFMU Network. The Preterm Prediction Study: association of mid-trimester genital chlamydia infection and subsequent spontaneous preterm birth [abstract]. Am J Obstet Gynecol 1997;176:151.
[130] Offenbacher S, Katz V, Fertik G, et al. Periodontal infection as a possible risk factor for preterm low birth weight. J Periodontol 1996;67(Suppl 10):1103–13.
[131] Jeffcoat MK, Hauth JC, Geurs NC, et al. Periodontal disease and preterm birth: results of a pilot intervention study. J Periodontol 2003;74:1214–8.
[132] Wong SF, Chow KM, Leung TN, et al. Pregnancy and perinatal outcomes of women with severe acute respiratory syndrome. Am J Obstet Gynecol 2004;191:292–7.
[133] Wenstrom KD, Andrews WW, Bowles NE, et al. Intrauterine viral infection at the time of second trimester genetic amniocentesis. Obstet Gynecol 1998;92(3):420–4.
[134] Klein JO, Remington JS. Current concepts of infections of the fetus and newborn infant. In: Klein JO, Remington JS, editors. Infectious diseases of the fetus and newborn infant. Philadelphia: Saunders; 2001. p. 1–22.
[135] Goldenberg RL, Andrews WW, Yuan A, et al. Pregnancy outcome related to sexually

transmitted diseases. In: Hitchcock PJ, MacKay HT, Wasserheit JN, et al, editors. Sexually transmitted diseases and adverse outcomes of pregnancy. Washington (DC): ASM Press; 1999. p. 1–24.
[136] Ramsey PS, Goldenberg RL. Maternal infections and their consequences. In: Newell ML, McIntyre J, editors. Congenital and perinatal infections. Cambridge, United Kingdom: Cambridge University Press; 2000. p. 32–63.
[137] Cohen I, Veille JC, Calkins BM. Improved pregnancy outcome following successful treatment of chlamydial infection. JAMA 1990;263:3160–3.
[138] Schachter J, Grossman M, Sweet RL, et al. Prospective study of perinatal transmission of *Chlamydia trachomatis*. JAMA 1986;255:3374–7.
[139] Hardy PH, Hardy JB, Nell EE, et al. Prevalence of six sexually transmitted disease agents among pregnant inner-city adolescents and pregnancy outcome. Lancet 1984;2:333–7.
[140] Sweet RL. Hepatitis B infection in pregnancy. Obstet Gynecol Rep 1990;2:128–39.
[141] Snydman DR. Hepatitis in pregnancy. N Engl J Med 1985;313:1398–401.
[142] Puranen M, Yliskoski M, Saarikoski S, et al. Vertical transmission of human papillomavirus from infected mothers to their newborn babies and persistence of the virus in childhood. Am J Obstet Gynecol 1996;174:694–9.
[143] Orjuela M, Castaneda VP, Ridaura C, et al. Presence of human papilloma virus in tumor tissue from children with retinoblastoma: an alternative mechanism for tumor development. Clin Cancer Res 2000;6:4010–6.
[144] Gwinn M, Pappaioanou M, George JR, et al. Prevalence of HIV infection in childbearing women in the United States. JAMA 1991;265:1704–8.
[145] Davis SF, Byers RH, Lindegren LM, et al. Prevalence and incidence of vertically acquired HIV infection in the United States. JAMA 1995;274:952–5.
[146] Mason PR, Brown IM. Trichomona*s* in pregnancy. Lancet 1980;2:1025–6.
[147] McGregor JA, French JI. *Chlamydia trachomatis* infection during pregnancy. Am J Obstet Gynecol 1991;164:1782–8.
[148] Stagno S, Pass RF, Cloud G, et al. Primary cytomegalovirus infection in pregnancy: incidence, transmission to fetus, and clinical outcome. JAMA 1986;256:1904–8.
[149] Stagno S. Cytomegalovirus. In: Remington JS, Klein JO, editors. Infectious diseases of the fetus and newborn infant. 4th edition. Philadelphia: W.B. Saunders; 1995. p. 312–53.
[150] Judson FN. Assessing the number of genital chlamydial infections in the United States. J Reprod Med 1985;30:269–72.
[151] Harrison HR, Alexander ER, Weinstein L, et al. Cervical *Chlamydia trachomatis* and mycoplasmal infections in pregnancy: epidemiology and outcomes. JAMA 1983;250:1721–7.
[152] Alger LS, Lovchik JC, Hebel JR, et al. The association of *Chlamydia trachomatis*, *Neisseria gonorrhoeae*, and group B streptococci with preterm rupture of the membranes and pregnancy outcome. Am J Obstet Gynecol 1988;159:397–404.
[153] McDonald HM, O'Loughlin JA, Jolly P, et al. Vaginal infection and preterm labour. Br J Obstet Gynaecol 1991;98:427–35.
[154] McDonald HM, O'Loughlin JA, Jolly P, et al. Prenatal microbiological risk factors associated with preterm birth. Br J Obstet Gynaecol 1992;99:190–6.
[155] Whitley RJ, Hutto C. Neonatal herpes simplex virus infections. Pediatr Rev 1985;7:119.
[156] Whitley R, Arvin A, Prober C, et al. Predictors of morbidity and mortality in neonates with herpes simplex virus infections. N Engl J Med 1991;324:450–4.
[157] Rouzioux C, Costagliola D, Burgard M, et al. Estimated timing of mother-to-child human immunodeficiency virus type I transmission by use of a Markov model. Am J Epidemiol 1995; 142:1330–7.
[158] Minkoff H, Burns DN, Landesman S, et al. The relationship of the duration of ruptured membranes to vertical transmission of human imunodeficiency virus. Am J Obstet Gynecol 1995;173:585–9.
[159] Mandelbrot L, Mayaux M-JA, Bongain A, et al. Obstetric factors and mother-to-child transmission of human immunodeficiency virus type 1: the French perinatal cohorts. Am J Obstet Gynecol 1996;175:661–7.

[160] Mayaux MJ, Blanche S, Rouzioux C, et al, and the French Pediatric HIV Infection Study Group. Maternal factors associated with perinatal HIV-1 transmission: the French cohort study—7 years of follow-up observation. J Acquir Immune Defic Syndr Hum Retrovirol 1995;8:188–94.
[161] Newell ML, and the European Collaborative Study. Perinatal findings in children born to HIV-infected mothers. Br J Obstet Gynaecol 1994;101:136–41.
[162] Clyde S. Crumpacker. In: Remington JS, Klein JO, editors. Infectious diseases of the fetus and newborn infant. Philadelphia: Saunders; 2001. p. 913–41.
[163] Newell ML, and the European Collaborative Study. Mother to child transmission of cytomegalovirus. Br J Obstet Gynaecol 1994;101:122–34.
[164] Romero R, Ovarzun E, Mazor M, et al. Meta-analysis of the relationship between asymptomatic bacteriuria and preterm delivery low birthweight. Obstet Gynecol 1989;73:576–82.

ELSEVIER
SAUNDERS

CLINICS IN
PERINATOLOGY

Clin Perinatol 32 (2005) 561–569

Pathophysiology of Preterm Birth: Emerging Concepts of Maternal Infection

Kim A. Boggess, MD

Department of Obstetrics and Gynecology, Division of Maternal Fetal Medicine, University of North Carolina School of Medicine, CB 7516, Chapel Hill, NC 27599-7516, USA

Preterm birth is a significant health concern

Annually over 400,000 infants are born prematurely as a result of preterm labor, preeclampsia, and other adverse events. It is well recognized that there are substantial morbidity, mortality, and societal costs associated with preterm delivery, and preterm birth is the leading cause of death in nonanomalous infants. Although vast improvements have been made in treating sick newborns, there has been little success in understanding and preventing the events that lead up to adverse pregnancy outcome. Today's challenge is to identify and understand factors contributing to preterm birth that may be amenable to prevention or intervention and treatment.

Preterm birth (less than 37 weeks' gestation) is the leading cause of neonatal mortality in the United States, affecting 11% of all live births. Preterm birth is responsible for three quarters of neonatal mortality and one half of long-term neurological impairments in children. Although preterm birth as a result of preterm labor contributes to approximately two thirds of the cases of preterm birth, the signals responsible for the initiation of parturition remain elusive. Both preventive and treatment efforts have been disappointing: the preterm birth rate remains unchanged in 30 years [1].

E-mail address: kboggess@med.unc.edu

doi:10.1016/j.clp.2005.05.002 **perinatology.theclinics.com**

Maternal infection is a risk factor for preterm birth

Maternal infections have long been recognized as risk factors for adverse pregnancy outcomes, and intrauterine infection and bacterial vaginosis have both been identified as risks for preterm birth. The mechanism by which maternal infection mediates early delivery is unclear, but likely involves both maternal and fetal inflammatory and humoral responses. It is possible that genetic variation [2] in response to these infections also plays a role in the risk for preterm birth.

There is epidemiological, microbiological, and clinical evidence of an association between infection and preterm birth [3–7]. Epidemiological studies of spontaneous preterm birth reveal that births at less than 34 weeks' gestation are much more frequently accompanied by clinical or subclinical infection than those at more than 34 weeks [8]. The strength of the association between both clinical and histologic infection increases as gestational age decreases, especially before 30 to 32 weeks. The frequency of positive amniotic fluid cultures is also inversely related to gestational age, and intrauterine infection is much less common after 34 weeks. Both maternal and neonatal infections are more common after preterm than term birth, with increasing risk as gestational age decreases. Infection not only contributes significantly to preterm birth, but most strongly with those very early preterm births that are responsible for significant infant morbidity and mortality.

Maternal genitourinary and reproductive tract infections have implicated as a main risk factor in 15% to 25% of preterm deliveries [3,9–11]. In a case control study of 380 women, Andrews and colleagues [12] assessed the role of *Chlamydia trachomatis* in preterm birth. Eleven percent of women were *C trachomatis* positive by urine ligase-chain reaction, and women who delivered preterm at less than 37 weeks were more likely to be *C trachomatis*-positive at 24 weeks than those who delivered at term (16% versus 6%, $P = 0.003$). Women with *C trachomatis* were more likely to deliver preterm at less than 37 and less than 35 weeks (odds ratio [OR] 2.2, 1.0–4.8; 3.2, 1.1–9.6 respectively) [12].

Another important reproductive tract infection associated with preterm birth is bacterial vaginosis [3,10,13]. Bacterial vaginosis is a gram-negative, anaerobic infection of the vagina that occurs in up to 20% of all pregnancies [10]. Studies have demonstrated a twofold to sixfold increased risk for preterm birth among women with bacterial vaginosis [3,10]. In a cohort study of over 10,000 pregnant women, Hillier and coworkers [10] found that the presence of bacterial vaginosis was related to preterm delivery of a low-birthweight infant (OR 1.4, 1.1–1.8). Among women with bacterial vaginosis, the highest risk of preterm delivery of a low-birthweight infant was found among those with both vaginal *Bacteroides* and *Mycoplasma hominis* (OR 2.1, 1.5–3.0).

Despite these findings, data have been conflicting on the role of antibiotic treatment of bacterial vaginosis to reduce preterm birth risk [14–17]. This controversy has stimulated research into other potential infectious mediators of preterm birth.

Oral infections and their role in systemic disease

Periodontal disease is a gram-negative anaerobic infection of the mouth that occurs commonly in women of childbearing age. Infection and inflammation of the gingiva and local support structures of the teeth occurs and results in the destruction of the tooth-supporting structures. Fluid that bathes the tooth at the gingival margin, known as gingival crevicular fluid, often contains inflammatory mediators and oral pathogens associated with periodontal disease.

The mechanisms underlying this destructive process involve both direct tissue damage resulting from plaque bacterial products, and indirect damage through bacterial induction of the host inflammatory and immune responses [18]. Periodontal disease affects up to 50% of the population, with a relatively high proportion of pregnant women demonstrating periodontal disease [19–21]. Advancing age, smoking, and diabetes are some risk factors for the development of periodontal disease [22]. Although periodontal disease is a chronic, local oral infection, there is evidence that both local and systemic inflammation may occur [18]. In addition, periodontal disease has recently been recognized as a risk factor for the development of atherosclerosis [23] and rheumatoid arthritis [24].

Maternal periodontal disease is associated with preterm birth

In 1996, Offenbacher and coworkers [19] first reported a potential association between maternal periodontal disease and delivery of a preterm/low birthweight infant. In a case-control study of 124 pregnant women, they observed that women who delivered at less than 37 weeks' gestation or delivered an infant weighing less than 2500 g had significantly worse periodontal disease than control women. The adjusted OR for delivery of a preterm, low birthweight infant was approximately 7. These data led the study authors to conclude that periodontal disease may represent a previously unrecognized and clinically significant risk factor for delivery of a preterm low birthweight infant [19]. Extrapolation from the data suggested that 18% of the preterm, low birthweight infants born annually might be attributable to periodontal disease, which may thus account for a significant proportion of the $5.5 billion annual hospital costs associated with the care of preterm/low birthweight infants. In a subsequent case-control study, Dasanayake and colleagues [25] studied 55 pairs of women. Logistic regression indicated that mothers with "healthy gingiva" were at lower risk for low birthweight infants. Women in both of these case-control studies were examined at the end of pregnancy or after delivery, which does not convincingly prove an antecedent exposure and thus causality. Despite this limitation, these early studies led to the hypothesis that periodontopathic bacteria, largely including gram-negative anaerobes, may serve as a source for endotoxin and lipopolysaccharides, which then increases local inflammatory mediators, including prostaglandin E2 (PGE_2), and cytokines, and that this increases systemic inflammatory mediators that can then lead to preterm birth [26].

Jeffcoat and coworkers [27] examined the relationship between maternal periodontal disease and spontaneous preterm birth among 1313 pregnant women. They found that moderate/severe maternal periodontal disease identified early in pregnancy was associated with an increased risk for spontaneous preterm birth, independent of other traditional risk factors [27]. Importantly, they noted increasing risk with decreasing gestational age. Table 1 shows adjusted risk ratio for spontaneous preterm birth.

Severe periodontal disease was more common among women with spontaneous preterm birth at less than 32 weeks compared with women who delivered due to medical indications (49% versus 25%, $P = 0.02$) [28]. Neither histologic chorioamnionitis, a positive placental culture, nor an elevated umbilical cord interleukin (IL)-6 level was associated with maternal periodontal disease among the women with preterm births at less than 32 weeks, however, leading the investigators to speculate that the potential mechanism of periodontal disease-associated preterm birth is not hematogenous spread of oral organisms to the placenta that results in colonization, infection, or placental inflammation [28].

Despite these compelling data, it is important to recognize that other studies have failed to demonstrate an association between maternal periodontal disease and preterm birth. In a case-control study conducted in London, Davenport and coworkers [29] examined 236 infants born at less than 37 weeks' gestation or weighing less than 2500 g, and compared them to a random sample of 507 control infants who were born at 38 weeks' or more gestation weighing 2500 g or more. They found no evidence for an association between delivery of a preterm, low birthweight infant and periodontal disease, and surprisingly found that deeper mean tooth pocket depths at delivery was associated with a reduction in the risk of delivery of a preterm, low birthweight infant [29]. Furthermore, they examined in detail other possible confounding demographic risk factors. The study authors surmised that these discrepant findings might be due at least in part to differences in study populations. In a follow-up longitudinal study of 3738 women, Moore and colleagues [30] found no association between maternal periodontal disease and preterm birth; however, there was an increase in second trimester fetal loss rates among women with periodontal disease [30].

In spite of the conflicting clinical data, there is microbiologic evidence supporting the role of clinical periodontal disease and adverse pregnancy outcome. Microbiologic investigation by culture or polymerase chain reaction (PCR) of the amniotic fluid, amniotic membranes, and placentas of women who experience spontaneous preterm birth reveals that a significant proportion of women who deliver following spontaneous preterm labor demonstrate presence of organisms, and the frequency of positive amniotic fluid cultures is inversely related to

Table 1

Adjusted risk ratio[a] for spontaneous preterm birth among women with periodontal disease

<37 weeks	<35 weeks	<32 weeks
4.45 (2.16 – 9.18)	5.28 (2.05 – 13.6)	7.07 (1.70 – 27.4)

[a] Adjusted for maternal age, race, parity, and smoking.

gestational age [5]. Some of the organisms commonly identified in the amniotic fluid or placenta of women who deliver preterm are oral in origin. *Fusobacterium nucleatum*, a common oral species, is the most frequently isolated species from amniotic fluid cultures among women with preterm labor and intact membranes [31]. Also, the species and subspecies of fusobacteria identified from amniotic fluid most closely match those reported from healthy and diseased subgingival sites, namely *F nucleatum* subspecies vincentii and *F nucleatum* subspecies nucleatum, compared with strains identified from the lower genital tract [31]. In a case-control study of 48 women undergoing elective cesarean delivery at term, amniotic fluid was positive for universal bacteria PCR, *Streptococcus spp* PCR, and *F nucleatum* PCR in 34/48, 20/48, and 7/48 of cases, respectively. *Streptococcus spp* and *F nucleatum* were cultured from the dental plaque, vaginas, and amniotic fluid of 48/48, 14/48, and 0/48; and 29/48, 6/48, and 0/48 subjects, respectively. These findings led the investigators to speculate that *Streptococcus spp* and *F nucleatum* in the amniotic fluid may be oral in origin [32]. These data provide further evidence that maternal periodontal disease represents a chronic oral microbial challenge to the mother that may mediate preterm birth risk.

In an effort to better understand the possible mechanism behind the association between periodontal disease and preterm delivery, Offenbacher and colleagues [26] measured gingival crevicular levels of PGE_2 and IL-1β in 48 mothers who delivered preterm, low birthweight infants compared with levels in control women. They discovered that gingival crevicular fluid levels of PGE_2 were significantly higher in case women compared with control women. Furthermore, among the primiparous women of preterm, low birthweight infants, a significant inverse association was demonstrated between birthweight and gestational age and gingival crevicular PGE_2 levels [26].

In addition to local inflammation, Madianos and coworkers [33] examined maternal and fetal humoral responses to oral pathogens as a possible risk factor/marker/mechanism for preterm delivery among pregnant women with periodontal disease [33]. There was a 2.9-fold higher prevalence of fetal IgM seropositivity for one or more oral pathogens among preterm babies, as compared with term babies (19.9% versus 6.9%, respectively; $P = 0.0015$). A lack of maternal IgG antibody to more pathogenic oral organisms was associated with an increased rate of preterm birth, (OR 2.2; 95% confidence interval [CI] 1.5–3.8). The highest rate of preterm birth (66.7%) was observed among those mothers without any protective IgG response to oral pathogens who delivered an infant that demonstrated an IgM response. These data led the study authors to conclude that maternal periodontal infection without a protective maternal antibody response is associated with systemic dissemination of oral organisms that may translocate to the fetus and result in preterm delivery [33], and they hypothesized the paradigm in Fig. 1.

Although periodontal disease and its association with preterm birth is exciting because it represents a potentially treatable cause of preterm birth, caution should be exercised as these data are interpreted. Maternal periodontal disease may also represent a surrogate for another maternal factor that predisposes

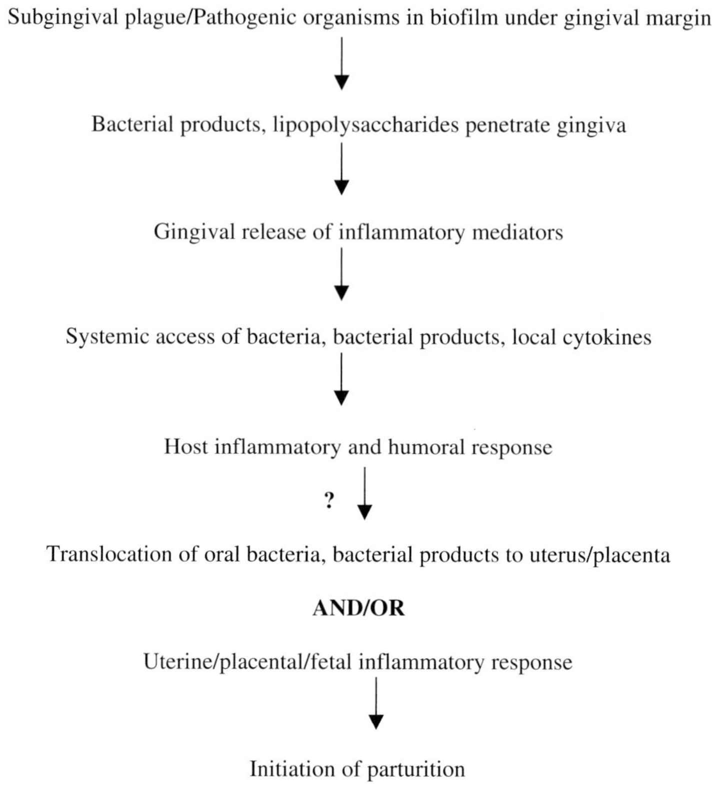

Fig. 1. Hypothetical translocation of periodontal infection to fetus resulting in preterm delivery. (*Data from* Madianos PN, Lieff S, Murtha AP, et al. Maternal periodontitis and prematurity. Part II: maternal infection and fetal exposure. Ann Periodontol 2001;6(1):175–82.)

preterm birth. Furthermore, although the model presented is interesting and biologically plausible, the underlying mechanism behind periodontal disease-associated preterm birth remains to be determined. Further study on the maternal and fetal inflammatory responses to chronic oral infection and on placental pathology in women with periodontal disease is ongoing to determine the relationship between periodontal disease and preterm birth.

Antepartum treatment of periodontal disease to reduce preterm birth risk

Three published studies of antepartum versus delayed (postpartum) treatment of maternal periodontal disease [34–36] demonstrate promise for this intervention for preterm birth prevention. In a prospective study designed to examine the relationship between periodontal disease and preterm low birthweight infants in a cohort of young, minority, pregnant and postpartum women [34], the effect of periodontal interventions on pregnancy outcome was assessed. Of 164 women for whom birth outcome data were available, 74 were subjected to oral prophylaxis during pregnancy, and 90 received no periodontal treatment. The preterm/low birthweight rate was lower among women who received periodontal treatment compared with those who did not (13.5% versus 18.9%). Lopez and colleagues [35] conducted a randomized clinical trial to assess the impact of periodontal treatment initiated during pregnancy versus delayed until postpartum on preterm/low-birthweight infant rates. The incidence of preterm/low-birthweight infants in the antepartum treatment group was 1.84% (3/163), and in the delayed/postpartum group it was 10.11% (19/188), (OR 5.49, 95% CI 1.65–18.22; P=0.001). Multivariable logistic regression analysis showed that periodontal disease was the strongest factor related to delivery of a preterm/low birthweight infant (OR 4.70, 95% CI 1.29–17.13). The data from these two studies [34,35] suggest that treatment of periodontal disease during pregnancy could reduce preterm/low-birthweight infant rates.

In a pilot intervention trial designed to assess the feasibility of conducting a trial to determine whether treatment of periodontal disease reduces the risk of spontaneous preterm birth, Jeffcoat and coworkers [36] found that among women at high risk for preterm birth and presence of periodontal disease, scaling and root planing therapy initiated during pregnancy is tolerated by pregnant women and may reduce spontaneous preterm birth.

Summary

In conclusion, data are emerging to support a role for maternal periodontal disease as another infectious risk factor for preterm birth. The prevalence of periodontal disease and the possibility of preterm birth prevention by treatment of oral infection make this a novel approach for preterm birth prevention. Further studies to better understand the mechanism of periodontal disease-associated preterm birth will enable us to tailor treatment to those women who might benefit the most.

References

[1] Guyer B, Strobino DM, Ventura SJ, et al. Annual summary of vital statistics—1994. Pediatrics 1995;96(6):1029–39.
[2] Genc MR, Gerber S, Nesin M, et al. Polymorphism in the interleukin-1 gene complex and spontaneous preterm delivery. Am J Obstet Gynecol 2002;187(1):157–63.
[3] McGregor JA, French JI, Richter R, et al. Antenatal microbiologic and maternal risk factors associated with prematurity. Am J Obstet Gynecol 1990;163:1465–73.
[4] Hillier SL, Krohn MA, Kiviat NB, et al. Microbiologic causes and neonatal outcomes associated with chorioamnion infection. Am J Obstet Gynecol 1991;165:955–61.
[5] Watts DH, Krohn MA, Hillier SL, et al. The association of occult amniotic fluid infection with gestational age and neonatal outcome among women in preterm labor. Obstet Gynecol 1992;79(3):351–7.
[6] Gibbs RS. Chorioamnionitis and bacterial vaginosis. Am J Obstet Gynecol 1993;169:460–2.

[7] Gibbs RS. The relationship between infections and adverse pregnancy outcomes: an overview. Ann Periodontol 2001;6(1):153–63.
[8] Hitti J, Tarczy-Hornoch P, Murphy J, et al. Amniotic fluid infection, cytokines, and adverse outcome among infants at 34 weeks' gestation or less. Obstet Gynecol 2001;98(6):1080–8.
[9] Meis PJ, Goldenberg RL, Mercer B, et al. The preterm prediction study: significance of vaginal infections. National Institute of Child Health and Human Development Maternal-Fetal Medicine Units Network. Am J Obstet Gynecol 1995;173(4):1231–5.
[10] Hillier SL, Nugent RP, Eschenbach DA, et al. Association between bacterial vaginosis and preterm delivery of a low-birth-weight infant. The Vaginal Infections and Prematurity Study Group. N Engl J Med 1995;333(26):1737–42.
[11] Kimberlin DF, Andrews WW. Bacterial vaginosis: association with adverse pregnancy outcome. Semin Perinatol 1998;22(4):242–50.
[12] Andrews WW, Goldenberg RL, Mercer B, et al. The Preterm Prediction Study: association of second-trimester genitourinary chlamydia infection with subsequent spontaneous preterm birth. Am J Obstet Gynecol 2000;183(3):662–8.
[13] McGregor JA, French JI. Bacterial vaginosis in pregnancy. Obstet Gynecol Surv 2000; 55(5 Suppl 1):S1–19.
[14] McGregor JA, French JI, Parker R, et al. Prevention of premature birth by screening and treatment for common genital tract infections: results of a prospective controlled evaluation. Am J Obstet Gynecol 1995;173(1):157–67.
[15] McDonald HM, O'Loughlin JA, Vigneswaran R, et al. Impact of metronidazole therapy on preterm birth in women with bacterial vaginosis flora (*Gardnerella vaginalis*): a randomised, placebo controlled trial. Br J Obstet Gynaecol 1997;104(12):1391–7.
[16] Carey JC, Klebanoff MA, Hauth JC, et al. Metronidazole to prevent preterm delivery in pregnant women with asymptomatic bacterial vaginosis. National Institute of Child Health and Human Development Network of Maternal-Fetal Medicine Units. N Engl J Med 2000;342(8): 534–40.
[17] Leitich H, Brunbauer M, Bodner-Adler B, et al. Antibiotic treatment of bacterial vaginosis in pregnancy: a meta-analysis. Am J Obstet Gynecol 2003;188(3):752–8.
[18] Genco RJ. Host responses in periodontal diseases: current concepts. J Periodontol 1992; 63(Suppl 4):338–55.
[19] Offenbacher S, Katz V, Fertik G, et al. Periodontal infection as a possible risk factor for preterm low birthweight. J Periodontol 1996;67(Suppl 10):1103–13.
[20] Davenport ES, Williams CE, Sterne JA, et al. The East London Study of Maternal Chronic Periodontal Disease and Preterm Low Birthweight Infants: study design and prevalence data. Ann Periodontol 1998;3(1):213–21.
[21] Moore S, Ide M, Wilson RF, et al. Periodontal health of London women during early pregnancy. Br Dent J 2001;191(10):570–3.
[22] Genco R. Risk factors for periodontal disease. Hamilton, Ontario, Canada: BC Decker; 2000.
[23] Beck JD, Pankow J, Tyroler HA, et al. Dental infections and atherosclerosis. Am Heart J 1999; 138:528–33.
[24] Mercado F, Marshall RI, Klestov AC, et al. Is there a relationship between rheumatoid arthritis and periodontal disease? J Clin Periodontol 2000;27(4):267–72.
[25] Dasanayake AP. Poor periodontal health of the pregnant woman as a risk factor for low birthweight. Ann Periodontol 1998;3(1):206–12.
[26] Offenbacher S, Jared HL, O'Reilly PG, et al. Potential pathogenic mechanisms of periodontitis associated pregnancy complications. Ann Periodontol 1998;3(1):233–50.
[27] Jeffcoat MK, Geurs NC, Reddy MS, et al. Periodontal infection and preterm birth: results of a prospective study. J Am Dent Assoc 2001;132(7):875–80.
[28] Goepfert AR, Jeffcoat MK, Andrews WW, et al. Periodontal disease and upper genital tract inflammation in early spontaneous preterm birth. Obstet Gynecol 2004;104(4):777–83.
[29] Davenport ES, Williams CE, Sterne JA, et al. Maternal periodontal disease and preterm low birthweight: case-control study. J Dent Res 2002;81(5):313–8.

[30] Moore S, Ide M, Coward PY, et al. A prospective study to investigate the relationship between periodontal disease and adverse pregnancy outcome. Br Dent J 2004;197(5):251–8 [discussion: 247].

[31] Hill GB. Preterm birth: associations with genital and possibly oral microflora. Ann Periodontol 1998;3(1):222–32.

[32] Bearfield C, Davenport ES, Sivapathasundaram V, et al. Possible association between amniotic fluid micro-organism infection and microflora in the mouth. BJOG 2002;109(5):527–33.

[33] Madianos PN, Lieff S, Murtha AP, et al. Maternal periodontitis and prematurity. Part II: maternal infection and fetal exposure. Ann Periodontol 2001;6(1):175–82.

[34] Mitchell-Lewis D, Engebretson SP, Chen J, et al. Periodontal infections and pre-term birth: early findings from a cohort of young minority women in New York. Eur J Oral Sci 2001;109(1):34–9.

[35] Lopez NJ, Smith PC, Gutierrez J. Periodontal therapy may reduce the risk of preterm low birthweight in women with periodontal disease: a randomized controlled trial. J Periodontol 2002;73(8):911–24.

[36] Jeffcoat MK, Hauth JC, Geurs NC, et al. Periodontal disease and preterm birth: results of a pilot intervention study. J Periodontol 2003;74(8):1214–8.

ELSEVIER
SAUNDERS

Clin Perinatol 32 (2005) 571–600

CLINICS IN
PERINATOLOGY

Preterm Labor, Preterm Premature Rupture of Membranes, and Chorioamnionitis

Edward R. Newton, MD

Department of Obstetrics and Gynecology, Brody School of Medicine, East Carolina University, Room 162, Teaching Annex, Pitt County Memorial Hospital, Greenville, NC 27834, USA

Because 60% to 70% of neonatal death, morbidity, and cost are linked to birth before 37 weeks, understanding the causes and developing effective management is critical. In the last 25 years, researchers have compiled a massive amount of data linking infection with preterm birth. Infection is associated directly or indirectly with 40% to 60% of preterm birth. In the last 10 years, the need to understand the links between infection and preterm birth has grown more important. Clinical and subclinical chorioamnionitis are linked to fetal brain injury and neurodevelopmental handicap [1].

In this article, the author reviews the etiology and biochemical links between infection and preterm birth, the problem of preterm birth, and the management of infection-related risks of preterm birth. The management section reviews current opinions regarding prophylactic antibiotic therapy in the prevention of preterm birth; adjunctive antibiotic therapy in the treatment of preterm labor, with and without rupture of membranes; and antibiotic therapy of intra-amniotic infection (clinical chorioamnionitis, IAI). Finally, the article reviews the risk of neurodevelopmental handicap potentially associated with IAI.

Etiology of preterm birth

Preterm birth is related to physician-initiated birth (indicated preterm birth) or spontaneous preterm birth. Indicated preterm births account for approximately 30% of preterm births. Indicated preterm delivery may result from maternal or fetal risks perceived to be greater than the neonatal risks of preterm birth. The

E-mail address: newtoned@mail.ecu.edu

0095-5108/05/$ – see front matter
doi:10.1016/j.clp.2005.05.001

most frequent reasons for indicated preterm birth are pre-eclampsia (40%), fetal distress (30%), intrauterine growth retardation (10%), abruption placenta or placenta previa (10%), and fetal death (5%). In 20% of cases, multiple indications are identified [2]. The risk factors for indicated preterm birth in from strongest to weakest are: mullerian duct abnormality, proteinuria less than 24 weeks, chronic hypertension, previous indicated preterm birth, lung disease, previous spontaneous preterm birth, maternal age greater than 30, black ethnicity, and work during pregnancy [2].

The remaining two thirds of preterm births are associated with preterm labor (PTL) or preterm premature rupture of membranes (PPROM) in approximately equal proportions [3–5]. Preterm labor tends to be a more frequent cause in more educated, more economically secure women; PPROM occurs more frequently in less educated and economically handicapped women. Table 1 lists the commonly recognized risk factors for PTL and PPROM.

In either complication, many of the risk factors suggest a genomic predisposition to an altered immune response, have epidemiologic links to genitourinary tract organisms and infections, or are associated with behaviors or conditions that reduce host resistance to infection.

Fig. 1 depicts a highly simplified framework which relates infection and host response to one of three common clinical scenarios: preterm labor, PPROM, and premature cervical dilation. Often, the clinical presentation is a confusing combination of all three. For example, a woman at 24 weeks gestational age complains of occasional uterine tightening. On cervical examination, she is 4 cm dilated. Shortly thereafter, she has gross rupture of membranes. Which clinical scenario is most prominent?

Different individuals and different populations vary considerably in their proclivity for preterm birth, despite their similarity in the degree of maternal stress or the frequency of genitourinary infection. Although behaviors and psychosocial stress may be similar from one pregnancy to the next, the strength of previous preterm birth as a risk factor for preterm labor or PPROM suggests a genomic relationship to the preterm births in the individual. On a population level, genetic polymorphisms are strongly linked to the changes in vaginal microflora consistent with bacterial vaginosis (BV), and to subsequent more

Table 1
Risk factors for preterm labor and preterm premature rupture of membranes

Preterm labor	Preterm premature rupture of membranes
Previous preterm birth	Infection
Low body mass	(STI, UTI)
Poor weight gain	Uterine distension
Heavy work load	Cervical incompetence
Uterine abnormalities	African-American
Psychosocial stress	Low socioeconomic class
Drug abuse (including smoking)	Drug abuse (including smoking)
Teenage pregnancy	First and/or second trimester bleeding

Abbreviations: STI, sexually transmitted infections; UTI, urinary tract infection.

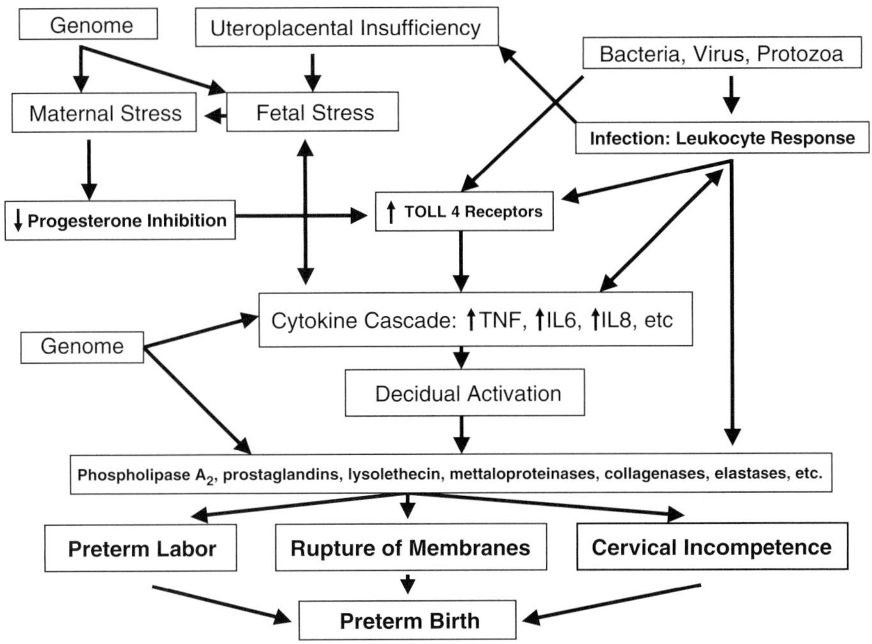

Fig. 1. Relation of infection and host response to preterm labor, preterm premature membrane rupture, and premature cervical dilation.

frequent low-birthweight neonates and preterm birth [6–9]. These factors and others may explain a portion of the excess frequency of preterm birth and low birthweight among patients who have a history of preterm birth or among African Americans, through changes in their vaginal microflora [10].

Pregnancy is a unique antigen-antibody phenomena. The fetus is an antigen to the mother. Only through natural immunosuppression and blocking antibodies does the mother allow the fetus to grow and prosper, rather than reject it with an overwhelming cytokine and leukocytic response. A group of surface receptors (Toll receptors) help modify the immune response to antigens [11]. In particular, Toll-4 receptor binds to the lipopolysaccharides of common genital tract organisms. The antigen-receptor binding initiates the cytokine response. High levels of glucocorticoids reduce Toll-4 receptors by nuclear interactions; progesterone increases the cytoplasmic degradation (post-transcriptional inhibition) of Toll-4 receptors. Local reduction of progesterone levels allows greater density Toll-4 receptors on decidual cell surfaces and greater likelihood for infection-related preterm birth [12].

The control of progesterone levels is not clear. A chronic stress response may change the hormonal mileu to reduce progesterone levels. This may explain the associations between social stresses and preterm birth. An individual's adaptation to stress, as determined by her nature (genomic) and her nurture (social upbringing and supports), may explain the complex relationship between social stress and preterm birth. On the other hand, recent clinical trials of progesterone supplementation are associated with a 30% to 50% reduction in preterm birth [13]. This observation supports the role of progesterone in labor suppression.

One unexplained observation relating infection to preterm birth is the strong association between infection and earlier preterm births (< 32 weeks gestation). Intermembrane cultures in women who delivered at less than 30 weeks are more than two times more likely to be positive than after 30 weeks [14]. Incidence of subclinical histologic chorioamnionitis is much more common in preterm gestation: 50% at 24 to 28 weeks, 30% at 28 to 32 weeks, 20% at 33 to 36 weeks, and 10% at more than 37 weeks [15]. The smaller the fetus at cesarean section delivery with intact membranes, the more likely the chorioamnion cultures are positive; 80% likely at less than 1000 g, 60% likely at 1000 to 1499 g, 35% likely at 1500 to 2499 g, and 30% likely at more than 2500 g [16]. Intra-amniotic infection (clinical chorioamnionitis) is more likely in pregnancies complicated by early PPROM than premature rupture of membranes at less than 37 weeks: 40% likely at less than 28 weeks, 20% likely at 28 to 34 weeks, and 5% likely at more than 37 weeks [17].

Another understudied observation is that different organisms have markedly different abilities to stimulate a host response. In a classic experiment, Bejar and colleagues [18] evaluated multiple species of bacteria in their ability to stimulate in-vitro prostaglandin production, as measured by arachodonic acid metabolites. The species that most researchers associate with preterm birth (BV organisms) had the highest ability to stimulate prostaglandin production. These correspond to the lower genital tract organisms that are associated epidemiologically with preterm birth: high concentrations of anaerobes, genital mycoplasmas, *Gardnerella vaginalis,* urinary group B streptococcus (GBS), high concentrations of aerobic gram-negative rods, active (IgM positive) *Chlamydia trachomatis* (Ct), and *Trichomonas vaginalis* (Tv). Hydrogen peroxide-producing *Lactobacilli spp* are associated with a significant reduction in preterm births. Few combinations (and varying concentrations) of organisms have been studied in relationship to preterm birth. Only one combination of organisms, BV, has undergone considerable clinical and epidemiologic analysis. BV is associated consistently with preterm birth [19,20]. Table 2 describes the frequency of organisms in patients at 23 to 26 weeks gestation (cervical-vaginal cultures) [21], amniotic fluid (AF) cultures (using amniocentesis) in preterm labor with intact membranes (PTL) [19], and AF (using amniocentesis) from women who have PPROM [22].

In addition, the Vaginal Infections and Prematurity Study (VIPS) [21] noted among 13,913 women sampled at 23 to 26 weeks gestation that Ct was present in 9%, *Neisseria gonorrhoeae* in 1.3%, Tv in 12.5%, and BV by Gram's stain in 16.2%. Among patients who had PPROM, amniocentesis revealed that 4.2% of cultures were positive for *N gonorrhoeae* [22].

Technical challenges account for the slow progress on the role of infection in preterm birth. Testing vaginal flora is only a proxy for the microflora of the upper genital tract in women who had threatened preterm birth. Researchers are most interested in the variety, combinations, and concentrations of organisms

Table 2
Microbiology of the female genital tract during pregnancy

Organism(s)	Cervix-vagina at 23–26 weeks (VIPS) [21]	PTL	PPROM
Aerobic gram-negative rods	1.2%	<1%	4.7%
Group B streptococcus	20.7%	3.7%	8.9%
Other streptococci	5.6%	3.1%	3.1%
Aerobic *Lactobacilli*	72.5%	3.7%	2.1%
Gardnerella vaginalis	56.2%	7.4%	11.5%
Ureaplasma urealyticum	75.2%	21.5%	—
Mycoplasma hominis	33.1%	9.2%	4.2%
Bacteroides/Prevotella spp	20%	3.1%	6.8%
Anaerobic cocci	6.6%	9.2%	13.6%
Fusobacterium spp	0.6%	1.8%	9.4%

infecting the decidua, membranes, or fetus. The decidua, membranes, and fetus are dangerous and difficult to sample in pregnant women. Only amniocentesis has a reasonable safety record; a risk of rupture of membranes is about 1% in the third trimester. On the other hand, it is twice as likely to isolate a greater variety of organisms at higher concentrations from intramembrane cultures than from simultaneously sampled AF [23].

In addition to the danger and difficulty of upper genital tract sampling, there are major questions related to the timing of the biochemical cascades leading to preterm birth. Sampling the decidua, placenta, and newborn after birth gives only the end results. Sampling the upper genital tract just prior to the onset of preterm labor will demonstrate significant differences from postbirth sampling. Currently, we have no easy and safe way to sample the upper genital tract, and no way of knowing the best time to sample prior to preterm labor.

Given that lower genital tract flora are the best, albeit poor, proxies for upper genital tract infection, major technical obstacles limit classic microbiologic methodology of lower genital tract microflora. The obstacles include isolation and concentration measurement in an ever-changing environment with many different bacterial species. Some of the most clinically important organisms (anaerobes and mycoplasmas) are the most difficult to isolate and identify in clinical microbiology laboratories. Adequate experience and methodology is limited to a handful of research laboratories. The concentration of an organism or organisms is an important predictor of clinical pathology. There are no universally accepted methods to measure concentrations of lower genital tract organisms. Most research relies on semi-quantitative measurement of concentration.

The problem of preterm birth

Preterm birth is one of the most common perinatal complications. Despite the enormous amount of research, medical intervention, and money, the incidence in the United States rose by 12% in the 11 years between 1992 and 2002 (Fig. 2)

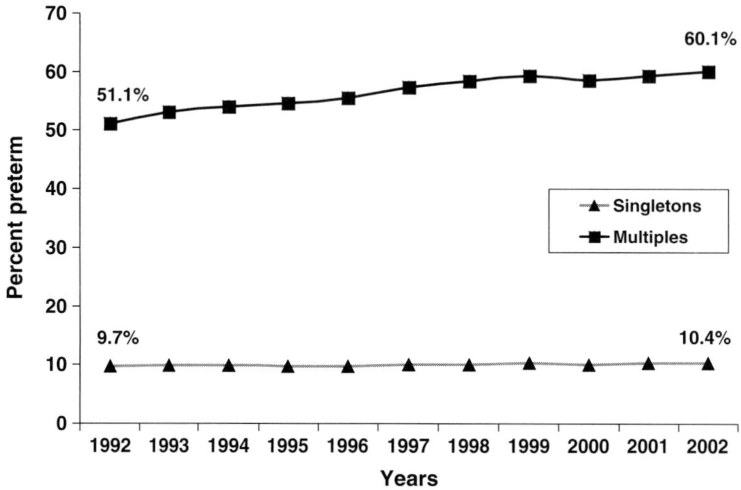

Fig. 2. US incidence of preterm birth 1992–2002. (*Data from* National Center for Health Statistics. Final 2002 natality data. Available at: www.marchofdimes.com/peristats.)

[24]. Approximately 12% of viable pregnancies deliver at less than 37 weeks; and, the incidence of the most vulnerable population (birth at less than 28 weeks) is about 1%. Three major factors have contributed to the rise in the preterm delivery rate: (1) dramatic increases in multiple births from assisted reproductive technologies; (2) changes in the obstetric management between 34 to 37 weeks gestation (ie, induction of labor in patients who have preterm rupture of membranes at greater of equal to 34 weeks); and (3) increased obstetric inventions at very early gestational ages (<28 weeks). The willingness to resuscitate the very premature neonate has profound implications.

These 30,000 vulnerable infants (born at <29 weeks) a year populate the level 3 neonatal intensive care units for 3 to 4 months with a swarm of caretakers and the most advanced technological resources committed to their intact survival. Hospital costs alone exceed $200,000 per surviving infant born at 25 to 26 weeks (Table 3).

Table 3
Hospital charges by gestational age of delivery—Pitt County Memorial Hospital, Greenville, North Carolina

Gestational age (number)	Mother charges	Baby charges	Mother-baby charges
25–26 weeks (40)	$11,102	$192,892	$203,994
27–28 weeks (58)	$9,765	$160,234	$169,999
29–30 weeks (76)	$10,882	$70,684	$81,566
31–32 weeks (127)	$9,500	$36,991	$46,490
33–34 weeks (208)	$9,016	$15,450	$24,447
35–36 weeks (240)	$6,091	$8,484	$14,457
>36 weeks (204)	$4,310	$2,276	$6,586

The professional fees for neonatalogists, pediatricians, neonatal nurse practitioners, radiologists, and other specialists (pediatric surgeons, neurologists, and infectious disease specialists) double the cost. Because 10% to 30% of these vulnerable infants have severe pulmonary complications (oxygen-dependent bronchopulmonary dysplasia), bowel resections (necrotizing enterocolitis), or severe neurological complications (nonambulatory cerebral palsy, mental retardation (IQ < 70), bilateral blindness), the lifelong burden of medical care and social costs is in the millions.

The neurological damage associated with early birth results from a baseline risk of prematurity, with added risks from maternal/neonatal complications. When a healthy baboon is delivered by elective hysterotomy at the equivalent of 26 to 28 weeks human gestation, immediately intubated and ventilated, and provided state-of-the-art neonatal intensive care, neurologic injury is clear when the infant baboon is sacrificed 15 days later [25]. Evidence of white matter injury is found in 50% of infants, accounting for 0.5% to 2.5% of total white matter. Twenty-five percent of neonates have enlarged cerebral ventricles and 40% have subarachnoid hemorrhage [25]. In human disease, maternal complications (ie, abruptio placenta or IAI), or neonatal complications (ie, respiratory distress, sepsis, hypotension) are associated with fetal hypoxic-ischemic injury or exaggerated fetal cytokine response. These complications increase the brain injury.

Whereas birth at less than 29 weeks is a neonatal disaster, birth between 29 and 34 weeks is associated with considerable short-term morbidity. On a population basis, preterm birth is most powerful complication that limits the potential of children and adults. Sixty to seventy percent of infant mortality, short-term morbidity, and perinatal costs are related to birth less that 37 weeks gestation. Table 4 describes the short term neonatal morbidity from 24 to 34 weeks gestation.

Several gestational age thresholds are associated with demonstrable decreases in short-term neonatal morbidity as gestational age progresses. The

Table 4
Neonatal morbidity and mortality by gestational age

Gestational age completed weeks	Survival	Respiratory distress syndrome	Intraventricular hemorrhage	Sepsis	Necrotizing enterocolitis	Intact survival
24	40%	70%	25%	25%	8%	25%
25	70%	90%	30%	29%	17%	50%
26	75%	93%	30%	30%	11%	60%
27	80%	84%	16%	36%	10%	70%
28	90%	65%	4%	25%	25%	80%
29	92%	53%	3%	25%	14%	85%
30	93%	55%	2%	11%	15%	90%
31	94%	37%	2%	14%	8%	93%
32	95%	28%	1%	3%	6%	95%
33	96%	34%	0%	5%	2%	96%
34	97%	14%	0%	4%	3%	97%

threshold of viability at 24 weeks dictates the willingness for the obstetrician to recommend cesarean section for fetal indications. Between 24 and 28 weeks, each day gained increases survival and reduces neonatal morbidity by 1% to 5%; the gain of 2 to 3 days is significant. The daily gain in survival and reduced morbidity between 29 and 32 weeks is also highly significant; a gain of 5 to 7 days has important benefits. After 32 weeks, maternal complications begin to alter the risk/benefit ratio for continued in-utero care. Some authors [26] advocate more aggressive fetal diagnosis in specific complications; for example, amniocentesis for fetal lung maturity studies in PPROM, between 32 and 34 weeks. After 34 0/7 weeks, many maternal-fetal medicine specialists in tertiary care centers will recommend delivery for PPROM, fetal growth restriction, monochorionic twin gestation, severe hypertensive disorders, even if fetal testing is reassuring. In addition, maternal and fetal therapy is often curtailed; most obstetricians will not give tocolytics for preterm labor or glucocorticoids for fetal lung maturity.

The relative rarity of neonatal death or serious short-term neonatal morbidity makes the choice for preterm delivery at 34 to 37 weeks deceptively easy for the obstetrician. Despite a low absolute risk, there is strong evidence that near-term delivery is risky for the infant. Infant mortality is threefold to fivefold higher with delivery at 34 to 36 weeks compared to delivery at 37 weeks [27]. Unfortunately, the average obstetrician has only anecdotal infant and childhood follow-up; perhaps the verbal report of the patient with her next pregnancy. The lack of accurate follow-up may lead to ill-advised obstetric decisions regarding timing of delivery.

Management of infection-related risks of preterm birth

Preconceptual care

The gynecologist can play an important role in the prevention of infection-related preterm birth in screening for high-risk sexual behavior, the identification and treatment of asymptomatic sexually transmitted infections (STI), and raising the patient's consciousness of the risks of genital tract infections and preterm birth. In the patient who has had a preterm birth associated with idiopathic preterm labor, PPROM, or idiopathic mid-trimester loss, the gynecologist provides anticipatory guidance with the next pregnancy.

The three major reasons that sexually active, nonpregnant, reproductive-aged women seek the care of a gynecologist are contraception, screening for STI (ie, cervical dysplasia), and the treatment of lower genital tract infections (ie, vaginitis). Several observations are important in considering the role of the gynecologist:

- Sixty percent of pregnancies are unintended, and 30% of women will become pregnant within 2 years of starting any contraceptive method.

- The rates of unintended pregnancy and STI are proportional to the context of the woman's relationships; rates with multiple concurrent partners are greater than short-term (3–12 month) relationships (ie, serial monogamous relationships), which are greater than a long-term monogamous relationship (ie, married).
- Most STI (60%–80%) are asymptomatic in women.
- At least 50% of women who have new yellow or brown vaginal discharge have an STI.
- The recurrence risk of STI in women is at least 25% within 12 months [28].
- If an STI (including BV) occurs during pregnancy, the risk of preterm birth is raised 50%–400% despite treatment.

The challenge of the gynecologist is to identify high-risk behaviors, screen at appropriate intervals (ie, with each new partner), treat to cure patient and partner, prevent unintended pregnancy, and educate the patient as to the infection-related risks of pregnancy.

Preconceptual counseling is critical during the gynecological visits between pregnancies. High-risk pregnancy history includes losses suggestive of an incompetent cervix or deliveries at less than 37 weeks or 2500 g. Of all the predictors of preterm birth, past obstetric history remains one of the strongest predictors of recurrent preterm birth. Given a baseline risk of 8% for first pregnancies, the risks of recurrent preterm birth after one, two, and three consecutive preterm births are 15%, 30%, and 45%, respectively [29]. Preconceptual counseling affects incidence of preterm birth by encouraging patients to make informed decisions concerning future pregnancies. Additionally, in case of infection-related births, preconceptual or early pregnancy identification and treatment of lower genital tract infection may reduce preterm birth.

First prenatal visit

At the first prenatal visit the obstetrician categorizes the patient as high or low risk for infection-related preterm birth. Table 5 lists the high risk factors for infection-related preterm birth.

In patients at low risk for infection-related preterm birth, many obstetricians (as required by state public health statute) sample their patient for STIs: gonorrhea, chlamydia, hepatitis B, human immunodeficiency virus, human papillomavirus (Pap smear), and syphilis. Most new obstetric patients will have a midstream, clean-catch urine culture to rule out asymptomatic bacteruria.

If any positive results are obtained, the patient is treated using the Centers for Disease Control *Guidelines* and reclassified as high risk for infection-related preterm birth. In addition to the testing for the above STIs, the high-risk patient should have an evaluation for BV (vaginal Gram's stain score of higher than 6 [30] or three of four positive Amsel's clinical criteria), trichomonas (wet smear or culture), and genital herpes (HSVII IgG antibody). Treatments are based on symptoms, public health indications, and the prevention of more serious

Table 5
Risk factors for infection-related preterm birth

Historical	Idiopathic preterm labor, preterm rupture of membranes, or incompetent cervix
	History of urinary tract infection
	History of STI within current relationship
	History of STI during current pregnancy
	STI within previous 5 years
Behavioral	Unintended pregnancy
	Unmarried
	New partner within 12 months
	Alcohol or drug abuse
	Uncertainty about partner fidelity
	Multiple current partners
Signs and symptoms	Vaginal discharge
	Dysuria
	Dypareunia
	Genital warts/dysplasia
	Genital ulcers
	Partner(s) with genitourinary symptoms
	Asymptomatic bacteruria

infection. Typically, patients who have symptoms of infection are treated. Asymptomatic STIs (including trichomonas) should be treated for public health indications. The issue of whether BV is have is not an STI is controversial; BV is found at much higher rates among populations that have high-risk sexual behavior than among populations that have no sexual activity or have long-term, mutually monogamous, and heterosexual relationships. The efficacy of prophylactic antibiotic therapy to prevent preterm birth is reviewed in the next section.

Prophylactic antibiotics to prevent preterm birth

Typically, patients who have infection symptoms should be treated. Depending on the organism, the asymptomatic high risk patient might benefit from prophylactic antibiotics.

Group B streptococcus

The incidence of vaginal GBS is about 20% to 25%; Mexican-Americans have a lower incidence (10% to 15%). Most epidemiologic studies have shown little or no association between vaginal GBS and preterm birth [31]. There are two randomized, placebo-controlled trials directed at group B streptococcal rectovaginal colonization and the prevention of preterm birth. An older study [32] demonstrated that treatment of GBS bacteruria reduced preterm birth and premature rupture of membranes. Antepartum treatment of GBS in the urine is standard of care. In a study of 938 patients who had vaginal GBS at 25 to 30 weeks and who were treated with oral erythromycin or placebo continuously for up to 10 weeks [33], no difference was seen in low birthweight, preterm delivery, or PPROM. Antenatal antibiotics are not indicated for recto-vaginal colonization of GBS.

Chlamydia trachomatis

The incidence of urogenital colonization and infection by Ct is 5% to 15%. Urogenital Ct prior to 24 weeks and immunoglobulin M seropositive (recent infection) [34] have been associated with preterm birth, despite treatment for public health reasons. In a study with a similar design to the latter GBS treatment trial [35], 414 patients were randomized to receive oral erythromycin or placebo. There were no differences in the incidence of low birthweight, preterm birth, or PPROM. Although CDC treatment regimens will cure Ct, no benefit is expected in reducing preterm birth.

Ureaplasma urealyticum

The isolation and differentiation of genital mycoplasmas from vaginal specimens is more complex than the average clinical laboratory can handle with accuracy. The incidence in pregnancy is 50% to 70%. The epidemiologic associations between *Ureaplasma urealyticum* (Uu) and preterm birth are inconsistent. In the Vaginal Infections in Pregnancy Study [36], 1181 patients were randomized to receive oral erythromycin or placebo. No difference was seen in low birthweight, preterm delivery, or PPROM.

Trichomonas vaginalis

The incidence of vaginal Tv in pregnancy is about 8%. Symptomatic Tv has been associated consistently with preterm birth; the associations with asymptomatic Tv are less clear. There have been two randomized controlled trials (total subjects 1469) [31]. Neither trial showed benefit in reducing preterm birth or low birthweight. In fact, Klebanoff and coworkers [37] showed an increase in preterm birth in the metronidazole treated group (relative risk, 1.8 (95% confidence interval [CI]1.2 – 2.7) among the 617 subjects. The current recommendation is not to screen or treat pregnant patients who have Tv with the purpose of reducing preterm birth.

Bacterial vaginosis

BV occurs in 10% to 25% of pregnant women. About 50% are asymptomatic. BV has been consistently associated with preterm birth. Leitich and colleagues [20] demonstrated in a large meta-analysis (number of subjects 20,232) a powerful association between first and second trimester BV and preterm birth, odds ratio (OR) (95% CI) = 2.19 (1.54–3.12). This association has been bolstered by the observations that certain genetic polymorphisms predict a greater incidence of vaginal microflora similar to BV and a greater incidence of preterm birth [6,9]. In addition, the presence of bacterial vaginosis in early labor is associated with maternal infections [10].

Unfortunately, there has been considerable inconsistency in the results of randomized controlled trials of prophylactic antibiotics to treat BV and prevent preterm birth. Meta-analyses of randomized controlled trials have not shown benefits when all patients and therapies are included [19,20]. The following considerations are suggested:

- Treatment before 20 weeks may be more effective in preventing preterm birth.
- The antibiotics effective against anaerobes are a better choice.
- Systemic antibiotics are more effective than topical antibiotics.
- Treatment duration needs to be 7 days or longer.
- Improvements in preterm birth rates occur primarily in patients who had a previous preterm birth.
- Patients who are undergoing cerclage should be screened and treated with perioperative antibiotics.

Asymptomatic bacteruria

The presence of asymptomatic bacteria is an indication for antibiotic therapy. Untreated asymptomatic bacteruria is associated with a 30% incidence of pyelonephritis later in pregnancy, and a 30% to 50% increase in preterm birth. Antibiotic treatment of asymptomatic bacteria reduces pyelonephritis, OR (95% CI) = 0.24 (0.19–0.32), and preterm birth, OR (95% CI) = 0.60 (0.45–0.85) [38]. The presence of group B streptococcus at any concentration in the urine is an indication for treatment during labor, regardless of treatment earlier in pregnancy [32].

Adjunctive therapeutic antibiotics for threatened infection-related preterm birth

Group B streptococcal prophylaxis

Early-onset GBS neonatal sepsis has a major impact on modern perinatal care. The overall incidence of GBS neonatal sepsis is 0.5 to 3 per 1000 live births. Maternal colonization, previous infant who had GBS sepsis, antenatal GBS asymptomatic bacteruria, rupture of membranes greater than 12 hours, intrapartum fever (probable IAI), and gestational age less than 37 weeks are recognized risk factors for GBS neonatal sepsis and meningitis. In these patients the risk of GBS neonatal sepsis is 20 to 70 per 1000 live births. For the infant, GBS sepsis is very dangerous—the case-fatality rate for term infants is 2% to 4%; for preterm infants, the case-fatality rate is 10% to 30%. Many of the survivors will have long-term neurodevelopmental handicaps.

Ten to twenty-five percent of laboring women are colonized by GBS. Colonization is determined by a specimen taken from the lower third of the vagina, perineal body, and the anal verge in one sweep. The GBS should be isolated in selective media, modified Todd-Hewitt or Lim broth. The results may be positive in 12 to 18 hours, and these are the women who transmit the GBS to their infant during the birth process. All colonized women or those who have the above risk factors should be treated. Because of the delay in the culture results, screening women at 34 to 36 weeks has become a standard of care. Unfortunately, threatened preterm birth often occurs in the absence of culture results. Patients in preterm labor (having cervical dilation >2 cm) or having PPROM should receive antibiotic prophylaxis against GBS before the culture results are available.

Penicillin (5 million units intravenous [IV] loading dose, then 2 million units IV every 4 hours) or ampicillin (2 g IV every 4 hours) are 90% to 95% effective in reducing infant colonization and neonatal sepsis. In patients who have anaphylaxis toward penicillins, the laboratory should determine the resistance of the GBS isolate to clindamycin (10% to 20%); if the isolate is resistant to clindamycin, IV vancomycin should be used. In patients who report a nonanaphylactic allergy to penicillin, IV cefazolin is the appropriate antibiotic choice.

Adjunctive antibiotics for inhibiting preterm labor with intact membranes

About twice as many women present having contractions as women who deliver early. Sometimes it is very difficult to diagnosis preterm labor. In a meta-analysis of all the well-designed antibiotic treatment trials [39], 58% (1215 of 2087) of patients who received placebo treatment delivered at more than 37 weeks. Did the patients have preterm labor at study entry?

The goals of initial management of preterm labor include: (1) to establish gestational age, 2) to make an accurate diagnosis of preterm labor, (2) to identify risk of infection-related preterm labor, (3) to document fetal well-being, (4) to provide prophylactic fetal therapy, then (5) to make a thoughtful choice to initiate tocolytic therapy.

The gestational age needs to be well established. Dates are determined by the first day of the last menstrual period (LMP) and confirmed by one or more of the following:

- A positive result from a pregnancy test (home or clinic) prior to the expected date of the second missed period
- Consistent uterine size at less than 12 weeks' gestation
- Electronically amplified fetal heart tones noted at 9–12 weeks' gestation
- A consistent ultrasound-based estimation of gestational age (ie, first trimester within 1 week, second trimester within 2 weeks, and third trimester within 3 weeks)

When the date of the LMP is not clear, the gestational age is determined by the results of the first ultrasound (preferably performed at <24 weeks). The first ultrasound-based estimation of gestational age is confirmed by consistent results from ultrasounds performed at 3- to 4-week intervals. Tocolytics are recommended for preterm labor between 23 and 34 weeks' gestation in an appropriately selected population.

The diagnosis of preterm labor is simple. Preterm labor is the presence of contractions of sufficient strength and frequency to effect progressive effacement and dilation of the cervix between 20 and 37 weeks' gestation. When the patient presents with advanced cervical dilation (>2 cm cervical dilation), therapy is not delayed until after the second pelvic examination.

Preterm labor has been associated with many factors, including infection, stress, fetal compromise, and the like [40–44]. Table 1 lists the commonly accepted risk factors for preterm labor with intact membranes. Of all the predictors of preterm birth, past obstetric history remains one of the strongest predictors of recurrent preterm birth. High-risk pregnancy history includes losses suggestive of an incompetent cervix or deliveries at less than 37 weeks or 2500 grams. Given a baseline risk of 8%, the risks of recurrent preterm birth after one, two, and three consecutive preterm births are 15%, 30%, and 45%, respectively [29].

Recently, the role of the fetus in the initiation of labor has been recognized. In a simplistic sense, the fetus recognizes a hostile intrauterine environment and precipitates labor. Fetal, decidual, or placental infection can initiate unstoppable labor, and may result in long-term neurodevelopmental handicap in excess of that expected by gestational age. Table 5 lists the risk factors for infection-related preterm birth. Tocolytics are contraindicated in the presence of asymptomatic or symptomatic intrauterine infection. The definition of IAI (chorioamnionitis) includes a temperature greater than 38.0°C (100.0°F) plus two of the five following signs:

WBC count greater than 15,000 cells/mm^3
Maternal tachycardia greater than 100 beats per minute (bpm)
Fetal tachycardia greater than 160 bpm
Tender uterus
Foul-smelling discharge

In the absence of IAI (clinical chorioamnitis), all patients having preterm labor need documentation of the presence or absence of lower genital tract infection. The following tests are recommended prior to the initiation of antibiotics or tocolytics:

Sterile speculum examination for ruptured membranes (ie, vaginal fluid pH [nitrazine test] and fern test)
Endocervical sampling for gonorrhea and chlamydia
Wet smear for BV and trichomonal infection
Potassium hydroxide smear for yeast and whiff test
Gram's stain of the upper lateral vaginal wall for BV score
GBS culture from the lower third of the vagina and anus (same swab) selective for GBS media (ie, Todd-Hewitt or Lim broth)
Urinalysis and culture on a specimen obtained by catheter

Fetal health is documented prior to inventions for preterm labor. An obstetric ultrasound and fetal monitoring are critical. The presence of fetal anomalies or hostile fetal environment requires more discrimination when initiating tocolytics. Hostile environments include the following:

Fetal growth restriction
Oligohydramnios
Nonreactive nonstress test results
Positive contraction stress test results
Absent or reversed diastolic flow upon Doppler examination of umbilical blood flow
Repetitive variable decelerations
Vaginal bleeding

The primary goal of tocolysis is to delay delivery for the 24 to 48 hours to allow the steroids to "mature" the fetal lungs. Prophylactic steroids (glucocorticoids) are the standard of care when the threat of delivery of a fetus at 24 to 34 weeks' gestation is present in the absence of clinical infection. Delivery must be delayed a minimum of 24 hours in order to observe the benefits of antenatal steroids. The benefits are proven to last 7 days. Betamethasone at 12.5 mg every 24 hours for two doses or dexamethasone at 6 mg every 6 hours for four doses is recommended. Special circumstances include the following:

In the presence of insulin-dependent, insulin-independent (adult-onset), or gestational diabetes, the provider must be prepared for aggressive control of blood sugars (including IV insulin drip) to maintain a blood sugar level of 70–110 mg/dL.
In the event of abnormal biophysical parameters (ie, nonreactive nonstress test result or positive contraction stress test result, biophysical profile >8 of 10, absent or reversed diastolic flow on Doppler evaluation of the umbilical blood flow, or oligohydramnios), the use of prophylactic steroids requires a thoughtful decision. Prophylactic steroids should not delay the delivery of an acutely distressed fetus.
Patients having advanced labor or having contractions plus cervical dilation greater than 6 cm do not benefit from prophylactic steroids.

In situations in which the diagnosis is not clear, an amniocentesis for fluid culture (aerobic/anaerobic bacteria), Gram's stain (bacteria present if Gram's stain is positive or if white blood cell [WBC] count is >30 cells/mm^3), glucose level (positive if <15 mg/dL), or leukocyte esterase evaluation may be indicated. Amniocentesis may result in a false-positive fetal fibronectin test. Tocolytics are not indicated in the presence of any positive test result involving AF.

Tocolytics have not been proven efficacious to help prevent preterm birth or to reduce neonatal mortality or morbidity [45]. The best outcome is a delay of delivery for 48 hours to allow the maximum benefit of glucocorticoids to take effect on the fetal lungs. Most tocolytics are able to affect this goal when membranes are intact; however, in some studies, the effectiveness of tocolytics is only slightly better than bed rest and hydration, both of which have fewer adverse effects compared with tocolytics. Preterm labor is often difficult to diagnose, and considerable potential exists for overtreatment of uterine irritability. Tocolytic agents, although generally safe in appropriate dosages and with monitoring, are potentially lethal medications, and should only be used after thoughtful consideration. Always keep in mind that the intrauterine environment may be more hostile to the fetus than the extrauterine environment.

The decision to use tocolytics must take into account the potential benefit for the fetus. Neonatal morbidity and mortality are greatly affected by gestational age (see Table 4). Prior to 23 weeks' gestation, the neonate has essentially no chance of survival and tocolysis should be used with caution. Similarly, the risk of neonatal mortality and morbidity is so low after 34 completed weeks of gestation that tocolytics are not recommended. Between 24 and 33 weeks' gestation, the neonate has a much better chance of benefiting from tocolysis.

Maternal condition can caution the use of tocolysis. Tocolysis is used with considerable caution in patients who have cardiac disease who require medication or have a history of congestive heart failure, cardiac surgery, significant pulmonary disease, renal failure, or maternal infection (eg, pneumonia, appendicitis, pyelonephritis). In these cases, it is prudent to consult with a maternal-fetal medicine specialist prior to the initiation of tocolytics.

Contraindications to the specific tocolytics are, for indomethacin, aspirin-induced asthma, coagulopathy, and significant liver disease; for magnesium sulfate, use of calcium channel blockers or gentamicin, myasthenia gravis, and neuromuscular disorders; and for beta-mimetics such as ritodrine and terbutaline, cardiac arrhythmia, valvular disease, and ischemic heart disease. Beta-mimetic tocolytics are relatively contraindicated in patients who have diabetes. No tocolytic agent should be used in the presence of known allergy to that agent.

The Cochrane Collaborative Group performs the best systematic review of treatment trials on many perinatal subjects [38,39]. They evaluate each published trial for selection bias (blinding of randomization), performance bias (blinding of intervention), attrition bias (complete follow-up), and detection bias (blinding of outcome assessment). The Cochrane Collaborative Group reviewed the trials regarding prophylactic antibiotics for inhibiting preterm labor [39]. Unfortunately, adjunctive antibiotics for inhibiting preterm labor with intact membranes have minimal efficacy. King and Flenady [39] reviewed 11 trials that included 7428 women who were randomized to receive antibiotics or placebo. Adjunctive antibiotics did not reduce preterm birth, delay in delivery until 48 hours or until 7 days, low birthweight, or perinatal mortality. Adjunctive antibiotics did not reduce neonatal morbidity. There were no differences in respiratory distress syndrome, days on a ventilator, more than 28 days of oxygen supplementation, necrotizing enterocolitis, or intraventricular hemorrhage. The only benefits were as a reduction in maternal infection, adjusted OR (95% CI) = 0.74 (0.64–0.87) and a clinically insignificant increase in gestational age at delivery, 0.29 weeks

(0.17–0.75 weeks). On subgroup analysis, use of antibiotics with anaerobic coverage (226 women) suggested benefit by lengthening randomization to delivery by 10.5 days (4.95–16.06 days), reducing delivery before 7 days—OR = 0.62 (0.42–0.90), and reducing admissions to the neonatal intensive care unit—OR = 0.63 (0.43–0.93).

In summary, adjunctive antibiotics are not recommended for patients in preterm labor with intact membranes. There are many unanswered questions: What is the right antibiotic? What is the right duration of therapy? What is the incidence of resistant organisms in mothers and babies after antibiotic exposure? Are there subgroups of patients who might benefit from a focused antibiotic regimen? The treatment effects are likely to be small and the necessary sample size precludes further study.

Adjunctive antibiotics for preterm premature rupture of membranes

The patient who arrives having preterm rupture of the membranes should receive the same risk assessment as that described for preterm labor with intact membranes: accurate gestational age, accurate diagnosis (positive history, positive nitrazine test, and positive fern test), assessment of infection-related preterm birth, documentation of fetal well-being, fetal therapy, and considered use of tocolysis. In PPROM, the risk of clinical infection is greater and the likelihood of preterm delivery is considerably greater. The risk of IAI is about 20% between 28 and 34 weeks; almost three times higher than in preterm labor patients who have intact membranes. About 80% of patients who have PPROM at 28 to 34 weeks will deliver within 1 week of ruptured membranes.

The use of tocolysis with PPROM is controversial. Because labor is an early consequence of subclinical infection and tocolysis may mask the early labor, many specialists argue against tocolysis. On the other hand, the fetal and neonatal benefits of maternal glucocorticoid therapy may warrant the risk. In the author's institution, magnesium tocolysis is used in asymptomatic women until maternal glucocorticoid therapy is completed. Regardless of ongoing adjunctive maternal or fetal therapies, delivery is warranted if clinical infection is apparent.

Adjunctive antibiotics are attractive in patients who have PPROM. Antibiotics seem to reduce maternal and fetal infections and inhibit subclinical infection and subsequent preterm labor. Multiple studies have demonstrated this hypothesis to be correct. Kenyon and coworkers [46] with the Cochrane Collaborative Group conducted a rigorous review of existing trials of adjunctive antibiotics for preterm rupture of membranes: 19 studies with over 6000 women assigned to antibiotics or placebo. Table 6 describes the beneficial results of their meta-analysis.

Antibiotic therapy showed nonsignificant trends toward reductions in respiratory complications and perinatal mortality. When comparing any penicillin versus placebo, there were significant reductions in maternal infections, neonatal infections, and central nervous system (CNS) abnormalities; and there were increased latent phase and higher birthweight. The use of erythromycin did not

Table 6
Adjunctive antibiotics for preterm rupture of membranes

Outcome	Number of women	Odds ratio (95% CI)
Intra-amniotic infection	1668	0.57 (0.37–0.86)
Birth within 48 hours	5927	0.71 (0.58–0.87)
Birth within 7 days	5860	0.80 (0.71–0.90)
Birthweight	6500	+52g (11.6–91.4 g)
Days in neonatal intensive care	225	−5.1 days (−9.8–−0.33 days)
CNS abnormality on ultrasound	67	0.82 (0.58–0.98)
Neonatal infections	1575	0.68 (0.53–0.87)

Data from Kenyon S, Boulvain M, Neilson J. Antibiotics for preterm rupture of membranes [review]. The Cochrane Database of Systematic Reviews 2004;4.

reduce maternal infections, but had similar neonatal benefits. One cautionary finding was that the use of oral amoxicillin plus clavulanic acid was associated with an increase in necrotizing enterocolitis—OR (95% CI) = 2.2 (1.1–4.3).

In summary, adjunctive antibiotics are recommended in the management of nonlaboring women who have PPROM; however, more answers are needed: What is the best type and duration of antibiotic therapy? Will improved anaerobic coverage help? Are the benefits the same for all gestational ages?

Intra-amniotic Infection

Background

Clinical infection of the intra-amniotic space, IAI, is an indication for immediate antibiotic treatment and delivery. The fetus and the mother are relatively unprotected from the evolving infection; maternal immune systems cannot completely penetrate to the fetus and the fetal immune system is immature, especially in preterm infants. Although infection initially stimulates the uterus to reject the infection (ie, labor), the concentration of cytokines or endotoxins reaches a point at which myometrial function is compromised. Fetal death, maternal sepsis, and maternal death will ensue. In addition, recent evidence demonstrates that IAI is associated with neurodevelopmental handicaps of childhood.

Subclinical infection

In patient who has asymptomatic threatened preterm birth from PTL or PPROM, the incidences of a positive AF culture are 17% and 49%, respectively [47]. These patients present often with a confusing physical examination or laboratory results. In study of 75 patients who had PPROM, Carrol and colleagues

Table 7
Predicting amniotic and fetal infection by maternal signs and laboratory tests in asymptomatic women with PPROM

Patients (N)	Tachycardia[a]	Fever[b]	Leukocytosis[c]	Elevated CRP[d]
Negative cultures (45)	2%	7%	0%	13%
Positive AF (18)	5%	11%	7%	28%
Positive FB (12)	25%	16%	16%	33%

Abbreviations: CRP, C-reactive protein; FB, fetal blood culture.
[a] Tachycardia >100 bpm.
[b] Oral temperature >38°C.
[c] Leukocytosis $>15 \times 10^9$/l.
[d] C-reactive protein >2mg/dl.
Data from Carroll SG, Papaloannou S, Davies ET, et al. Maternal assessment in the prediction of intrauterine infection in preterm prelabor amniorrhexis. Fetal Diagn Ther 1995;10:290–6.

[48] performed simultaneous measurement of maternal vital signs, maternal white cell count, maternal serum c-reactive protein, AF culture, and fetal blood culture. Forty-five had negative amniotic and fetal blood cultures, 18 had a positive AF culture, and 12 had a positive fetal blood culture. Table 7 describes the frequency of findings across there latter groups.

Yoon and coworkers [49] asked a similar question concerning the association between funisitis and subsequent clinical infection, positive AF cultures, and IL-6 levels in 315 consecutive patients between 20 and 35 weeks. Table 8 describes the results.

After control for gestational age, the OR for funisitis and the incidence of congenital neonatal sepsis was 7.2 (1.8–29.0).

Amniocentesis for AF culture is the gold standard for documentation of subclinical IAI. This procedure has been used in women who have refractory preterm labor to determine whether continued tocolysis is appropriate. Additionally, amniocentesis is performed to discriminate between IAI and other causes of abdominal pain, uterine tenderness, or maternal fever (eg, maternal viral syndrome, abruption, appendicitis).

In most cases the clinician cannot wait the 24 to 48 hours for the culture result. He or she must use proxies for the culture result. These proxies include Gram's stain, glucose concentration, WBC concentration, leukocyte esterase

Table 8
The relationship between funisitis and clinical findings or amniotic fluid in preterm gestations

Findings	Funisitis	No funisitis[a]
Positive AF culture	53%	12%
Intra-amniotic infection	18%	4%
Congenital neonatal sepsis	12%	1%
Maternal IL-6 (median ng/dl)	52.4%	4.6%

Abbreviation: IL, interleukin.
[a] All comparisons <0.001.

level, and measurement of cytokines (eg, interleukin [IL]-6). Tests and significant thresholds include

Gram's stain is performed on an unspun specimen of AF; centrifugation does not significantly improve the sensitivity of the technique. Twenty to 30 high power fields should be examined. The presence of any bacteria and leukocytes (at least six leukocytes per high-power field) is suspicious for infection.

Glucose concentration is measured with an autoanalyzer (abnormal result <15 mg/dL).

WBC concentration can be determined using a Coulter counter (abnormal result >30 cells/mm^3).

Leukocyte esterase activity is evaluated with Chemstrip 9 Reagent Strips (Roche Diagnostics, Pleasanton, California). Abnormal result = trace or greater.

All of these tests have relatively low predictive value for predicting a positive AF culture (25% to 50%), and an even lower ability to predict neonatal sepsis [47,50]. There is also great variability in findings among studies because of diverse patient populations, dissimilar microbiologic techniques, and different definitions of preterm labor. Table 9 depicts the ability of AF Gram's stain to predict a positive AF culture.

In patients who have preterm labor, the combined result of positive Gram's stain, positive leukocyte esterase, low glucose concentration, and elevated WBC concentration has sensitivity of 90% and specificity of 80% for predicting positive results of AF culture; however, because the prevalence of IAI is relatively low (about 15%–20%), this combination of tests has a false positive rate of 60%. Thus the clinician should use caution in acting prior to obtaining culture results, particularly when the intervention involves delivery of a very immature fetus. Some clinicians perform amniocentesis to exclude subclinical IAI in patients who have preterm labor or cervical insufficiency before attempts are made to prolong pregnancy. The author does not recommend amniocentesis because of the poor predictive value of the combined test, the 48-hour delay in obtaining culture results, and the lack of data proving that this approach reduces maternal/neonatal morbidity.

Cytokines, such as IL-6, IL-1, IL-8, matrix metalloproteinase-8, and tumor necrosis factor-alpha, can be measured in AF and fetal blood by immunoassay,

Table 9
Efficacy of A. Gram's stain in predicting a positive AF culture

Diagnosis (N)	+AF cultures	Sensitivity	Specificity	+PPV	−PPV
PTL (667)	17%	40%	50%	45%	49%
PPROM (765)	49%	33%	49%	44%	44%

Abbreviations: +PPV, positive predictive value; −PPV, negative predictive value.
Adapted from Gomez R, Ghezzi F, Romero R, et al. Premature labor and IAI. Clinical aspects and role of the cytokines in diagnosis and pathophysiology. Clin Perinatol 1995;22:281.

although these tests are not generally available outside of research laboratories. Elevations are associated with infection, preterm birth, and systemic fetal inflammatory syndrome (see below). IAI has been associated with an increased risk of preterm delivery even when AF cultures are negative [51,52].

Clinical infection

IAI refers to infection of the AF, membranes, placenta, or uterus. Other terms used to describe this condition include chorioamnionitis, amnionitis, AF infection, and intrapartum fever. The term "chorioamnionitis" refers to clinical infection rather than histologic chorioamnionitis. IAI accounts for 10% to 40% of cases of maternal febrile morbidity in the peripartum period, and 50% of preterm deliveries before 30 weeks of gestation [17]. IAI is also associated with 20% to 40% of cases of early neonatal sepsis and pneumonia [53].

Diagnosis of IAI is typically based upon the presence of maternal fever of greater than 38°C (100.4°F) and at least two of the following conditions [52]:

- Maternal leukocytosis (greater than 15,000 cells/cubic millimeter)
- Maternal tachycardia (greater than 100 bpm)
- Fetal tachycardia (greater than 160 bpm)
- Uterine tenderness
- Foul odor of the AF

IAI complicates 0.5% to 10.5% of deliveries [17]. Prospective studies report higher rates than retrospective studies. Differences between reports reflect center-based differences in prevalence of risk factors, differing diagnostic criteria, and changes in obstetric practice over time and among centers (eg, conservative management of rupture of membranes at term, use of internal pressure catheters for amnioinfusion, active management of labor).

The incidence of IAI is highest in preterm deliveries. IAI occurs in one third of cases of preterm labor with intact membranes. IAI occurs in 40% of women who have preterm premature rupture of membranes (PPROM) admitted having contractions and 75% of those who develop labor after admission for PPROM [52].

Obstetric risk factors for IAI include nulliparity, meconium-stained AF, longer duration of internal fetal or uterine monitoring, longer length of labor, presence of genital tract pathogens (eg, gonorrhea, GBS, BV), and a greater number of digital vaginal examinations. IAI can be either a risk factor for or a result of preterm labor or rupture of the fetal membranes. Early gestational age at membrane rupture is a related factor. As an example, the incidences of IAI in women who have PPROM at less than 27 weeks of gestation, 28 to 36 weeks of gestation, and term are 41%,15%, and 2%, respectively [17].

AF culture in pregnancies complicated by IAI has revealed multiple organisms from the vaginal flora. Two thirds of women who have IAI have at least two isolates per specimen of AF. Table 10 shows the microflora of AF of 404 patients who have IAI.

Table 10
The microflora of amniotic fluid of 404 patients with intraamniotic infection

Organism(s)	Percent
Group B streptococcus	14.6
E coli	8.2
Enterococci	5.4
Gardnerella vaginalis	24.5
Prevotella bivia	29.5
Bacteroides fragilis	3.5
Peptostreptococcus spp	9.4
Fusobacterium spp	5.4
Any gram-negative anaerobe	38.4
Mycoplasma hominis	30.4
Ureaplasma urealyticum	47.7

Adapted from Sperling RS, Newton E, Gibbs RS. Intra-amniotic infection in low-birth-weight infants. J Infect Dis 1988;157:113.

The diagnosis of IAI is not always confirmed by histological or microbiological studies. In one study of 139 pregnancies who had clinical findings of chorioamnionitis [54], histologic examination of the placenta did not support the clinical diagnosis in approximately one third of cases. The investigators suggested that noninflammatory events (eg, epidural anesthesia, abruption) could be responsible for maternal fever, tachycardia, uterine tenderness, or foul-smelling AF. In addition, histologic evidence of placental inflammation may not always be associated with microbiological evidence of an infectious organism. Cultures of the AF or membranes did not document a bacterial infection in 25% to 30% of placentas that had histologic chorioamnionitis [54–56]. Negative cultures in the presence of histologic inflammation may be due to suboptimal microbiological techniques for fastidious organisms such as *Mycoplasma spp* or administration of intrapartum antibiotics.

The maternal risks of septic shock, coagulopathy, or adult respiratory distress syndrome related to IAI are low in areas where broad-spectrum antibiotics and modern medical facilities are available. More common maternal complications include bacteremia, labor abnormalities, need for cesarean delivery, and hemorrhage. Bacteremia occurs in 5% to 10% of women who have IAI, but is more common with IAI associated with GBS or *Escherichia coli* (bacteremia in 18% and 15% of cases, respectively). In addition, cesarean delivery in the presence of IAI increases the risk of surgical complications, such as hemorrhage, wound infection, and endomyometritis [56–59].

The pathophysiologic mechanisms for labor abnormalities related to IAI are poorly understood [56–59]. Endotoxins or exotoxins produced by bacteria seem to have a biphasic effect on cytokine and prostaglandin production by the amnion, chorion, and decidua. Initially, there is an increase in cytokine and prostaglandin synthesis, thus confirming a relationship between IAI and preterm labor. As the concentration of toxins or cytokines increase, myometrial function is impaired and labor abnormalities become manifest.

The effect of IAI on labor was illustrated by large retrospective series using multivariate analysis to control for potential confounders [57–59]. The authors found that IAI was associated with an increased need for oxytocin, epidural analgesia, and cesarean delivery, as well as an increased incidence of first- and second-stage labor abnormalities. The type of infection also plays a role. Women who have persistent high-virulence organisms in their AF have more labor abnormalities and more severe IAI than women who have low-virulence organisms [60].

Hemorrhage associated with IAI is due to impaired myometrial contraction, or atony. As an example, the large retrospective series described above showed that postpartum hemorrhage was almost twice as likely after both vaginal and cesarean delivery when IAI was present [58,59].

Maternal management of intra-amniotic infection

Early administration of broad-spectrum antibiotic therapy reduces both maternal and neonatal infectious morbidity [61–64]. As an example, a randomized trial of intrapartum versus postpartum antibiotic therapy for IAI [61] found that intrapartum therapy (ampicillin plus gentamicin) was associated with a lower rate of neonatal sepsis and shorter maternal and neonatal hospital stays than postpartum treatment.

Administration of broad spectrum parenteral antibiotics with coverage for beta-lactamase–producing anaerobes is the preferred therapy of both chorioamnionitis There are few comparative trials of antibiotic regimens on which to base treatment recommendations.

- The standard treatment of ampicillin (2 g IV every 6 hours plus gentamicin (1.5 mg/kg every 8 hours for patients who have normal renal function) has been found to be safe and effective.
- Some alternative antibiotic regimens include ampicillin-sulbactam (3 grams IV every 6 hours), ticarcillin-clavulanate (3.1 grams IV every 4 hours), or cefoxitin (2 grams IV every 6 hours).
- Anaerobes play a major role in the pathogenesis of preterm birth, the AF flora of IAI (see Table 10), and complications associated with postcesarean endometritis. The addition of anaerobic coverage has reduced failure rates in postcesarean endometritis and, because of this finding, the author's group adds clindamycin (900 mg IV every 8 hours) after cord clamping to the primary antibiotic regimen if the patient is undergoing a cesarean delivery [65].

Treatment should continue until the woman is clinically improved and afebrile for 24 to 48 hours. Oral antibiotic therapy is not necessary after successful parenteral treatment, unless staphylococcal bacteremia is present [66]. Modifications in therapy may be necessary if there is no response to the initial antibiotic regimen after 48 to 72 hours postpartum. Approximately 20% of treatment failures are due to resistant organisms, such as enterococci, which are not covered by cephalosporins or clindamycin plus gentamicin. The addition of ampicillin (2 g every 4 hours) to the regimen can improve the response rate. Metronidazole (500 mg orally or IV every 8 hours) may be more effective than clindamycin against gram-negative anaerobes.

The potential neonatal risks of IAI are well-recognized. Some clinicians believe that the longer the fetus stays in an infected environment, the greater the likelihood of developing neonatal infection and short- and long-term complications. This concern may be reflected in a greater rate of cesarean birth; however, an urgent delivery does not appear warranted. Intrapartum antimicrobial chemotherapy will provide bactericidal concentrations of antibiotics to the fetus, membranes, and AF within 0.5 to 1.0 hours after infusion. Because the average time between diagnosis of IAI and delivery is 3 to 5 hours [57], it is unlikely that shortening this period will affect neonatal outcome if the fetus is receiving adequate antibiotic therapy transplacentally and labor is progressing. Finally, there is no evidence that the duration of infection correlates with adverse neonatal outcome [17,57]. Therefore, cesarean delivery should be reserved for standard obstetrical indications.

These conclusions were supported by a large multicenter study by the Maternal-Fetal Medicine Network [57] that compared pregnancy outcome in women who had (n = 1965) and did not have (n = 14,685) chorioamnionitis and who underwent cesarean delivery at term. The major findings from this study were:

- Chorioamnionitis significantly increased the risk of maternal and fetal morbidity. The risks of uterine atony, blood transfusion, pelvic abscess, thromboembolism, and wound complications were increased in the mother; the risks of neonatal sepsis, neonatal seizures, and low 5-minute Apgar scores (< 3) were increased in the infant. The prevalence of cerebral palsy, an important potential complication associated with IAI, was not determined, however.
- The duration of chorioamnionitis did not significantly increase the risk of maternal or neonatal complications, with the exception of uterine atony, low 5-minute Apgar score, and mechanical ventilation within 24 hours of birth, all of which were mildly elevated with longer durations of infection.
- The use of continuous electronic fetal monitoring is appropriate for detecting the development of fetal compromise in cases of IAI. The combination of villous edema, hyperthermic stress, and fetal infection can lead to fetal acidosis. Although no particular pattern of periodic heart rate changes signifies fetal infection, a nonreassuring tracing (eg, one with absent variability and late decelerations) is predictive of fetal acidosis and poor short-term outcomes.

Fetal tachycardia is a predictor of fetal sepsis or pneumonia [67,68], but may be due only to fetal hyperthermia. The use of an antipyretic (eg, 625 mg acetaminophen rectal suppository every 4 hours) is therapeutic, and may be diagnostic [69]. The lowering of maternal temperature reduces the metabolic stress of fetal hyperthermia and thereby decreases the fetal heart rate. If the tachycardia is not due to maternal fever, the acetaminophen will not reduce the fetal heart rate. In these cases of persistent fetal tachycardia, health care providers must prepare for delivery of a hemodynamically unstable neonate.

The risk of fetal infection associated with maternal IAI is 10% to 20%. Complications are more common in premature and low birthweight infants. As an example, one study [68] stratified 404 neonates whose mothers had AF-culture–documented IAI into those who weighed <2500 g (n=37) and those weighing >2500 g (n=367). The low-birthweight neonates had a significantly higher incidence of sepsis (16% versus 4%) and death from sepsis (10.8% versus 0%). Gram-negative anaerobes were a common pathogen among these infants. In another series [57], multivariate analysis showed that prematurity, preterm labor, fetal tachycardia, and sexually transmitted disease in the index pregnancy were independent risk factors for early neonatal pneumonia and/or sepsis.

IAI can lead to perinatal asphyxia. Possible mechanisms include villous edema [70], abruptio placentae [71,72], an increase in oxygen consumption related to hyperthermia, or a primary endotoxin effect on the fetus. In addition, in animal models, maternal hyperthermia and subsequent hyperventilation led to a reduction in uterine blood flow and fetal acidosis [69]. These observations support the adjunctive use of antipyretics in IAI.

Neurodevelopmental delay and cerebral palsy are potential long-term disabilities resulting from IAI [73–76]. Among infants weighing less than 2000 g, IAI is associated with a lower mental developmental index (Bayley Scales of Infant Development), and children exposed to IAI in utero are less likely to develop normally than unexposed children (64% versus 80%) [74]. This relationship was illustrated by data from the Collaborative Perinatal Project of the National Institute of Neurological and Communicative Disorders and Stroke (NCPP) [75] that showed chorioamnionitis was associated with a 4.8-fold increased risk of cerebral palsy (2.6-fold when limited to infants >2500 g). Similar findings have subsequently been reported by others. In 2003, a case-control nested cohort study of over 230,000 singleton infants born at more than 36 weeks of gestation [74] found that cerebral palsy could be attributed to chorioamnionitis in 11% of cases, and the OR for developing cerebral palsy after a diagnosis of chorioamnionitis was 4.1 (95% CI, 1.6–10.1) in multivariable analysis. In addition, a meta-analysis evaluating the association between IAI/clinical chorioamnionitis or histologic chorioamnionitis and periventricular leukomalacia (PVL) or cerebral palsy [76] reported that IAI was associated with both PVL (relative risk [RR] 3.0, 95% CI 2.2–4.0) and cerebral palsy (preterm neonates RR 1.9, 95% CI 1.4–2.5; term neonates RR 4.7; 95% CI 1.3–16.2). These complications were still observed, but at a slightly lower rate, with histologic chorioamnionitis: cerebral palsy (RR 1.6; 95% CI 0.9–2.7), PVL (RR 2.1, 95% CI 1.5–2.9). This analysis was limited by many potential biases, however, including differences in the definitions of IAI, histologic chorioamnionitis, cerebral palsy, and PVL across studies; extent of blinding in determining exposure status; and whether the study controlled for potential confounders.

Three mechanisms have been proposed to explain the association between IAI and neurodevelopmental disability: aberrant fetal cytokine response, asphyxia, and toxic injury by bacterial products.

The term systemic fetal inflammatory syndrome (also known as fetal inflammatory response syndrome) refers to the fetal immune response to intrauterine infection and the consequences of this response: preterm labor, fetal growth restriction, severe neonatal morbidity, brain injury, and chronic lung disease in the child [77–80]. High levels of fetal/neonatal cytokines, especially tumor necrosis factor [81], appear to mediate the fetal/neonatal brain injury [77–82]. These inflammatory cytokines can cause cerebral ischemia and damage, ultimately leading to intraventricular hemorrhage and periventricular leukomalacia.

Funisitis and chorionic vasculitis appear to be the placental histological manifestations of fetal inflammatory response syndrome [83–87]. An elevated fetal plasma (>10 pg/mL) or AF IL-6 concentration is the laboratory finding characteristic of this process [84–87]. One group that followed preterm infants for 18 months after birth [81] found that funisitis was an independent risk factor for a lower median Bayley Psychomotor Development Index—94 versus 99 in infants without funisitis. The study authors postulated that funisitis might be a marker for vascular inflammation elsewhere in the fetus.

References

[1] Willoughby RE, Nelson KB. Chorioamnionitis and brain injury. Clin Perinatol 2002;29: 603–21.

[2] Meis PJ, Goldenberg RL, Mercer BM, et al. The Preterm Prediction Study: risk factors for indicate preterm births. Am J Obstet Gynecol 1998;178(3):562–7.

[3] Meis PJ, Ernest JM, Moore ML. Causes of low birth weight births in public and private patients. Am J Obstet Gynecol 1987;156(5):1165–8.

[4] Moutquin JM. Classification and heterogeneity of preterm birth. BJOG 2003;110(Suppl 20): 30–3.

[5] Iams J. The epidemiology of preterm birth. Clin Perinatol 2003;30(4):651–64.

[6] Genc MR, Vardhana S, Delaney ML, et al. Relationship between a Toll-like receptor-4 gene polymorphism, bacterial vaginosis-related flora and vaginal cytokine responses in pregnant women. Eur J Obstet Gynecol Rep Biology 2004;116(2):152–6.

[7] Romero R, Chaiworapongsa T, Kuivaniemi H, et al. Bacterial vaginosis, the inflammatory response and the risk of preterm birth: a role for genetic epidemiology in the prevention of preterm birth. Am J Obstet Gynecol 2004;190:1509–19.

[8] Lorenz E, Hallman M, Riitta H, et al. Association between the Asp299Gly polymorphisms in the Toll-like receptor 4 and premature births in the Finnish population. Pediatr Res 2002;52(3): 373–6.

[9] Macones G, Parry S, Elkousy M, et al. A polymorphism in the promoter region of TNF and bacterial vaginosis: preliminary evidence of gene-environment interaction in the etiology of spontaneous preterm birth. Am J Obstet Gynecol 2004;190:1504–8.

[10] Newton ER, Piper J, Peairs W. Bacterial vaginosis and IAI. Am J Obstet Gynecol 1997;176(3): 672–7.

[11] Janssens S, Beyaert R. Role of Toll-like receptors in pathogen recognition. Clin Microbiol Rev 2003;16(4):637–46.
[12] Pawelczyk E. Toll-like receptor 4 (TLR4) in gestational infection and preterm birth [PhD dissertation]. Galveston (TX): University of Texas Medical Branch at Galveston; 2004.
[13] Meis P, Connors N. Progesterone treatment to prevent preterm birth. Clin Obstet Gynecol 2004; 47(4):784–95.
[14] Hillier SL, Joachim M, Kraohn M, et al. A case-control study of chorioamnionic infection and histologic chorioamnionitis in prematurity. N Engl J Med 1988;319(15):972–8.
[15] Cassell G, Haugh JC, Andrews WW, et al. Chorioamnion colonization: correlation with gestational age in women delivered following spontaneous labor versus indicated delivery. Am J Obstet Gynecol 1993;168–425.
[16] Salafia CM, Vogel CA, Vintzileos AM, et al. Placental pathological findings in preterm birth. Am J Obstet Gynecol 1991;165:934–8.
[17] Newton ER. Chorioamnionitis and IAI. Clin Obstet Gynecol 1993;36:795.
[18] Bejar R, Curbelo V, Davis C, et al. Premature labor. II. Bacterial sources of phospholipase. Obstet Gynecol 1981;57(4):479–82.
[19] McDonald H, Brocklehurst P, Parsons J. Antibiotics for treating bacterial vaginosis in pregnancy. McDonald: The Cochrane Library 2005;1.
[20] Leitich H, Bodner-Adler B, Brunbauer M, et al. Bacterial vaginosis as a risk factor for preterm delivery: a meta-analysis. Am J Obstet Gynecol 2003;189(1):139–47.
[21] Carey JC, Sumner JY, Catz C. The vaginal infections and prematurity study: an overview. Clin Obstet Gynecol 1993;36(4):809–20.
[22] Ehrenberg H, Mercer B. Antibiotics and the management of preterm premature rupture of the fetal membranes. Clin Perinatol 2001;28(4):807–19.
[23] Cassell G, Andrews WW, Haugh JC, et al. Isolation of microorganisms from the chorioamnion is twice that from amniotic fluid at cesarean delivery in women with intact membranes. Am J Obstet Gynecol 1993;168:424.
[24] National Center for Health Statistics. Final 2002 natality data. Available at: www.marchofdimes.com/peristats.
[25] Inder T, Neil J, Yoder B, et al. Non-human primate models of neonatal brain injury. Semin Perinatol 2004;28(6):396–404.
[26] Mercer B, Crocker L, Boe N, et al. Induction versus expectant management in premature rupture of the membranes with mature amniotic fluid at 32 to 36 weeks: a randomized trial. Am J Obstet Gynecol 1993;169:775–81.
[27] Kramer MS, Demissie K, Yang H, et al. The contribution of mild and moderate preterm birth to infant mortality. JAMA 2000;284(7):843–9.
[28] Shain RN, Piper JM, Newton ED, et al. A randomized, controlled trial of a behavioral intervention to prevent sexually transmitted disease among minority women. N Engl J Med 1999;340(2):93–100.
[29] Bakketieg LS, Hoffman HJ. Epidemiology of preterm birth: results of a longitudinal study in Norway. In: , editors. Preterm labor. London: Butterworths; 1981. p.
[30] Nugent RP, Krohn MA, Hillier SL. Reliability of diagnosing bacterial vaginosis is improved by a standardized method of gram stain interpretation. J Clin Microbiol 1991;29:297–301.
[31] Riggs M, Klemanoff M. Treatment of vaginal infections to prevent preterm birth: a meta-analysis. Clin Obstet Gynecol 2004;47(4):796–807.
[32] Thomsen AC, Morup L, Hansen KB. Antibiotic elimination of group B streptococci in urine in prevention of preterm labor. Lancet 1987;1(8533):591–3.
[33] Klebanoff MA, Regan JA, Rao AV, et al. Outcome of the vaginal infections and prematurity study: results of a clinical trial of erythromycin among pregnant women colonized with group B streptococci. Am J Obstet Gynecol 1995;172:1540–5.
[34] Klein L, Gibbs R. Use of microbial cultures and antibiotics in the prevention of infection-associated preterm birth. Am J Obstet Gynecol 2004;190:1493–502.
[35] Martin DH, Eschenback DA, Cotch FA, et al. Double-blind placebo-controlled treatment trial

of *Chlamydia trachomatis* endocervical infections in pregnant women. Infect Dis Obstet Gynecol 1997;5:10–7.

[36] Eschenbach DA, Nugent RP, Rao AV, et al. A randomized placebo-controlled trial of erythromycin for the treatment of *Ureaplasma urealyticum* to prevent premature delivery. Am J Obstet Gynecol 1991;164:734–42.

[37] Klebanoff M, Carey J, Hauth J, et al. Failure of metronidazole to prevent preterm delivery among pregnant women with asymptomatic *Trichomonas vaginalis* infection. N Engl J Med 2001; 345(7):487–93.

[38] Smaill F. Antibiotics for asymptomatic bacteriuria in pregnancy. Smaill: The Cochrane Database of Systematic Reviews 2005;1.

[39] King J, Flenady V. Phroylactic antibiotics for inhibiting preterm labour with intact membranes. King:The Cochrane Database of Systematic Reviews 2005;1.

[40] Meis PJ, Michielutte R, Peters TJ, et al. Obstetrics: factors associated with preterm birth in Cardiff, Wales. I. Univariable and multivariable analysis. Am J Obstet Gynecol 1995;173(2): 590–6.

[41] Meis PJ, Michielutte R, Peters TJ, et al. Obstetrics: factors associated with preterm birth in Cardiff, Wales. II. Indicated and spontaneous preterm birth. Am J Obstet Gynecol 1995; 173(2):597–602.

[42] Mercer BM, Goldenberg RL, Das A, et al. The preterm prediction study: a clinical risk assessment system. Am J Obstet Gynecol 1996;174(6):1885–93 [discussion: 1893–5].

[43] Mercer B, Goldenberg R, Moawad A, et al. The Preterm Prediction Study: effect of gestational age and cause of preterm birth on subsequent obstetric outcome. Am J Obstet Gynecol 1999; 181:1216–21.

[44] Iams JD, Goldenberg RL, Mercer BM, et al. The Preterm Prediction Study: recurrence risk of spontaneous preterm birth. National Institute of Child Health and Human Development Maternal-Fetal Medicine Units Network. Am J Obstet Gynecol 1998;178(5):1035–40.

[45] Higby K, Xenakis EM, Pauerstein CJ. Do tocolytic agents stop preterm labor? A critical and comprehensive review of efficacy and safety. Am J Obstet Gynecol 1993;168(4):1247–56 [discussion: 1256–9].

[46] Kenyon S, Boulvain M, Neilson J. Antibiotics for preterm rupture of membranes [review]. The Cochrane Database of Systematic Reviews 2004;4.

[47] Gomez R, Ghezzi F, Romero R, et al. Premature labor and IAI. Clinical aspects and role of the cytokines in diagnosis and pathophysiology. Clin Perinatol 1995;22:281–342.

[48] Carroll SG, Papaloannou S, Davies ET, et al. Maternal assessment in the prediction of intrauterine infection in preterm prelabor amniorrhexis. Fetal Diagn Ther 1995;10:290–6.

[49] Yoon BH, Romero R, Park JS, et al. The relationship among inflammatory lesions of the umbilical cord (funisitis), umbilical cord plasma interleukin 6 concentration, amniotic fluid infection, and neonatal sepsis. Am J Obstet Gynecol 2000;183(5):1124–9.

[50] Gomez R, Romero R, Ghezzi F, et al. The fetal inflammatory response syndrome. Am J Obstet Gynecol 1998;179:194–202.

[51] Shim SS, Romero R, Hong JS, et al. Clinical significance of intra-amniotic inflammation in patients with preterm premature rupture of membranes. Am J Obstet Gynecol 2004;191: 1339–45.

[52] Gibbs RS, Duff P. Progress in pathogenesis and management of clinical IAI. Am J Obstet Gynecol 1991;164:1317–26.

[53] Morales WJ, Washington 3rd SR, Lazar AJ. The effect of chorioamnionitis on perinatal outcome in preterm gestation. J Perinatol 1987;7:105–10.

[54] Smulian JC, Schen-Schwarz S, Vintzileos AM, et al. Clinical chorioamnionitis and histologic placental inflammation. Obstet Gynecol 1999;94:1000–5.

[55] Dong Y, St. Clair PJ, Ramzy I, et al. A microbiologic and clinical study of placental inflammation at term. Obstet Gynecol 1987;70:175.

[56] Hillier SL, Martius J, Krohn M, et al. A case-control study of chorioamnionic infection and histologic chorioamnionitis in prematurity. N Engl J Med 1988;319:972–8

[57] Rouse DJ, Landon M, Leveno KJ, et al. The Maternal-Fetal Medicine Unit's cesarean registry: chorioamnionitis at term and its duration-relationship to outcomes. Am J Obstet Gynecol 2004;191:211–6.
[58] Satin AJ, Maberry MC, Leveno KJ, et al. Chorioamnionitis: a harbinger of dystocia. Obstet Gynecol 1992;79:913–5.
[59] Mark SP, Croughan-Minihane MS, Kilpatrick SJ. Chorioamnionitis and uterine function. Obstet Gynecol 2000;95:909.
[60] Yoder PR, Gibbs RS, Blanco JD, et al. A prospective, controlled study of maternal and perinatal outcome after IAI at term. Am J Obstet Gynecol 1983;145:695–707.
[61] Gibbs RS, Dinsmoor MJ, Newton ER, et al. A randomized trial of intrapartum versus immediate postpartum treatment of women with IAI. Obstet Gynecol 1988;72:823–8.
[62] Gilstrap 3rd LC, Leveno KJ, Cox SM, et al. Intrapartum treatment of acute chorioamnionitis: impact on neonatal sepsis. Am J Obstet Gynecol 1988;159:579–83.
[63] Maberry MC, Gilstrap 3rd LC. Intrapartum antibiotic therapy for suspected IAI: impact on the fetus and neonate. Clin Obstet Gynecol 1991;34:345–51.
[64] Hopkins L, Smaill F. Antibiotic regimens for management of IAI. Cochrane Database Syst Rev 2002;CD003254.
[65] French LM, Smaill FM. Antibiotic regimens for endometritis after delivery. Cochrane Database Syst Rev 2000;CD001067.
[66] Dinsmoor MJ, Newton ER, Gibbs RS. A randomized, double-blind, placebo-controlled trial of oral antibiotic therapy following intravenous antibiotic therapy for postpartum endometritis. Obstet Gynecol 1991;77:60–2.
[67] Spaans WA, Knox AJ, Koya HB, et al. Risk factors for neonatal infection. Aust N Z J Obstet Gynaecol 1990;30:327–30.
[68] Sperling RS, Newton E, Gibbs RS. Intra-amniotic infection in low-birth-weight infants. J Infect Dis 1988;157:113–7.
[69] Kirshon B, Moise Jr KJ, Wasserstrum N. Effect of acetaminophen on fetal acid-base balance in chorioamnionitis. J Reprod Med 1989;34:955–9.
[70] Ilagan NB, Elias EG, Liang KC, et al. Perinatal and neonatal significance of bacteria-related placental villous edema. Acta Obstet Gynecol Scand 1990;69:287–90.
[71] Rana A, Sawhney H, Gopalan S, et al. Abruptio placentae and chorioamnionitis-microbiological and histologic correlation. Acta Obstet Gynecol Scand 1999;78:363–6.
[72] Darby MJ, Caritis SN, Shen-Schwarz S. Placental abruption in the preterm gestation: an association with chorioamnionitis. Obstet Gynecol 1989;74:88–92.
[73] Gilstrap 3rd LC, Ramin SM. Infection and cerebral palsy. Semin Perinatol 2000;24:200–3.
[74] Wu YW, Escobar GJ, Grether JK, et al. Chorioamnionitis and cerebral palsy in term and near-term infants. JAMA 2003;290:2677–84.
[75] Nelson KB, Ellenberg JH. Antecedents of cerebral palsy. I. Univariate analysis of risks. Am J Dis Child 1985;139:1031–8.
[76] Wu YW, Colford JM. Chorioamnionitis as a risk factor for cerebral palsy. A meta-analysis. JAMA 2000;284:1417–24.
[77] Yoon BH, Jun JK, Romero R, et al. Amniotic fluid inflammatory cytokines (interleukin-6, interleukin-1 beta and tumor necrosis factor-alpha), neonatal brain white matter lesions, and cerebral palsy. Am J Obstet Gynecol 1997;177:19–26.
[78] Williams MC, O'Brien WF, Nelson RN, et al. Histologic chorioamnionitis is associated with fetal growth restriction in term and preterm infants. Am J Obstet Gynecol 2000;183:1094–9.
[79] Kadhim H, Tabarki B, Verellen G, et al. Inflammatory cytokines in the pathogenesis of periventricular leukomalacia. Neurology 2001;56:1278–84.
[80] Perlman JM. White matter injury in the preterm infant: an important determination of abnormal neurodevelopment outcome. Early Hum Dev 1998;53:99–120.
[81] Mittendorf R, Montag AG, MacMillan W, et al. Components of the systemic fetal inflammatory response syndrome as predictors of impaired neurologic outcomes in children. Am J Obstet Gynecol 2003;188:1438–40.

[82] Debillon T, Gras-Leguen C, Verielle V, Winer N. Intrauterine infection induces programmed cell death in rabbit periventricular white matter. Pediatr Res 2000;47:736–42.
[83] Pacora P, Chaiworapongsa T, Maymon E, et al. Funisitis and chorionic vasculitis: the histological counterpart of the fetal inflammatory response syndrome. J Matern Fetal Med 2002;11:18–25.
[84] Yoon BH, Romero R, Park JS, et al. The relationship among inflammatory lesions of the umbilical cord (funisitis), umbilical cord plasma interleukin 6 concentration, amniotic fluid infection, and neonatal sepsis. Am J Obstet Gynecol 2000;183:1124–9.
[85] Harirah H, Donia SE, Hsu CD. Amniotic fluid matrix metalloproteinase-9 and interleukin-6 in predicting IAI. Obstet Gynecol 2002;99:80–4.
[86] Yoon BH, Romero R, Moon JB, et al. Clinical significance of intra-amniotic inflammation in patients with preterm labor and intact membranes. Am J Obstet Gynecol 2001;185:1130–6.
[87] Naccasha N, Hinson R, Montag A, et al. Association between funisitis and elevated interleukin-6 in cord blood. Obstet Gynecol 2001;97:220–4.

ELSEVIER
SAUNDERS

Clin Perinatol 32 (2005) 601–615

CLINICS IN
PERINATOLOGY

Prevention of Neonatal Sepsis

Stephanie Schrag, D Phil[a], Anne Schuchat, MD[b,*]

[a]*Division of Bacterial and Mycotic Diseases, National Center for Infectious Diseases, Mailstop, C-23 Centers for Disease Control and Prevention, Atlanta, GA 30333, USA*
[b]*Office of the Director, National Center for Infectious Diseases, Mailstop, C-23 Centers for Disease Control and Prevention, Atlanta, GA 30333, USA*

Traditionally, neonatal sepsis has been a focus of concern for pediatric caregivers; however, obstetric practitioners can have a tremendous impact on reducing the burden of this serious disease through interventions that are applied during pregnancy or childbirth. In the last decade, the use of intrapartum antimicrobial prophylaxis has increased in the United States, primarily for group B streptococcal (GBS) disease prevention, and to a lesser extent for preterm premature rupture of membranes (pPROM). During the 1990s, the incidence of laboratory-confirmed GBS infections in newborns declined dramatically. Although neonatal sepsis is a leading cause of neonatal mortality around the world, and the neonatal period contributes disproportionately to child mortality in resource-poor countries [1], this article focuses on prevention of neonatal sepsis in industrialized countries. The scope of the article also is restricted to infections that develop in the first days of life, because perinatal interventions may have the most impact on these infections.

Burden of neonatal sepsis

Severe bacterial infections (ie, sepsis or meningitis) during the neonatal period typically are divided into early- and late-onset syndromes. Early-onset sepsis is acquired through vertical transmission by ascending spread from the lower genital tract, through transplacental transmission after maternal bacteremia (eg, *Listeria monocytogenes*), or through neonatal acquisition during passage through the birth canal. Early-onset sepsis becomes clinically evident within the first few

* Corresponding author.
E-mail address: aschuchat@cdc.gov (A. Schuchat).

0095-5108/05/$ – see front matter. Published by Elsevier Inc.
doi:10.1016/j.clp.2005.05.005

days of life, and has been defined in most reports as occurring within the first week or the first 72 hours of life. Late-onset sepsis presents thereafter, with an outer limit of 28, 30, or 90 days in various reports. Late-onset infections may be acquired intrapartum during passage through the birth canal, through horizontal spread within hospital settings, or from maternal or other sources in the home or community. Prevention strategies have not been identified to reduce late-onset sepsis.

The pathogens that are identified most frequently from early-onset sepsis have varied over the past 60 years and may differ from hospital to hospital or country to country [2,3]. The relative contribution of the leading etiologies of neonatal sepsis from four multicenter U.S. reports from the past decade is shown in Fig. 1 [4–7]. Since its emergence in the 1970s, GBS has ranked consistently as the leading cause of early-onset sepsis in U.S. surveillance populations. Before prevention efforts were adopted in the United States, rates of laboratory-confirmed early-onset GBS disease ranged from 1.4 [4] to 1.7 [8] per 1000 live births in the general population. The case fatality ratio was influenced strongly by gestational age. Rates in the very low birth weight (<1500 g) population in the early 1990s were 5.9 per 1000 births [2,7]. *Escherichia coli* and other gram negatives accounted for a large proportion of non-GBS cases. One multicenter study that was performed in the mid-1990s reported a case fatality ratio of 6.7% for cases of early-onset GBS cases compared with 22.3% for non-GBS cases [4]. Prematurity was linked closely to the higher case fatality ratio for non-GBS cases in that report.

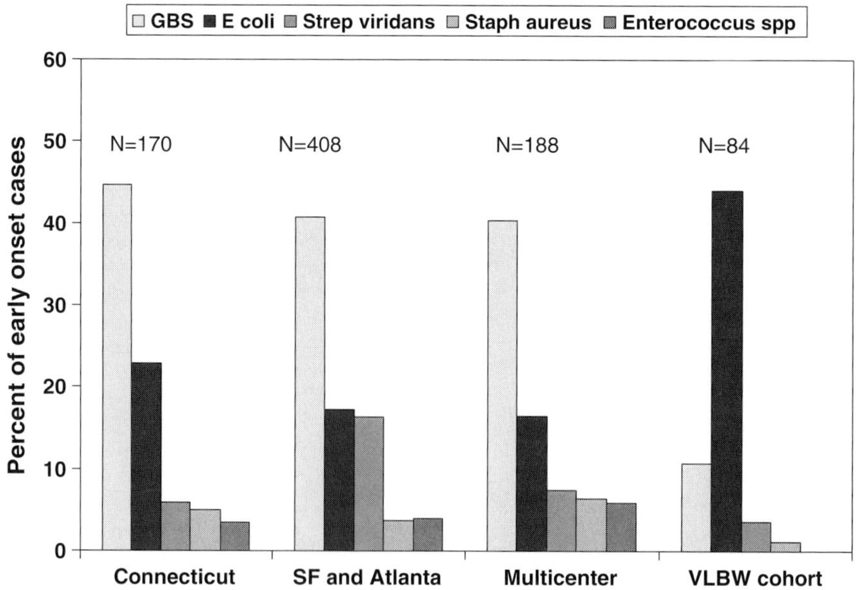

Fig. 1. Leading etiologies of neonatal sepsis from four U.S. reports. SF, San Francisco; Staph, *Staphylococcus*; Strep, *Streptococcus*; VLBW, very low birth weight. (*Data from* Refs. [1–4].)

The incidence of early-onset GBS disease declined by 81% from 1993 through 2003, with a 60% narrowing of the black:white disparity in disease [8,9]. During this time period, trends in overall neonatal sepsis have been difficult to gauge, but most data point to no significant increase or decrease in other causes of early-onset sepsis in the general population. In contrast, the rate of non-GBS sepsis seems to have increased among very low birth weight infants [7,10].

Many episodes of suspected clinical sepsis in newborns are not confirmed through isolation of pathogens from blood cultures. Although some clinical episodes may have falsely negative cultures as a result of limitations in sample collection, processing, or the interference of antimicrobial agents, other culture-negative sepsis episodes may reflect an inflammatory response that mimics sepsis but without active bacterial involvement. Although clinically-defined sepsis is nonspecific in its etiologies, trends in U.S. deaths and hospitalizations that are attributed to neonatal sepsis generally have paralleled those observed for laboratory-confirmed GBS disease. Lukacs and colleagues [11] reported a significant decline in early newborn deaths that were assigned *International Classification of Diseases, Ninth Revision* codes that were consistent with neonatal sepsis. The rate of early death from neonatal sepsis averaged 24.9 per 100,000 live births from 1985 through 1991, but decreased to 15.6 per 100,000 live births in 1995 through 1998. The annual percent decreased from a 3.0% annual decline for 1985 through 1991 to a 5.0% annual decline from 1995 through 1998. The rate of decrease in early sepsis deaths in 1995 through 1998 was steeper than trends for other causes of death, consistent with the declines being attributable to increased antimicrobial prophylaxis for GBS disease prevention. Similar declines were not seen for late neonatal sepsis deaths in the U.S. population. Declines in early sepsis deaths occurred in all gestational age categories. A similar analysis aimed at tracking trends in hospitalizations for neonatal sepsis using the National Hospital Discharge Survey. Investigators found that national hospitalizations decreased by 23% between 1990 and 2002, with more than 20,000 fewer neonatal sepsis hospitalizations occurring in 2002 compared with 1990 [12]. These analyses suggest the full impact of intrapartum prophylaxis may be greater than that estimated by measurement of laboratory-confirmed cases of early-onset sepsis alone.

Risk factors for neonatal sepsis

Risk factors for early-onset GBS disease have been well-characterized and include maternal GBS colonization, prolonged rupture of membranes, preterm delivery, GBS bacteriuria during pregnancy, delivery of a previous infant with invasive GBS disease, maternal chorioamnionitis as evidenced by intrapartum fever, young maternal age, black race, Hispanic ethnicity, low levels of antibody to type-specific capsular polysaccharide antigens, and frequent vaginal examinations during labor [13–16]. A multivariable analysis of a large multistate birth cohort in 1998 and 1999 found that intrapartum fever and previous infant with GBS disease were associated with a greater than fivefold increased risk; maternal age younger than 20 years, black race, and preterm delivery each were associated independently with a 1.5 to twofold increased risk of having an infant who had GBS disease [17]. A cohort analysis in Atlanta showed that black race remained an independent risk factor after controlling for birth weight and maternal age [18].

Risk factors for non-GBS sepsis have not been studied as intensively. Preterm delivery is identified consistently as a strong risk factor. Compared with early-onset GBS disease where approximately 80% of cases in the United States occur in infants born at 37 or more weeks of gestation, a multicenter study found that only 40% of cases of early-onset non-GBS sepsis occurred in term infants; in contrast, 46% of cases occurred among preterm infants who were born at less than 34 weeks of gestation [4]. Other important risk factors that were identified by multiple studies include intra-amniotic infection and prolonged membrane rupture. Among infants who are born preterm, prelabor rupture of membranes has been associated with up to a threefold risk of sepsis [19]. Non-GBS neonatal sepsis occurs more commonly in black infants and sepsis-related perinatal mortality rates are disproportionately higher among black neonates; however, because preterm delivery is such a strong risk factor for non-GBS sepsis, it is challenging to identify independent risk factors that are not confounded by prematurity.

Prevention of perinatal group B streptococcal disease

Intrapartum antimicrobial prophylaxis

Although GBS infections during pregnancy can result in stillbirth, most newborns acquire GBS infections during the intrapartum period, either through ascending spread of the bacteria into the amniotic fluid or through exposure to the bacteria during passage through the birth canal. Several clinical trials have demonstrated that the use of intravenous antibiotics during the intrapartum period is highly effective at preventing early-onset neonatal GBS infections [20–23]. The use of intrapartum prophylaxis also was shown to be cost-effective in the United States [24–26].

Despite the availability of an effective intervention, agreement on a strategy for identifying candidates for chemoprophylaxis has proved challenging. In the 1990s, guidelines recommended late antenatal culture-based screening of pregnant women for GBS colonization or a risk-based approach that monitored for obstetric factors associated with increased risk of neonatal GBS disease during the intrapartum period. The first U.S. consensus guidelines for perinatal GBS disease prevention, issued in 1996, recommended a risk-based or a culture-based screening approach [27]. Active multistate surveillance for invasive GBS disease in neonates documented a 70% decline in early-onset GBS disease during the 1990s [8,28]. During this same time period, invasive GBS disease among pregnant women (primarily intra-amniotic infections) declined by 20%.

A recent large, multistate, retrospective evaluation of the effectiveness of these two strategies found that late antenatal culture-based screening for GBS was greater than 50% more effective than the alternative, risk-based approach at preventing neonatal early-onset GBS disease [17]. This benefit derived largely from the identification and prophylaxis of culture-positive women who did not present with risk factors (18% of delivering women in the population-based retrospective study and up to 45% of women who gave birth to infants who had early-onset GBS disease in the preprevention era), as well as improved compliance with the screening-based approach.

These findings were the basis of new perinatal GBS disease prevention guidelines that were released by the Centers for Disease Control and Prevention (CDC), American Academy of Pediatrics, and American College of Obstetricians and Gynecologists in 2002 that recommend universal late antenatal screening of all pregnant women [29,30]. An algorithm for identifying candidates for chemoprophylaxis is shown in Fig. 2, and recommended prophylaxis agents are summarized in Box 1. Multistate data from 2003 showed a 34% decline in early-onset disease incidence in the year after the issuance of these new guidelines [9].

Postnatal penicillin

Universal administration of single-dose intramuscular penicillin to neonates at birth has been considered as an alternative strategy for prevention of early-onset GBS disease. Randomized trials have shown that this intervention alone [31–33], or in combination with a risk-based intrapartum prophylaxis approach [34], can result in significant prevention of early-onset invasive GBS disease. A large delivery center in Texas was able to achieve a rate of GBS disease that approached the one that was attained by late antenatal screening using a combined risk-based and universal postnatal penicillin approach [35].

This strategy has not been implemented widely, in part because of concerns about potential adverse consequences of such widespread use of antibiotics in neonates, including increased risk of nosocomial acquisition of resistant organisms and masking of culture-confirmed infections. From a prevention perspective, intrapartum prophylaxis has the opportunity to protect the neonate from in utero and birth canal acquisition of GBS colonization; postnatal penicillin does not have the same scope for prevention because it is administered after the newborn has been delivered.

Group B streptococcal vaccine research

Intrapartum antimicrobial prophylaxis has been viewed as an interim strategy for neonatal GBS disease prevention, in part because of concerns that β-lactam resistance may emerge in GBS or other important sepsis pathogens in neonates, and also because an adolescent or maternal immunization strategy holds promise

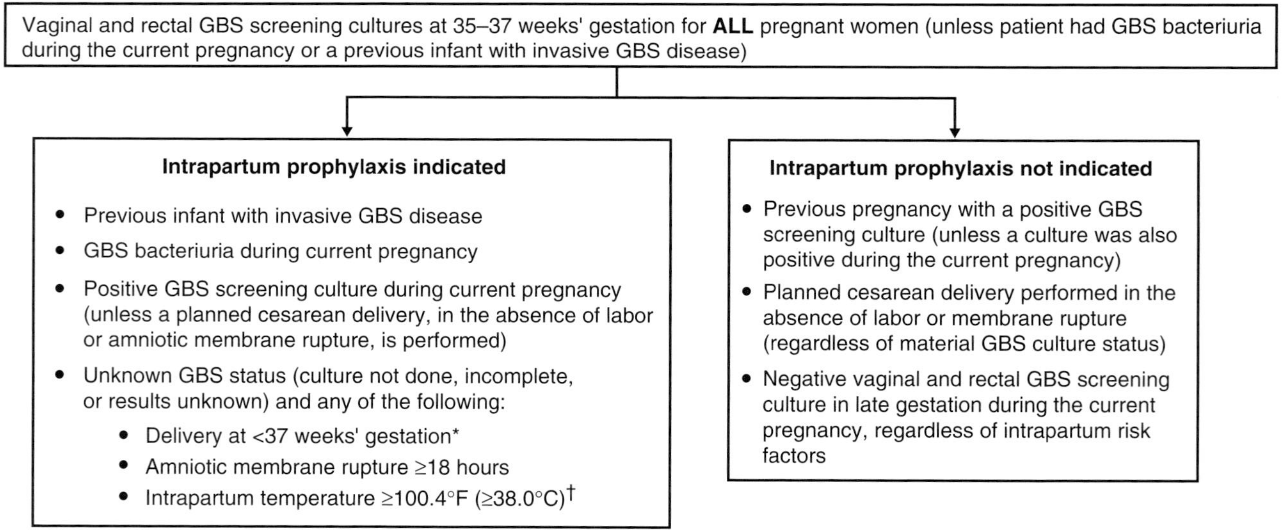

* If onset of labor or rupture of amniotic membranes occurs at <37 weeks' gestation and there is a significant risk for preterm delivery (as assessed by the clinician), a suggested algorithm for GBS prophylaxis management is provided.
† If amnionitis is suspected, broad-spectrum antibiotic therapy that includes an agent known to be active against GBS should replace GBS prophylaxis.

Fig. 2. Indications for intrapartum antibiotic prophylaxis to prevent perinatal GBS disease under a universal prenatal screening strategy based on combined vaginal and rectal cultures collected at 35–37 weeks' gestation from all pregnant women. (*From* Centers for Disease Control and Prevention. Prevention of Perinatal Group B Streptococcal Disease. MMWR 2002;51(RR-11):8.)

Box 1. Recommended regimens for intrapartum antimicrobial prophylaxis for perinatal GBS disease prevention

Recommended:
Penicillin G, 5 million units IV initial dose, then 2.5 million units IV every 4 hours until delivery
Alternative:
Ampicillin, 2 g IV initial dose, then 1 g IV every 4 hours until delivery
If penicillin allergic[b]:
Patients not at high risk for anaphylaxis
Cefazolin, 2 g IV initial dose, then 1 g IV every 8 hours until delivery
Patients at high risk for anaphylaxis[c]
1. GBS susceptible to clindamycin and erythromycin[d]
Clindamycin, 900 mg IV every 8 hours until delivery
OR
Erythromycin, 500 mg IV every 6 hours until delivery
2. GBS resistant to clindamycin or erythromycin or susceptibility unknown
Vancomycin,[e] 1 g IV every 12 hours until delivery

[a] Broader-spectrum agents, including an agent active against GBS, may be necessary for treatment of chorioamnionitis.
[b] History of penicillin allergy should be assessed to determine whether a high risk for anaphylaxis is present. Penicillin-allergic patients at high risk for anaphylaxis are those who have experienced immediate hypersensitivity to penicillin including a history of penicillin-related anaphylaxis; other high-risk patients are those with asthma or other diseases that would make anaphylaxis more dangerous or difficult to treat, such as persons being treated with beta-adrenergic–blocking agents.
[c] If laboratory facilities are adequate, clindamycin and erythromycin susceptibility testing should be performed on prenatal GBS isolates from penicillin-allergic women at high risk for anaphylaxis.
[d] Resistance to erythromycin is often but not always associated with clindamycin resistance. If a strain is resistant to erythromycin but appears susceptible to clindamycin, it may still have inducible resistance to clindamycin.
[e] Cefazolin is preferred over vancomycin for women with a history of penicillin allergy other than immediate hypersensitivity reactions, and pharmacologic data suggest it achieves effective intraamniotic concentrations. Vancomycin should be reserved for penicillin-allergic women at high risk for anaphylaxis.
(*From* Centers for Disease Control and Prevention. Prevention of perinatal Group B streptococcal disease. MMWR 2002;51(RR-11):10.)

to prevent a larger burden of disease, including GBS-associated spontaneous abortions and stillbirths, maternal bacteremias, and late-onset neonatal GBS disease. Phase I and II trials of candidates for capsular polysaccharide-protein conjugate GBS vaccines have been conducted in healthy, nonpregnant adults, and phase I safety and immunogenicity trials were conducted in pregnant women and yielded promising results [36–38]. Recent animal studies that explored a GBS vaccine that is based on a conserved surface protein which is expressed by all GBS serotypes found that it induced a strong systemic and mucosal antibody response in mice. This raises the hope that a protein vaccine that would be effective against all serotypes also may prevent maternal colonization with GBS and protect neonates against invasive disease [39]. One obstacle in proceeding to phase III licensure trials is that large trials are needed in the context of intrapartum prophylaxis; the use of immunologic correlates may be necessary. Liability concerns of researching a vaccine with an indication for use in pregnant women may pose the larger obstacle, and may be impeding progress toward phase III trials.

Toward prevention of non-group B streptococcal sepsis

Effectiveness of intrapartum agents

Theoretically, intrapartum chemoprophylaxis might be an effective strategy for preventing non-GBS sepsis, just as it has proven efficacious against GBS sepsis; however, there are few evaluations of effectiveness against the non-GBS end point. A multicenter case-control study of infants who had culture-confirmed early-onset neonatal sepsis found that receipt of intrapartum antibiotics had an efficacy of 63% against sepsis that was caused by non-GBS organisms when potential confounders, such as maternal fever, were controlled for; the efficacy of intrapartum prophylaxis against GBS sepsis in the same study was 85% [4]. The trends of incidence of non-GBS sepsis before and after widespread implementation of GBS prevention may shed light indirectly on the efficacy of intrapartum antibiotics against non-GBS sepsis. A multicenter population-based surveillance for early-onset neonatal sepsis in very low birth weight infants found significant declines in GBS sepsis incidence in the era of intrapartum prophylaxis and no overall change in non-GBS sepsis incidence. This suggested that if intrapartum prophylaxis has any efficacy against non-GBS sepsis, the impact is much smaller than that observed for GBS sepsis [7]; however, the population of very low birth weight infants makes up less than 2% of all births. Population-based non-GBS sepsis trends in the broader population might shed more light on the impact of intrapartum antibiotics but data are limited. Data from sentinel hospitals in Australia in the 1990s suggested decreasing trends of non-GBS sepsis [40]; population-based data in three U.S. states in the late 1990s suggested stable trends of non-GBS sepsis [5,41].

If intrapartum prophylaxis were pursued for non-GBS sepsis, adaptation of the current GBS prevention policy to this new outcome would require new evidence and decision making. Whether penicillin or ampicillin—the first-line agents for GBS prophylaxis—would be the appropriate prophylactic agents for non-GBS sepsis is debatable, particularly because the leading cause of non-GBS sepsis is *Escherichia coli*, an organism with increasing β-lactam resistance. The identification of candidates for chemoprophylaxis also would pose challenges. The current GBS prevention strategy that is based on late antenatal maternal colonization with GBS is unlikely to be the best strategy for non-GBS sepsis. A more intensive characterization of risk factors for non-GBS sepsis might be necessary if this avenue of prevention were pursued.

Effectiveness of intrapartum antibiotics in the context of preterm labor

Because maternal infections are implicated in preterm delivery, and infants who are born preterm are at increased risk for neonatal sepsis, several trials have attempted to evaluate whether antenatal and intrapartum antibiotic regimens can be used to prolong pregnancy latency in the context of threatened preterm delivery, and whether these antibiotic regimens can improve neonatal outcomes. A small multicenter, randomized trial of women who had pPROM remote from term—a group at elevated risk for non-GBS sepsis—evaluated the efficacy of a 2-day intravenous antimicrobial regimen (ampicillin plus erythromycin) followed by a 5-day oral course of amoxicillin and erythromycin in the prevention of non-GBS sepsis among GBS-negative women (GBS-positive women received intrapartum prophylaxis for GBS) [42]. In this trial, documented sepsis in the first 72 hours of life and pneumonia were reduced significantly in the group that received antibiotics. These results were influential in the U.S. obstetric community and led to pPROM management guidelines that recommended maternal antibiotics.

At the time of this trial, however, corticosteroids were not a standard of care; now that there is widespread use of corticosteroids for preterm infants, debate has focused on whether antibiotics confer any benefits beyond those that result from corticosteroids. Two recent large, multicenter, randomized trials in the United Kingdom attempted to resolve controversies by evaluating three different oral antibiotic regimens and a placebo group with sufficient power to evaluate separately a population of women who had preterm, prelabor rupture of fetal membranes, and one with spontaneous preterm labor in the era of corticosteroids [43,44]. The trials had a composite neonatal outcome measure as the primary end point. Neither trial found a significant benefit of any of the antibiotic regimens on the composite neonatal outcome. Positive blood culture indicative of clinical neonatal infections was one of several secondary end points that were evaluated. Regarding pPROM, the group that received erythromycin alone had a significantly lower rate of positive blood culture (5.7% versus 8%); this benefit was not evident in the group that received erythromycin plus co-amoxiclav or co-amoxiclav alone. For spontaneous preterm labor, no protective effect of oral antibiotic regimens against neonatal positive blood culture was observed. Additionally, in both groups there was no overall significant benefit of antibiotics for the primary composite neonatal end point or prolongation of pregnancy, and an elevated risk of neonatal necrotizing enterocolitis was observed in the co-amoxiclav groups. Thus, well-designed large trials do not suggest clear efficacy of antibiotics against neonatal sepsis in the context of threatened preterm delivery. Current clinical opinion favors focusing on aggressive intravenous antibiotic regimens combined with oral regimens for pPROM remote from term (<32 weeks' gestation) [45].

Vaginal antisepsis

A pathogen-specific approach to non-GBS sepsis prevention, such as a targeted vaccine, poses challenges because a wide array of bacterial pathogens can cause sepsis, and often, leading causes of non-GBS sepsis are not well-documented. Broad-spectrum antimicrobials might overcome this limitation, but emerging resistance may threaten any sustained impact that these agents achieve. One intervention that has appeal in this regard is disinfection of the birth canal during labor or the newborn at birth with topical microbicide with broad antimicrobial activity. In vitro studies showed strong activity of some microbicides against GBS and other gram-positive and gram-negative sepsis-causing pathogens. Several clinical trials that evaluated the disinfectant chlorhexidine suggested that application to the birth canal during labor or wiping of the newborn at birth can protect newborns from colonization with GBS and other sepsis pathogens and reduce newborn disease [46–48] A trial at a large hospital in Malawi found significant reductions in neonatal morbidity and mortality and maternal postpartum infections in the chlorhexidine arm of the trial [46]. There was no microbiologic component to this trial so the leading sepsis-causing pathogens are unknown and the generalizability to other populations remains uncertain. Other studies found no beneficial effects of chlorhexidine [49]. Trials have used different methodologies that prevent direct comparisons and, without a pivotal trial, the efficacy against neonatal sepsis remains debatable. Although this intervention holds the most promise for developing countries where intravenous intrapartum antibiotics often are not affordable or feasible, it also is of renewed interest in some developed countries as a mode of GBS prevention to retard emerging infections with ampicillin-resistant *E coli* [50].

Unintended consequences of intrapartum prophylaxis

A particular concern with current strategies for neonatal sepsis prevention is their reliance on the provision of intrapartum antimicrobial agents to large numbers of women. Approximately 25% to 30% of deliveries receive intrapartum antimicrobial agents, either for GBS prophylaxis or other indications [17,51]. Unintended consequences of widespread antibiotics are being monitored in some populations.

The development of resistance among GBS has been limited to certain clinically relevant agents (ie, macrolides and clindamycin). No penicillin resistance has occurred despite testing of thousands of GBS isolates from sterile sites and colonization surveys. Resistance to erythromycin occurs in up to 25% of invasive or colonization strains, and a slightly lower proportion (up to 15%) of clinical isolates are clindamycin resistant [52–54]. Because the prevalence of resistance to these agents seemed to increase during the 1990s, GBS prevention guidelines that were issued in 2002 recommended an alternate approach to prophylaxis for women with penicillin allergy. Those without life-threatening allergies who are GBS colonized should receive cefazolin, whereas those who are at high risk for anaphylaxis ideally should have GBS screening performed with susceptibility testing if GBS is isolated. If the GBS strain is not susceptible to clindamycin and erythromycin, the colonized woman who has a penicillin allergy should receive vancomycin. The clinical efficacy of agents other than penicillin or ampicillin is not known, and the CDC plans to monitor adherence to the new recommendations in selected populations.

Emergence of antimicrobial resistance in other perinatal pathogens also is a concern in the context of increasing GBS prophylaxis. To date, the incidence of ampicillin resistance among *E coli* populations seems to be increasing. This is evident in *E coli* detected from patients who had community-acquired urinary tract infections and among nosocomial infections, and not simply among neonatal sepsis infections. The role of intrapartum prophylaxis in these general trends is not clear. In terms of neonatal disease, the prevalence of ampicillin-resistant *E coli* infections seems to have increased among cases of sepsis that occur in preterm infants, but not among infections in term infants [6,10]. The benefit-to-risk ratio for the use of antimicrobial prophylaxis in the case of preterm delivery still seems to be favorable, but requires continued monitoring.

In addition to the potential for changes in the proportion of sepsis cases that is caused by drug-resistant pathogens, increased use of prophylactic antibiotics may lead to changes in the general ecology of neonatal sepsis (ie, the ecological niche previously occupied by GBS might be filled by other organisms). If sepsis that is caused by gram-negative pathogens increases in the wake of GBS declines, the net effect might be to replace treatable infections with infections that are more virulent and frequently fatal. There is no evidence that gram-negative organisms are causing sepsis increasingly in the general newborn population. Although the incidence of *E coli* sepsis increased among very low birth weight infants in one report (from 3.2 to 6.8 cases per 1000 births), the occurrence of other gram-negative sepsis declined in the same report (from 5.1 to 2.6 per 1000 births) [7]. A thorough review of this issue was published recently [10]. A more recent report failed to find an association between GBS maternal prophylaxis and any increased risk of non-GBS infection [55].

Future priorities

Although reductions in neonatal sepsis that are attributable to prenatal screening for GBS and the use of intrapartum antimicrobial prophylaxis represent a major perinatal success story, infections remain a major contributor to perinatal morbidity. The greatest impact on the remaining burden of neonatal bacterial infections in industrialized countries would be achieved through strategies that can reduce preterm delivery. Research in this area is a critical priority, but is likely to be slow to bear fruit in terms of broad implementation.

The large-scale use of intrapartum antimicrobial prophylaxis requires continued assessment, because the emergence of resistance in GBS or other organisms eventually might shift the benefit-to-risk ratio that is associated with the strategy. In this context, continued prevention studies of other modalities, including vaccines and vaginal antisepsis, are important priorities that could yield results in the midrange timeline, or potentially sooner than breakthroughs in the prevention of prematurity.

While research on these newer approaches to prevention continues, public health and clinical researchers should continue to carry out surveillance of the incidence, causes, and health service burden that are associated with neonatal sepsis. Detecting important trends in the occurrence of gram-negative infections or drug resistance among GBS or other gram-positive pathogens will be important sentinels to the need for revision in prophylaxis recommendations. Tracking adherence to the 2002 guidelines can help to direct future educational programs and determine whether overuse of intrapartum prophylaxis is occurring. In particular, the recent guidelines that suggested the use of vancomycin in certain limited circumstances require follow-up to assure that excessive use is not occurring.

Beyond the setting of industrialized countries, the burden of neonatal sepsis in developing countries represents a major challenge and opportunity. A concerted effort should be made to measure disease burden, identify etiologies and risk factors for neonatal sepsis or death, and explore promising interventions for applicability to the complex circumstances of childbirth in developing countries. The Safe Motherhood Initiative promoted by the World Health Organization and other partners raises awareness of the need for clean deliveries with skilled birth attendants. Identifying simple, low-cost, and sustainable strategies for the prevention and improvement of early treatment of neonatal sepsis is a global concern.

References

[1] Black R, Morris S, Boyce J. Where and why are 10 million children dying every year? Lancet 2003;361:2226–34.

[2] Stoll B. Neonatal infections: a global perspective. In: Remington J, Klein J, editors. Infectious diseases of the fetus and newborn infant. 5th edition. Philadelphia: W.B. Saunders; 2001. p. 139–68.

[3] Freedman R, Ingram D, Gross I, et al. A half century of neonatal sepsis at Yale, 1928 to 1978. Am J Dis Child 1981;135:140–4.
[4] Schuchat A, Zywicki SS, Dinsmoor MJ, et al. Risk factors and opportunities for prevention of early-onset neonatal sepsis: a multicenter case-control study. Pediatrics 2000;105(1):21–6.
[5] Baltimore RS, Huie SM, Meek JI, et al. Early-onset neonatal sepsis in the era of group B streptococcal prevention. Pediatrics 2001;108(5):1094–8.
[6] Hyde TB, Hilger TM, Reingold A, et al. Trends in incidence and antimicrobial resistance of early-onset sepsis: population-based surveillance in San Francisco and Atlanta. Pediatrics 2002;110(4):690–5.
[7] Stoll BJ, Hansen N, Fanaroff AA, et al. Changes in pathogens causing early-onset sepsis in very-low-birthweight infants. N Engl J Med 2002;347:240–7.
[8] Schrag SJ, Zywicki S, Farley MM, et al. Group B streptococcal disease in the era of intrapartum antibiotic prophylaxis. N Engl J Med 2000;342:15–20.
[9] Centers for Disease Control and Prevention. Diminishing racial disparities in early-onset neonatal group B streptococcal disease - United States, 2000–2003. MMWR 2004;53(23): 502–5.
[10] Moore MR, Schrag SJ, Schuchat A. Effects of intrapartum antimicrobial prophylaxis for prevention of group-B-streptococcal disease on the incidence and ecology of early-onset neonatal sepsis. Lancet Infect Dis 2003;3(4):201–13.
[11] Lukacs S, Schoendorf K, Schuchat A. Trends in sepsis-related neonatal mortality in the United States, 1985–98. Pediatr Inf Dis J 2004;23:599–603.
[12] Lukacs S, Schuchat A, Schoendorf KC. National estimates of newborn sepsis: United States, 1990–2002. Presented at the Society for Pediatric and Perinatal Epidemiologic Research. Salt Lake City, June 14–15, 2004.
[13] Schuchat A, Deaver-Robinson K, Plikaytis BD, et al. Multistate case-control study of maternal risk factors for neonatal group B streptococcal disease. Pediatr Inf Dis J 1994;13:623–9.
[14] Schuchat A, Wenger JD. Epidemiology of group B streptococcal disease: risk factors, prevention strategies, vaccine development. Epidemiol Rev 1994;16(2):374–402.
[15] Boyer KM, Gadzala CA, Burd LI, et al. Selective intrapartum chemoprophylaxis of neonatal group B streptococcal early-onset disease. I. Epidemiologic rationale. J Infect Dis 1983; 148:795–801.
[16] Yancey M, Duff P, Kubilis P, et al. Risk factors for neonatal sepsis. Obstet Gynecol 1996; 87:188–94.
[17] Schrag SJ, Zell ER, Lynfield R, et al. A population-based comparison of strategies to prevent early-onset group B streptococcal disease in neonates. N Engl J Med 2002;347:233–9.
[18] Schuchat A, Oxtoby M, Cochi S, et al. Population-based risk factors for neonatal group B streptococcal disease: results of a cohort study in metropolitan Atlanta. J Infect Dis 1990; 162:672–7.
[19] Martius J, Roos T, Gora B, et al. Risk factors associated with early-onset sepsis in premature infants. Eur J Obstet Gynecol Reprod Biol 1999;85:151–8.
[20] Boyer KM, Gotoff SP. Prevention of early-onset neonatal group B streptococcal disease with selective intrapartum chemoprophylaxis. N Engl J Med 1986;314(26):1665–9.
[21] Tuppurainen N, Hallman M. Prevention of neonatal group B streptococcal disease: intrapartum detection and chemoprophylaxis of heavily colonized parturients. Obstet Gynecol 1989;73: 583–7.
[22] Matorras R, Garcia-Perea A, Omenaca F, et al. Intrapartum chemoprophylaxis of early-onset group B streptococcal disease. Eur J Obstet Gynecol Reprod Biol 1991;40:57–62.
[23] Garland SM, Fliegner JR. Group B streptococcus (GBS) and neonatal infections: the case for intrapartum chemoprophylaxis. Aust NZ J Obstet Gynecol 1991;31(2):119–22.
[24] Rouse DJ, Goldenberg RL, Cliver SP, et al. Strategies for the prevention of early-onset neonatal group B streptococcal sepsis: a decision analysis. Obstet Gynecol 1994;83:483–94.
[25] Mohle-Boetani JC, Schuchat A, Plikaytis BD, et al. Comparison of prevention strategies for neonatal group B streptococcal infection: a population-based economic approach. JAMA 1993;270(12):1442–8.

[26] Mohle-Boetani JC, Lieu TA, Ray GT, et al. Preventing neonatal group B streptococcal disease: cost-effectiveness in a health maintenance organization and the impact of delayed hospital discharge for newborns who received intrapartum antibiotics. Pediatrics 1999;103(4):703–10.
[27] Centers for Disease Control and Prevention. Prevention of perinatal group B streptococcal disease: a public health perspective. MMWR Morb Mortal Wkly Rep 1996;45(RR-7):1–24.
[28] Centers for Disease Control and Prevention. Early-onset group B streptococcal disease, United States, 1998–1999. MMWR Morb Mortal Wkly Rep 2000;49(35):793–6.
[29] Centers for Disease Control and Prevention. Prevention of perinatal group B streptococcal disease: Revised guidelines from CDC. MMWR Morb Mortal Wkly Rep 2002;51(RR-11):1–22.
[30] Committee on Obstetric Practice American College of Obstetricians and Gynecologists. Prevention of early-onset group B streptococcal disease in newborns. Washington, DC: American College of Obstetricians and Gynecologists; 2002.
[31] Siegel JD, McCracken GHJ, Threlkeld N, et al. Single dose penicillin prophylaxis against neonatal group B streptococcal infections: a controlled trial in 18,738 newborn infants. N Engl J Med 1980;303:769–75.
[32] Siegel JD, McCracken GHJ, Threlkeld N, et al. Single-dose penicillin prophylaxis of neonatal group B streptococcal disease. Lancet 1982;i:1426–30.
[33] Pyati SP, Pildes RS, Jacobs NM, et al. Penicillin in infants weighing two kilograms or less with early-onset group B streptococcal disease. N Engl J Med 1983;308:1383–9.
[34] Patel D, Rhodes P, LeBlanc M, et al. Role of postnatal penicillin prophylaxis in prevention of neonatal group B streptococcus infection. Acta Paediatr 1999;88:874–9.
[35] Wendel GD, Leveno KJ, Sanchez PJ, et al. Prevention of neonatal group B streptococcal disease: a combined intrapartum and neonatal protocol. Am J Obstet Gynecol 2002;186(4):618–26.
[36] Kasper DL, Paoletti LC, Wessels MR, et al. Immune response to type III group B streptococcal polysaccharide-tetanus toxoid conjugate vaccine. J Clin Invest 1996;98:2308–14.
[37] Baker C, Rench M, McInnes P. Immunization of pregnant women with group B streptococcal type III capsular polysaccharide-tetanus toxoid conjugate vaccine. Vaccine 2003;21:3468–72.
[38] Baker CJ, Edwards MS. Group B streptococcal conjugate vaccines. Arch Dis Child 2003;88(5):375–8.
[39] Hunter SK, Andracki M. Univalent GBS vaccine utilizing C5A peptidase encapsulated within biodegradable polymeric microspheres. Presented at the Infectious Diseases Society of Obstetricians and Gynecologists. San Diego, August 5–7, 2004.
[40] Isaacs D, Royle JA. Intrapartum antibiotics and early onset neonatal sepsis caused by group B streptococcus and by other organisms in Australia. Pediatr Inf Dis J 1999;18:524–8.
[41] Hyde TB, Hilger TM, Reingold A, et al. Trends in the incidence and antimicrobial resistance of early-onset sepsis: population-based surveillance in San Francisco and Atlanta. Pediatrics 2002;110(4):690–5.
[42] Mercer BM, Miodovnik M, Thurnau G, et al. Antibiotic therapy for reduction of infant morbidity after preterm premature rupture of the membranes: a randomized controlled trial. JAMA 1997;278(12):989–95.
[43] Kenyon SL, Taylor DJ, Tarnow-Mordi W. ORACLE Collaborative Group: broad-spectrum antibiotics for preterm, prelabour rupture of fetal membranes: the ORACLE I randomised trial. Lancet 2001;357:979–88.
[44] Kenyon SL, Taylor DJ, Tarnow-Mordi W. ORACLE Collaborative Group: broad-spectrum antibiotics for spontaneous preterm labour: the ORACLE II randomised trial. Lancet 2001;357(9261):989–94.
[45] Mercer B, Goldenberg R, Das A, et al. What we have learned regarding antibiotic therapy for the reduction of infant morbidity after preterm premature rupture of the membranes. Semin Perinatol 2003;27(3):217–30.
[46] Taha TE, Biggar RJ, Broadhead RL, et al. Effect of cleansing the birth canal with antiseptic solution on maternal and newborn morbidity in Malawi: clinical trial. BMJ 1997;315:216–20.
[47] Stray-Pedersen B, Bergan T, Hafstad A, et al. Vaginal disinfection with chlorhexidine during childbirth. Int J Antimicrob Agents 1999;12(3):245–51.
[48] Burman LG, Christensen P, Christensen K, et al. Prevention of excess neonatal morbidity

associated with group B streptococci by vaginal chlorhexidine disinfection during labour. Lancet 1992;340:65–9.

[49] Rouse DJ, Hauth JC, Andrews WW, et al. Chlorhexidine vaginal irrigation for the prevention of peripartal infection: a placebo-controlled randomized clinical trial. Am J Obstet Gynecol 1997; 176:617–22.

[50] Facchinetti F, Piccinini F, Mordini B, et al. Chlorhexidine vaginal flushings versus systemic ampicillin in the prevention of vertical transmission of neonatal group B streptococcus, at term. J Matern Fetal Neonatal Med 2002;11:84–8.

[51] Davis RL, Hasselquist MB, Cardenas V, et al. Introduction of the new Centers for Disease Control and Prevention group B streptococcal prevention guideline at a large West Coast health maintenance organization. Am J Obstet Gynecol 2001;184(4):603–10.

[52] Andrews JJ, Diekema DJ, Hunter SK, et al. Group B streptococci causing neonatal bloodstream infection: antimicrobial susceptibility and serotyping results from SENTRY centers in the Western hemisphere. Am J Obstet Gynecol 2000;183:859–62.

[53] Fernandez M, Hickman ME, Baker CJ. Antimicrobial susceptibilities of group B streptococci isolated between 1992 and 1996 from patients with bacteremia or meningitis. Antimicrob Agents Chemother 1998;42:1517–9.

[54] Heelan J, Hasenbein M, McAdam A. Resistance of group B streptococcus to selected antibiotics, including erythromycin and clindamycin. J Clin Microbiol 2004;42:1263–4.

[55] Sinha A, Yokoe D, Platt R. Intrapartum antibiotics and neonatal invasive infections caused by organisms other than group B streptococcus. J Pediatr 2003;142(5):492–7.

ELSEVIER
SAUNDERS

Clin Perinatol 32 (2005) 617–627

CLINICS IN
PERINATOLOGY

Bacterial Vaginosis in Pregnancy: Diagnosis, Screening, and Management

Mark H. Yudin, MD, MSc

Department of Obstetrics and Gynecology, St. Michael's Hospital, University of Toronto, 15 Cardinal Carter Wing, 30 Bond Street, Toronto, ON M5B 1W8, Canada

Bacterial vaginosis is the most common lower genital tract infection among women of reproductive age, and the most common cause of vaginitis in both pregnant and nonpregnant women [1]. It is estimated that over 3 million symptomatic cases occur annually in the United States [2], and it is the most prevalent cause of vaginal discharge and malodor. Historically, this infection was regarded as a bothersome, but not very serious problem. More recently, however, it has been associated with a number of significant obstetric and gynecologic complications, such as preterm labor and delivery, preterm premature rupture of membranes, spontaneous abortion, chorioamnionitis, postpartum endometritis, postcesarean delivery wound infections, postsurgical infections, and subclinical pelvic inflammatory disease [3–11]. This review will focus on bacterial vaginosis in pregnancy, and will discuss approaches to diagnosis, screening, and management.

History and microbiology

Bacterial vaginosis was first recognized in the late nineteenth century. Descriptive microbiology for vaginal infections began in 1894, when Doderlein [12] described the presence of lactobacilli in normal vaginal flora. In 1914 Curtis [13] reported an association between abnormal anaerobic vaginal flora and vaginal discharge, and Gardner and Dukes [14] first described the organism *Gardnerella vaginalis* in 1955. The syndrome of bacterial vaginosis was initially referred to as nonspecific vaginitis, which was well-characterized in many

E-mail address: yudinm@smh.toronto.on.ca

0095-5108/05/$ – see front matter
doi:10.1016/j.clp.2005.05.007 *perinatology.theclinics.com*

studies [15]. Several changes in nomenclature occurred over the years. In 1984, the term bacterial vaginosis was proposed and became widely accepted.

The normal vaginal flora consists of both aerobic and anaerobic bacteria. The predominant microorganisms are *Lactobacillus spp*, accounting for greater than 95% of all bacteria present [16,17]. These organisms are believed to provide defense against infection by maintaining an acidic pH in the vagina. The lactobacilli of normal women tend to contain more hydrogen peroxide-producing species, which damage organisms lacking free radical scavengers such as many of the bacterial vaginosis-associated organisms, thereby inhibiting vaginal colonization by these organisms [17–19]. Both pregnant and nonpregnant women colonized with adequate numbers of hydrogen peroxide-producing lactobacilli have decreased acquisition of bacterial vaginosis compared with women not having these bacteria [20,21]. In contrast, bacterial vaginosis is a polymicrobial syndrome resulting in a decreased concentration of lactobacilli and an increase in pathogenic bacteria. These organisms include *G vaginalis*, *Mobiluncus spp*, *Bacteroides* and *Prevotella spp*, and *Mycoplasma spp* [18,22].

Prevalence and epidemiology

As already noted, bacterial vaginosis is very common. Studies have revealed that the prevalence varies widely depending on the patient population. In private offices, the prevalence has ranged from 4% to 17%, whereas in gynecology clinic populations, the prevalence has been higher, at 23% [23,24]. In college students, the prevalence has ranged from 4% to 25%, and it has been as high as 61% in women attending sexually transmitted disease clinics [15,16,25,26]. Studies of pregnant women have documented similar prevalence rates to those seen in nonpregnant populations, ranging from 6% to 32% [3,27–30].

Epidemiologic studies have identified several risk factors for the acquisition of bacterial vaginosis. It has been associated with racial origin, smoking, sexual activity, contraceptive practice, and vaginal douching. Bacterial vaginosis is more common in women of black race [31], women who smoke [32], women who are sexually active (although it has been isolated in virginal women as well) [33], and women who use vaginal douches [21].

Diagnosis

Bacterial vaginosis is a syndrome that can be diagnosed both clinically and microbiologically. In 1983, Amsel and colleagues [15] published a paper outlining clinical diagnostic criteria, and these are still in use today. The clinical diagnosis of bacterial vaginosis is made if three of the four following signs are present [15]:

1) An adherent and homogenous vaginal discharge
2) Vaginal pH greater than 4.5

3) Detection of clue cells (vaginal epithelial cells with such a heavy coating of bacteria that the peripheral borders are obscured) on saline wet mount
4) An amine odor after the addition of potassium hydroxide (positive whiff test)

Although these criteria are widely used, they have been criticized because of inherent difficulties with such a diagnostic scheme. With the exception of pH, the remainder of the criteria are either subjective (appearance of discharge, whiff test) or potentially technically difficult (appearance of clue cells in the saline wet mount examined by microscopy) [17,34,35].

Four laboratory methods have been used to diagnose bacterial vaginosis: (1) culture of vaginal fluid for *G vaginalis*, (2) biochemical tests for metabolic by-products of vaginal bacteria (gas-liquid chromatography), (3) assays for proline aminopeptidase, and (4) direct Gram's stain of vaginal secretions. *G vaginalis* is found in high concentrations in almost all women who have bacterial vaginosis, but is also often found in the vaginal flora of normal women [36]. Also, the isolation of any one specific organism on culture does not reliably predict bacterial vaginosis, so culture is not felt to be valuable in the diagnosis [15,25]. Chromatography equipment is not readily available in many laboratories. Therefore, Gram's stain of vaginal fluid is the most widely used and evaluated diagnostic method for bacterial vaginosis. To perform a Gram's stain, vaginal discharge is collected on a glass slide, allowed to air-dry, stained in the laboratory, and examined under oil immersion for the presence of bacteria. This diagnostic method has several advantages, including a permanent record, a high frequency of interpretable results, low cost, and ease of transport and storage [35].

Over the past 2 decades, there have been two main Gram's stain diagnostic schemes used for the evaluation of vaginal infections. In 1983, Spiegel and colleagues [37] published a paper describing an objective way to diagnose bacterial vaginosis by Gram's stain. Bacterial vaginosis was present by the Spiegel criteria if *Lactobacillus* morphotypes were fewer than five per oil immersion field, and if there were five or more other morphotypes (gram-positive cocci, small gram-negative rods, curved gram-variable rods, or fusiforms) per oil immersion field. If five or more lactobacilli and fewer than five other morphotypes were present per oil immersion field, the Gram's stain was considered to be normal. Although used for many years, the Spiegel system was criticized because there was no

Table 1
Scoring system (0 to 10) for Gram-stained vaginal smears

Score	*Lactobacillus* morphotypes	*Gardnerella* and *Bacteroides spp* morphotypes	Curved gram-variable rods
0	4+	0	0
1	3+	1+	1+ or 2+
2	2+	2+	3+ or 4+
3	1+	3+	
4	0	4+	

account for the spectrum of severity [38]. In 1991, Nugent and colleagues [38] addressed this problem and developed a scoring system. This system is presented in Table 1. Each morphotype on the stain is quantitated from 1+ to 4+ with regard to the number of morphotypes per oil immersion field, and a corresponding score is assigned. The scoring system allows for gradations in severity. The criterion for bacterial vaginosis is a score of 7 or higher. A score of 4 to 6 is considered intermediate, and a score of 0 to 3 is considered normal.

Although there can be great variability in intraobserver and interobserver interpretation of Gram's-stained specimens from other body sites [39], the reliability and validity of using the Gram's stain for the diagnosis of bacterial vaginosis have been well documented. Spiegel and coworkers [37] demonstrated high intraobserver reliability for 20 specimens examined by three separate microbiologists, and Nugent and colleagues [38] showed high intercenter and intracenter reliability for 250 vaginal Gram's stains of pregnant women. In this study, the Nugent scoring system had a higher intercenter reliability using Spearman rank correlation coefficients than the Spiegel criteria ($r=0.82$ versus $r=0.61$), and it is largely due to these results that the scoring system is more widely used. Finally, Mazulli and coworkers [40] had three different microbiologists examine a total of 240 slides: 80 original slides, 80 duplicate slides of the same specimen, and the 80 original slides again, in a blinded fashion. Intraobserver and interobserver reproducibility was high, as assessed by the weighted kappa statistic for the interpretation of lactobacilli (kappa range 0.755–0.937), *G vaginalis* (kappa range 0.730–0.955), clue cells (kappa range 0.701–0.953), and bacterial vaginosis (kappa range 0.750–1.000) [40].

Validity studies examining the Gram's stain have also been encouraging. Krohn and colleagues [35] compared the sensitivity, specificity, and positive and negative predictive values of Gram's stain, culture, and gas-liquid chromatography with clinical signs of bacterial vaginosis in 593 pregnant women. They found that an elevated pH, clue cells, and amine odor were all independently related to bacterial vaginosis diagnosed by Gram's stain. Gram's stain had a moderate sensitivity (62%) and positive predictive value (76%), but excellent specificity (95%) and negative predictive value (92%). Similarly, Schwebke and coworkers [34] found a significant correlation between Gram's stain scores (by the Nugent scoring system) and clinical signs of bacterial vaginosis in 617 women.

Screening and management

Bacterial vaginosis has consistently been shown to be a risk factor for adverse obstetric outcomes such as preterm labor and delivery, preterm premature rupture of membranes, spontaneous abortion, chorioamnionitis, and postpartum infections such as endometritis and cesarean section wound infections [3–8]. Despite these associations, it is still not clear whether screening for and treatment of bacterial vaginosis in pregnancy can reliably reduce the incidence of these complications. Further, for clinicians who elect to screen pregnant women, the optimal time to screen, screening test to use, and treatment to administer are all uncertain. The United States Preventive Services Task Force (USPSTF) published a statement in 2001 [41] concluding that the available evidence was insufficient to recommend for or against routinely screening women at high risk for preterm birth for bacterial vaginosis, and recommending against screening average-risk asymptomatic pregnant women. If one chooses to treat this syndrome in pregnancy, the 2002 Centers for Disease Control and Prevention sexually transmitted diseases treatment guidelines [42] recommends using either metronidazole 250 mg orally three times daily for 7 days or clindamycin 300 mg orally twice a day for 7 days. There is no evidence that metronidazole is teratogenic or mutagenic, and it is considered safe for use in pregnancy [43,44]. Topical agents are not recommended.

There have been many trials over the past 2 decades exploring the treatment of bacterial vaginosis in pregnant women. These trials have evaluated the efficacy of various treatment regimens in achieving and maintaining cure. Oral and vaginal metronidazole and clindamycin have been used in various treatment trials. The studies have also investigated whether the treatment of abnormal vaginal flora can reduce the incidence of prematurity and the other bacterial vaginosis-associated adverse pregnancy outcomes. The varying results of these trials can be difficult to interpret, and the aim of this section is to summarize and consolidate this body of literature for the reader.

Cure rates following treatment

Definitions of cure vary widely among published trials on treatment of bacterial vaginosis, which may account for variation in reported treatment efficacy rates. As well, studies of the natural history of this syndrome have shown that it gradually recurs with longer follow-up in pregnant and nonpregnant women, and rates of cure depend on the timing of follow-up evaluations [23,29,33,45,46].

In oral treatment trials, cure rates have consistently been greater than 70%. Several trials have used oral metronidazole. Hauth and colleagues [46] demonstrated resolution of bacterial vaginosis (defined as less than three of four clinical signs and normal flora on Gram's stain) in 70% of women 2 to 4 weeks after treatment with oral metronidazole and erythromycin; McDonald and coworkers [47] showed cure rates (by Gram's stain or culture of *G* vaginalis) of 76% 4 weeks following two 2-day courses of metronidazole 400 mg twice daily; Carey and colleagues [48] reported normalization of vaginal flora on Gram's stain in 78% of women after two 2 gram doses of oral metronidazole; and Klebanoff and coworkers[49] found cure (defined as a Nugent score of <7 on Gram's stain) in 78% of patients following two 2-gram doses of oral metronidazole. In studies employing oral clindamycin, McGregor and colleagues [50] published cure rates of 92.5% 2 to 4 weeks after treatment, and a recent study completed by Ugwumadu and coworkers [51] using oral clindamycin 300 mg taken twice daily for 5 days resulted in cure rates (defined as a Gram's stain Nugent score of 0 to 3) of 90%.

In addition to oral treatment trials, there have been many studies using vaginal preparations, most commonly clindamycin cream, with cure rates ranging from 33% to 86%. In randomized controlled trials of clindamycin cream versus placebo, Joesef and coworkers [52] demonstrated a cure rate (defined as a Nugent Gram's stain score of less than 7 with a normal pH) of 85.5% 2 weeks after treatment in 340 pregnant women; Kekki and colleagues [53] reported normalization of vaginal flora (defined by Spiegel criteria) in 66% of 187 patients 1 week following treatment; Kurkinen and coworkers [54] found cure rates (on Gram's stain) of 33% in 51 women 2 weeks after treatment; and Lamont and colleagues [55] demonstrated a range of cure rates (71% to 78%) using several different criteria for cure in over 200 pregnant women 3 and 6 weeks post-treatment. A study by McGregor and coworkers [45] clearly showed that cure depends on the timing of follow-up, with rates of 90% at 1 week and 60% to 70% at 4 weeks post-treatment.

There are very few studies including both oral and vaginal treatment. In a study by Yudin and colleagues [56], pregnant women who had bacterial vaginosis were randomized to receive either oral metronidazole for 7 days or vaginal metronidazole gel for 5 days. Cure rates were defined in three ways: (1) microbiologic cure—Gram's stain score of 0 to 3, (2) clinical cure—absence of all four clinical signs, and (3) therapeutic cure—combination of both microbiologic and clinical cure. The results demonstrated that at 4 weeks after treatment, cure rates were greater than 70% for any of the three criteria, and were equivalent for oral and vaginal therapy.

Effects of treatment on adverse obstetric outcomes

There have been many trials designed to determine whether treatment of bacterial vaginosis in pregnancy can impact on the frequency with which adverse outcomes, especially premature delivery, are encountered. Despite the consistent association between bacterial vaginosis and preterm birth, the results of these treatment trials have not been consistent. The reason for this lack of clarity in the literature may be that studies have used mixed populations (women at both low and high risk for preterm birth) and different treatment modalities (systemic and local therapy).

In trials enrolling women from the general population who are at average risk for preterm birth, there does not seem to be any benefit to screening for and treating bacterial vaginosis. Studies involving this category of women have used both oral and vaginal treatment regimens. McGregor and colleagues [45] randomized women who had bacterial vaginosis from 16 to 27 weeks' gestation to receive intravaginal clindamycin or placebo. There were no significant differences in adverse outcomes such as preterm birth, preterm labor, or low birthweight between the two groups, despite adequate treatment and eradication of bacterial vaginosis. Similarly, Joesef and coworkers [52] found no difference in preterm delivery rates between women who had bacterial vaginosis at 14 to 26 weeks' randomized to topical clindamycin or placebo. A study from Finland

[54] found no difference in rates of preterm birth or puerperal infections among women enrolled at 12 weeks' gestation and receiving vaginal clindamycin versus placebo; and an Italian group [57] reported no difference in the frequencies of preterm delivery, low birthweight, or gestational age at birth in women enrolled between 14 and 25 weeks' gestation and randomized to topical clindamycin or placebo. Oral treatment trials in women at low risk for preterm birth have had similar results. In two large trials, McDonald and colleagues [47] found no difference in preterm delivery rates in 879 women randomized to oral metronidazole or placebo at 24 and 29 weeks' gestation; and Carey and coworkers [48] reported no differences in rates of preterm birth, low birthweight, or preterm premature rupture of membranes among 1953 pregnant women randomized to oral metronidazole or placebo from 8 to 22 weeks' gestation.

Although trials of women at low risk for preterm birth have failed to show a benefit in treating bacterial vaginosis in pregnancy, studies enrolling women who are at higher risk for premature delivery have had more promising results. Morales and colleagues [58] enrolled 80 women at 13 to 20 weeks' gestation with bacterial vaginosis and a history of preterm delivery, and randomized them to oral metronidazole or placebo. Women in the treatment group had a significantly decreased incidence of hospital admissions for preterm labor, premature births, infants who had low birthweights, and preterm premature rupture of membranes compared with those in the placebo group. Hauth and coworkers [46] showed that women who had bacterial vaginosis and either a history of preterm birth or low prepregnancy weight that were treated with oral metronidazole and erythromycin had a lower incidence of preterm birth than those receiving placebo. In the trials by McDonald and colleagues [47] and Carey and coworkers [48] described above, two groups of women were enrolled: those at average risk for preterm birth, and those deemed to be at higher risk because of a history of premature delivery in the past. As already noted, women at low risk did not benefit from treatment; however, in the study by McDonald and colleagues [47], the subgroup of women who had a history of preterm delivery that was randomized to oral metronidazole had an approximate 50% reduction in premature birth. In the trial by Carey and colleagues [48], there was no benefit of treatment for either the low-risk or high-risk population of women. In a Cochrane Collaboration review of ten treatment trials involving 4249 women [59], there was a statistically significant decrease in the rate of preterm premature rupture of membranes and low birthweight in treated women who had a history of previous preterm birth, but no effect on preterm delivery rates.

When evaluating treatment trials of bacterial vaginosis in pregnancy, in addition to stratifying patients by risk factors for prematurity, one must also consider the route of treatment. The body of evidence quite consistently shows that vaginal treatment regimens are ineffective in preventing preterm birth, even though they are efficacious in eradicating bacterial vaginosis [45,52–54,57,60]. The one published exception to this is a recent trial by Lamont and coworkers [61] showing a statistically significant reduction in preterm birth (4% versus 10%) in women randomized to clindamycin vaginal cream at 13 to 20 weeks' gestation compared with placebo. As noted above, some oral treatment trials have been successful in showing a decreased rate of prematurity in women treated for bacterial vaginosis, but only in those who had a previous history of a preterm birth [46,47,58,59]. A recent meta-analysis by Leitich and coworkers [62] attempted to further explore the issue of oral or vaginal treatment in low-risk versus high-risk women. In this analysis, there was no significant reduction in preterm delivery by treatment of all women, women who had a previous preterm birth, or women at low risk for prematurity; however, in the subgroup of women who had both a previous preterm delivery and received oral treatment for at least 7 days, there was a highly significant decrease in preterm delivery (odds ratio, 0.42; 95% CI 0.27, 0.67). There was no benefit seen in the group of women receiving vaginal treatment. Similarly, in the Cochrane review [59], there was no effect of vaginal antibiotics on any measure of preterm birth. It is still unclear why topical therapy might not be as effective as systemic treatment for the prevention of preterm birth, although some authors have hypothesized that systemic therapy might be required to fully eradicate bacterial vaginosis-associated organisms from both the lower and the upper genital tract, thereby preventing preterm labor and delivery [45,53].

Summary

Bacterial vaginosis is the most common lower genital tract infection among women of reproductive age, and has been associated with a number of significant obstetric and gynecologic complications. Treatment regimens recommended by the Centers for Disease Control and Prevention in pregnant women include metronidazole 250 mg orally three times daily for 7 days or clindamycin 300 mg orally twice a day for 7 days. Cure rates vary in published studies, and this syndrome tends to recur after treatment in both pregnant and nonpregnant women. There is currently no consensus as to whether to screen for and treat bacterial vaginosis in pregnancy. Treatment has not been shown to decrease adverse obstetric outcomes in the general population at low risk for prematurity, although oral treatment for at least 7 days may be effective in decreasing preterm birth rates in women who have a history of a prior preterm delivery. Further study is required in order to advance our knowledge and understanding of the effects of this syndrome in pregnant women, and to make definite conclusions regarding the role of treatment in pregnancy.

References

[1] Rein MF, Holmes KK. Non-specific vaginitis, vulvovaginal candidiasis, and trichomoniasis: clinical features, diagnosis and management. Curr Clin Top Infect Dis 1983;4:281–315.
[2] Fleury FJ. Adult vaginitis. Clin Obstet Gynecol 1987;24:407–38.
[3] Hillier SL, Nugent RP, Eschenbach DA, et al for the Vaginal Infections and Prematurity Study

Group. Association between bacterial vaginosis and preterm delivery of a low-birth-weight infant. N Engl J Med 1995;333:1737–42.
[4] Gravett MG, Hammel D, Eschenbach DA, et al. Preterm labor associated with subclinical amniotic fluid infection and with bacterial vaginosis. Obstet Gynecol 1986;67:229–37.
[5] Minkoff H, Brunebaum AN, Schwartz RH, et al. Risk factors for prematurity and premature rupture of membranes: a prospective study of the vaginal flora in pregnancy. Am J Obstet Gynecol 1984;150:965–72.
[6] Leitich H, Bodner-Adler B, Brunbauer M, et al. Bacterial vaginosis as a risk factor for preterm delivery: a meta-analysis. Am J Obstet Gynecol 2003;189:139–47.
[7] Hillier SL, Martius J, Krohn MA, et al. A case-control study of chorioamnionic infection and histologic chorioamnionitis in prematurity. N Engl J Med 1988;319:972–8.
[8] Watts DH, Krohn MA, Hillier SL, et al. Bacterial vaginosis as a risk factor for postcesarean endometritis. Obstet Gynecol 1990;75:52–8.
[9] Soper DE, Bump RC, Hunt WG. Bacterial vaginosis and *Trichomonas* vaginitis are risk factors for cuff cellulites after abdominal hysterectomy. Am J Obstet Gynecol 1990;163:1016–23.
[10] Korn AP, Bolan G, Padian N, et al. Plasma cell endometritis in women with symptomatic bacterial vaginosis. Obstet Gynecol 1995;85:387–90.
[11] Wiesenfeld HC, Hillier SL, Krohn MA, et al. Lower genital tract infection and endometritis: insight into subclinical pelvic inflammatory disease. Obstet Gynecol 2002;100:456–63.
[12] Doderlein A. Die scheidensekretuntersuchugen. Zentralb Gynakol 1894;18:10–4 [German].
[13] Curtis AH. On the etiology and bacteriology of leucorrhoea. Surg Gynecol Obstet 1914;18: 299–306.
[14] Gardner HL, Kukes CD. *Haemophilus vaginalis* vaginitis: a newly defined specific infection previously classified "non-specific vaginitis". Am J Obstet Gynecol 1955;69:962–76.
[15] Amsel R, Totten PA, Spiegel CA, et al. Nonspecific vaginitis: diagnostic criteria and microbial and epidemiologic associations. Am J Med 1983;74:14–22.
[16] Spiegel CA, Amsel R, Eschenbach D, et al. Anaerobic bacteria in nonspecific vaginitis. N Engl J Med 1980;303:601–7.
[17] Eschenbach DA. Bacterial vaginosis: emphasis on upper genital tract complications. Obstet Gynecol Clin North Am 1989;16:593–610.
[18] Hill GB, Eschenbach DA, Holmes KK. Bacteriology of the vagina. Scand J Urol Nephrol Suppl 1985;86:23–39.
[19] Eschenbach DA, Davick PR, Williams BL, et al. Prevalence of hydrogen peroxide-producing *Lactobacillus* species in normal women and women with bacterial vaginosis. J Clin Microbiol 1989;27:251–6.
[20] Hillier SL, Krohn MA, Rabe LK, et al. The normal vaginal flora, H_2O_2-producing lactobacilli, and bacterial vaginosis in pregnant women. Clin Infect Dis 1993;16(Suppl 4):S273–81.
[21] Hawes SE, Hillier SL, Benedetti J, et al. Hydrogen peroxide-producing lactobacilli and acquisition of vaginal infections. J Infect Dis 1996;174:1058–63.
[22] Hillier SL. Diagnostic microbiology of bacterial vaginosis. Am J Obstet Gynecol 1993;169: 455–9.
[23] Bump RC, Zuspan FP, Buesching 3rd WJ, et al. The prevalence, six-month persistence, and predictive values of laboratory indicators of bacterial vaginosis (nonspecific vaginitis) in asymptomatic women. Am J Obstet Gynecol 1984;150:917–24.
[24] Hill LH, Ruperalia H, Embil JA. Nonspecific vaginitis and other genital infections in three clinic populations. Sex Transm Dis 1983;10:114–8.
[25] Eschenbach DA, Hillier S, Critchlow C, et al. Diagnosis and clinical manifestations of bacterial vaginosis. Am J Obstet Gynecol 1988;158:819–28.
[26] Embree J, Caliando JJ, McCormack WM. Nonspecific vaginitis among women attending a sexually transmitted diseases clinic. Sex Transm Dis 1984;11:81–4.
[27] Paavonen J, Heinonen PK, Aine R, et al. Prevalence of nonspecific vaginitis and other cervicovaginal infections during the third trimester of pregnancy. Sex Transm Dis 1986;13:5–8.
[28] Kurki T, Sivonen A, Renkonen O-V, et al. Bacterial vaginosis in early pregnancy and pregnancy outcome. Obstet Gynecol 1992;80:173–7.

[29] Platz-Christensen JJ, Pernevi P, Hagmar B, et al. A longitudinal follow-up of bacterial vaginosis during pregnancy. Acta Obstet Gynecol Scand 1993;72:99–102.
[30] Meis PJ, Goldenberg RL, Mercer B, et al. The Preterm Prediction Study: significance of vaginal infections. Am J Obstet Gynecol 1995;173:1231–5.
[31] Goldenberg R, Klebanoff M, Nugent R, et al for the Vaginal Infections and Prematurity Study Group. Bacterial colonization of the vagina during pregnancy in four ethnic groups. Am J Obstet Gynecol 1996;174:1618–21.
[32] Jonsson M, Karlsson R, Rylander E, et al. The associations between risk behavior and reported history of sexually transmitted diseases, among young women: a population based study. Int J STD AIDS 1997;8:501–5.
[33] Bump R, Buesching III WB. Bacterial vaginosis in virginal and sexually active adolescent females: evidence against exclusive sexual transmission. Am J Obstet Gynecol 1988;158:935–9.
[34] Schwebke JR, Hillier SL, Sobel JD, et al. Validity of the vaginal Gram's stain for the diagnosis of bacterial vaginosis. Obstet Gynecol 1996;88:573–6.
[35] Krohn MA, Hillier SL, Eschenbach DA. Comparison of methods for diagnosing bacterial vaginosis among pregnant women. J Clin Microbiol 1989;27(6):1266–71.
[36] Totten PA, Amsel R, Hale J, et al. Selective differential human blood bilayer media for isolation of *Gardnerella* (*Haemophilus*) *vaginalis*. J Clin Microbiol 1982;15:141–7.
[37] Spiegel CA, Amsel R, Holmes KK. Diagnosis of bacterial vaginosis by direct Gram's stain of vaginal fluid. J Clin Microbiol 1983;18(1):170–7.
[38] Nugent RP, Krohn MA, Hillier SL. Reliability of diagnosing bacterial vaginosis is improved by a standardized method of Gram's stain interpretation. J Clin Microbiol 1991;29(2):297–301.
[39] Valenstein PN. Semiquantitation of bacteria in sputum Gram's stains. J Clin Microbiol 1988; 26:1791–4.
[40] Mazzuli T, Simor AE, Low DE. Reproducibility of interpretation of Gram-stained vaginal smears for the diagnosis of bacterial vaginosis. J Clin Microbiol 1990;28(7):1506–8.
[41] Guise JM, Mahon SM, Aickin M, et al. Screening for bacterial vaginosis in pregnancy. Am J Prev Med 2001;20(Suppl 3):62–72.
[42] Centers for Disease Control and Prevention. Sexually transmitted diseases treatment guidelines 2002. MMWR Morb Mortal Wkly Rep 2002;51:1–80.
[43] Caro-Paton T, Carvajal A, Martin de Diego I, et al. Is metronidazole teratogenic: a meta-analysis. Br J Clin Pharmacol 1997;44:179–82.
[44] Burtin P, Taddio A, Ariburnu O, et al. Safety of metronidazole in pregnancy: a meta-analysis. Am J Obstet Gynecol 1995;172:525–9.
[45] McGregor JA, French JI, Jones W, et al. Bacterial vaginosis is associated with prematurity and vaginal fluid mucinase and sialidase: results of a controlled trial of topical clindamycin cream. Am J Obstet Gynecol 1994;170:1048–60.
[46] Hauth JC, Goldenberg RL, Andrews WW, et al. Reduced incidence of preterm delivery with metronidazole and erythromycin in women with bacterial vaginosis. N Engl J Med 1995;333: 1732–6.
[47] McDonald HM, O'Loughlin JA, Vigneswaran R, et al. Bacterial vaginosis in pregnancy and efficacy of short-course oral metronidazole treatment: a randomized controlled trial. Obstet Gynecol 1994;84(3):343–8.
[48] Carey JC, Klebanoff MA, Hauth JC, et al. Metronidazole to prevent preterm delivery in pregnant women with asymptomatic bacterial vaginosis. N Engl J Med 2000;342(8):534–40.
[49] Klebanoff MA, Hauth JC, MacPherson CA, et al. Time course of the regression of asymptomatic bacterial vaginosis in pregnancy with and without treatment. Am J Obstet Gynecol 2004;190(2): 363–70.
[50] McGregor JA, French JI, Parker R, et al. Prevention of premature birth by screening and treatment for common genital tract infections: results of a prospective controlled evaluation. Am J Obstet Gynecol 1995;173:157–67.
[51] Ugwumadu A, Reid F, Hay P, et al. Natural history of bacterial vaginosis and intermediate flora in pregnancy and effect of oral clindamycin. Obstet Gynecol 2004;104(1):114–9.

[52] Joesef MR, Hillier SL, Wiknjosastro G, et al. Intravaginal clindamycin treatment for bacterial vaginosis: effects on preterm delivery and low birth weight. Am J Obstet Gynecol 1995;173: 1527–31.
[53] Kekki M, Kurki T, Pelkonen J, et al. Vaginal clindamycin in preventing preterm birth and peripartal infections in asymptomatic women with bacterial vaginosis: a randomized, controlled trial. Obstet Gynecol 2001;97:643–8.
[54] Kurkinen-Raty M, Vuopala S, Koskela M, et al. A randomized controlled trial of vaginal clindamycin for early pregnancy bacterial vaginosis. Br J Obstet Gynaecol 2000;107(11):1427–32.
[55] Lamont RF, Jones BM, Mandal D, et al. The efficacy of vaginal clindamycin for the treatment of abnormal genital tract flora in pregnancy. Infect Dis Obstet Gynecol 2003;11(4):181–9.
[56] Yudin MH, Landers DV, Meyn L, et al. Clinical and cervical cytokine response to treatment with oral or vaginal metronidazole for bacterial vaginosis during pregnancy: a randomized trial. Obstet Gynecol 2003;102:527–34.
[57] Guaschino S, Ricci E, Franchi M, et al. Treatment of asymptomatic bacterial vaginosis to prevent pre-term delivery: a randomized trial. Eur J Obstet Gynecol Reprod Biol 2003;110(2):149–52.
[58] Morales WJ, Schorr S, Albritton J. Effect of metronidazole in patients with preterm birth in preceding pregnancy and bacterial vaginosis: a placebo-controlled, double-blind study. Am J Obstet Gynecol 1994;171(2):345–7.
[59] McDonald H, Brocklehurst P, Parsons J, et al. Antibiotics for treating bacterial vaginosis in pregnancy. Cochrane Database Syst Rev 2003;2:CD000262. p. 1–36.
[60] Vermeulen G, Bruinse H. Prophylactic administration of clindamycin 2% vaginal cream to reduce the incidence of spontaneous preterm birth in women with an increased recurrence risk: a randomized placebo controlled double blind trial. Br J Obstet Gynaecol 1999;106:652–7.
[61] Lamont RF, Duncan SLB, Mandal D, et al. Intravaginal clindamycin to reduce preterm birth in women with abnormal genital tract flora. Obstet Gynecol 2003;101(3):516–22.
[62] Leitich H, Brunbauer M, Bodner-Adler B, et al. Antibiotic treatment of bacterial vaginosis in pregnancy: a meta-analysis. Am J Obstet Gynecol 2003;188:752–8.

ELSEVIER
SAUNDERS

Clin Perinatol 32 (2005) 629–656

CLINICS IN
PERINATOLOGY

Treatment of Sexually Transmitted Infections in Pregnancy

Lisa M. Hollier, MD, MPH[a,*],
Kimberly Workowski, MD[b,c]

[a]*Department of Obstetrics, Gynecology and Reproductive Sciences, University of Texas Houston Medical School, Lyndon Baines Johnson General Hospital, 5656 Kelly Street, Houston, TX 77026, USA*
[b]*Division of Infectious Diseases, Emory University, Atlanta, GA 30322, USA*
[c]*Guidelines Unit, Epidemiology and Surveillance Branch, Division of STD Prevention, Centers for Disease Control and Prevention, Atlanta, GA 30333, USA*

Sexually transmitted infections remain a major public health concern in the United States. An estimated 19 million infections occur each year [1]. The economic burden imposed by sexually transmitted infections is impressive: direct medical costs have been estimated as high as $15.5 billion annually [2]. Sexually transmitted infections are relatively common during pregnancy, especially in indigent, urban populations effected by drug abuse and prostitution. Education, screening, treatment, and prevention are important components of prenatal care for women at increased risk for these infections. Treatment of these sexually transmitted infections is clearly associated with improved pregnancy outcome and reductions in perinatal mortality [3–5].

Syphilis

Syphilis is caused by the spirochete *Treponema pallidum*. The rate of primary and secondary (P & S) syphilis in women continues to decrease and fell 27% to 0.8 cases per 100,000 women, with a total of 1217 cases reported in 2003 [6]. The rate of P & S syphilis increased 13.5% among men between 2002

* Corresponding author.
E-mail address: lisa.m.hollier@uth.tmc.edu (L.M. Hollier).

doi:10.1016/j.clp.2005.04.007 *perinatology.theclinics.com*

and 2003. The rate of P & S syphilis among African Americans (7.8 cases/ 100,000) was 5.2 times greater than among non-Hispanic whites (1.5 cases/ 100,000). Although important ethnic disparity still exists, this proportion reflects an important decline in the rates of syphilis among African Americans from 2002 to 2003 [7]. Syphilis is primarily acquired through sexual contact, though approximately 1000 cases of vertically acquired congenital infections occur each year in the United States.

Antepartum syphilis can profoundly affect pregnancy outcome by causing preterm labor, fetal death, and neonatal infection by transplacental or perinatal infection [8,9]. Fortunately, of the many congenital infections, syphilis is not only the most readily prevented but also the most susceptible to therapy.

Diagnosis

Diagnostic testing involves a two-step process, beginning with a nonspecific test and concluding with a treponeme-specific test for patients screening positive. The non-treponemal screening tests include the VDRL (Venereal Disease Research Laboratory), RPR (rapid plasma reagin), or ART (automated reagin test). Nontreponemal test antibody titers usually correlate with disease activity and should be reported with a quantitative titer. On the other hand, other disease states or physiologic states, such as pregnancy, can yield false-positive results. Because the current incidence of syphilis is so low, the majority of positive screening tests are not due to treponemal infection. Treponemal-specific tests including fluorescent treponemal antibody absorption test (FTA-ABS) or *Treponema pallidum* particle agglutination (TP-PA) are necessary to confirm the diagnosis of syphilis after a positive nontreponemal test. These tests are specific for *T pallidum* antigens and are reported as positive or negative.

Nontreponemal screening during pregnancy is recommended at the first prenatal visit, and again in the third trimester, particularly in high-risk populations [10–12]. Laws also mandate serologic screening at delivery in many states.

Treatment

Penicillin G, in benzathine, aqueous procaine, or aqueous crystalline form, is the drug of choice for treatment of all stages of syphilis, and is the only effective treatment for the prevention of congenital syphilis in pregnancy. Erythromycin may be curative in the mother, but may not prevent congenital syphilis because of the variability of transplacental passage of the antibiotic [13]. Thus, it is not currently recommended as a penicillin alternative. Ceftriaxone may prove useful in adults as an alternative regimen for patients who have penicillin allergy; however, there is insufficient information on its use in pregnancy [14,15]. The efficacy of azithromycin in the penicillin-allergic pregnant woman has not been adequately evaluated [16]. In addition, recent treatment failures with azithromycin have been reported [17]. Tetracyclines, including doxycy-

Table 1
Oral penicillin desensitization protocol

Dose[a]	Penicillin V suspension (units/ml)	Amount[b] (ml)	(units)	Cumulative dose (units)
1	1000	0.1	100	100
2	1000	0.2	200	300
3	1000	0.4	400	700
4	1000	0.8	800	1500
5	1000	1.6	1600	3100
6	1000	3.2	3200	6300
7	1000	6.4	6400	12,700
8	10,000	1.2	12,000	24,700
9	10,000	2.4	24,700	48,700
10	10,000	4.8	48,000	96,700
11	80,000	1.0	80,000	176,000
12	80,000	2.4	164,000	336,700
13	80,000	4.8	320,000	656,700
14	80,000	8.0	640,000	1,296,700

Patients will be desensitized as above. After desensitization, patients will be observed for 30 minutes before parenteral injection of benzathine penicillin. Patients who have been desensitized previously, have received their benzathine IM, and are returning for their second shot will not require additional desensitization. While desensitization is usually lost within 2 days of terminating the penicillin therapy, long acting benzathine penicillin will sustain the sensitized state for periods up to 3 weeks.

[a] Interval between doses: 15 minutes; elapsed time: 3 hours and 45 minutes; cumulative dose: 1.3 million units.

[b] The specific amount of drug is diluted in approximately 30 ml of water and then given orally. *Adapted from* Wendel Jr GD, Stark BJ, Jamison RB, et al. Penicillin allergy and desensitization in serious infections during pregnancy. N Engl J Med 1985;312:1229–32.

cline, are effective for treatment of syphilis in the nonpregnant woman, but are generally not recommended during pregnancy because of the risk of yellow-brown discoloration of the fetal deciduous teeth.

Because of the high rate of failure and insufficient data for alternative treatment modalities, patients who have known penicillin allergy should undergo desensitization with subsequent administration of penicillin [10]. In the past, pregnant women who had a history of penicillin allergy were skin-tested to confirm the risk of IgE-mediated anaphylaxis before desensitization [18]. Unfortunately, the necessary reagents for skin testing, including benylpenicilloyl polylysine injection, are in limited supply. Desensitization is recommended in all women describing a probable history of penicillin allergy. For one oral desensitization protocol, see Table 1 [18]. The first dose of benzathine penicillin should be given at the completion of the oral protocol. A recommended dosage regimen for pregnant women is as follows:

- Primary, secondary, or early latent stage: benzathine penicillin G, 2.4 million units intramuscularly (IM) in a single dose
- Late latent stage or syphilis of unknown duration: benzathine penicillin G, 2.4 million units IM once a week for 3 consecutive weeks

- Neurosyphilis: aqueous crystalline penicillin G, 3–4 million units intravenously (IV) every 4 hours, or 18–24 million units daily as continuous infusion, for 10–14 days

The rate of treatment failure may be increased in pregnant patients who have secondary syphilis, therefore some experts recommend the use of a second injection of benzathine penicillin G 2.4 million units IM 1 week after the first to treat early syphilis in pregnancy [19]. In a study of 340 pregnant women who had syphilis, six (1.8%) fetal treatment failures with maternal benzathine penicillin G therapy were reported [19]. Four of these six treatment failures occurred in women who had secondary syphilis, and the other 2 women had early latent syphilis. Treatment failures were generally confined to women treated after 26 weeks' gestation, probably related to the duration and severity of fetal infection.

Within hours after treatment, patients can develop an acute complication called the Jarisch-Herxheimer reaction. Symptoms include fever, chills, myalgias, headache, tachycardia, hyperventilation, vasodilation, and mild hypotension. Uterine contractions and fetal heart rate decelerations may occur. Although the reaction occurs in 10% to 25% of patients overall, it is most common in the treatment of early syphilis. A recent report [20] noted an incidence of 40% among treated pregnant women. Symptoms last for 12 to 24 hours and are usually self-limiting. Patients can be treated symptomatically with antipyretics. Routine hospitalization is not recommended for treatment during pregnancy, though this has not been systematically evaluated [16].

Consideration should be given to ultrasound evaluation of the fetus before therapy when syphilis is diagnosed after 24 weeks. Ultrasound abnormalities associated with syphilis include polyhydramnios, hepatosplenomegaly, ascites, and hydrops [21]. Fetuses that have physical evidence of severe disease discovered on ultrasound have also been shown to have biochemical evidence of severe disease. Treatment failure and other complications are more common among these fetuses [22]. When the fetal ultrasound is abnormal, consultation with specialists in maternal-fetal medicine and neonatology should occur. Complications such as preterm labor, preterm premature rupture of the membranes, fetal heart rate decelerations, and stillbirth may be precipitated by treatment. In the severely affected fetus, particularly with preexisting fetal heart rate abnormalities, consideration may be given to an untreated preterm or term delivery followed by neonatal treatment [16,23]. Despite the advantages of ultrasound assessment, maternal treatment should not be delayed unduly to obtain imaging.

Response to therapy should be monitored with clinical and serologic examination in the third trimester and at delivery [16]. Women who have a high risk of reinfection during pregnancy should be followed with monthly titers [10]. Titers decrease more quickly in earlier stages of disease, when titers are low, and in patients who have no previous history of syphilis. Failure of nontreponemal antibody titers to decrease fourfold at 6 months is indicative of probable treatment failure in primary or secondary syphilis [10]. A fourfold rise in the antibody titer (eg, 1:4 to 1:16) usually signifies failed treatment or recurrent infection. These patients should be retreated based on their stage of syphilis and evaluated for HIV infection [10]. Risks for failure of maternal treatment include high maternal serologic titers, preterm delivery, and delivery shortly after antepartum therapy [24]. Sexual contacts within the last 3 months should be evaluated for syphilis and treated presumptively, even if seronegative.

Herpes simplex virus

Approximately 5 million adults in the United States report a history of genital herpes infection. Based on very large serologic studies, however, the number of infected Americans is probably much closer to 45 million [25]! Genital herpes simplex infection can be caused by either herpes simplex virus type 1 (HSV-1), also associated with oral/facial lesions, and HSV type 2 (HSV-2). In many teens and young adults, HSV-1 infection causes more than half of new cases of genital herpes [26]. Both HSV-1 and 2 can be transmitted to other sites by direct contact with infected secretions or autoinoculation. Additionally, both can be transmitted vertically and cause symptomatic neonatal disease. Asymptomatic shedding is very common, especially in the first year after a primary episode, and probably represents the major source of sexual transmission.

Approximately 2% of susceptible women acquire HSV during pregnancy [27]. Among women who have recurrent disease, 16% to 82% may have a recurrence during pregnancy [28,29]. Because of the potential for neonatal morbidity and mortality with vertically acquired infection, herpes infection in pregnancy is especially important.

A primary outbreak in the first trimester of pregnancy has been associated with chorioretinitis, microcephaly, and skin lesions in rare cases [30]. Although HSV has been associated with an increased risk for spontaneous abortion, recent studies do not support such a risk [31].

The risk of neonatal transmission risk is influenced by the maternal antibody status and the timing of maternal infection. The risk of vertical transmission to the neonate when a primary outbreak occurs at the time of delivery is approximately 30% to 50% [27]. Among women who have recurrent lesions at the time of delivery, the rate of transmission is approximately 3%, and for women who have recurrent disease and no visible lesions at delivery, the transmission risk has been estimate to be 2/10,000 [32].

Diagnosis

One important step in reducing the burden of HSV is improvement in methods for the diagnosis of genital herpes simplex virus infection. The herpes virus has a characteristic protein coat, and each of the types has identifiable proteins.

Glycoprotein G2 is associated with type 2 and glycoprotein G1 is associated with type 1. Type-specific antibodies to the viral proteins develop within the first several weeks of infection and persist [25,33].

For patients who do not present with active lesions or whose lesions are culture negative, type-specific serologic assays are now commercially available. Because HSV-2 is an uncommon cause of oral infection, detection of HSV-2 antibodies is virtually diagnostic of genital HSV infection [34]. There are currently several US Food and Drug Administration (FDA)-approved type-specific tests, and others are under development. All are laboratory-based assays and include the HerpeSelect-1 enzyme-linked immunosorbent assay (ELISA) IgG and HerpeSelect-2 ELISA IgG, HerpeSelect 1 and 2 Immunoblot IgG (Focus Technologies, Cypress, California) and the Captia ELISA (Trinity Biotech, Bray, County Wicklow, Ireland). Recently, the FDA approved the rapid test formerly known as the POCkit test. It is being marketed as the BiokitHSV-2 Rapid Test (Biokit USA, Lexington, Massachusetts) and as the Sure-Vue HSV-2 (Fisher Scientific, Pittsburgh, Pennsylvania).

Despite the availability of truly type-specific testing, many laboratories continue to use older assays. It may be necessary to call the laboratory to confirm the type of testing to be used before submitting a specimen, and to request glycoprotein G-based serologic testing. Although serologic screening for HSV-2 should be available for persons who request testing, screening for HSV-1 or HSV-2 infection in the general population is not indicated [10].

Serologic screening of couples for HSV-2 antibodies during pregnancy has been proposed to identify both women who have serologic evidence of disease and women who are negative and have seropositive partners (discordant couples) [35,36]. This recommendation is controversial, and there is no clinical evidence to support the efficacy of such a policy to prevent HSV transmission and neonatal infection [37,38]. The cost-effectiveness of prenatal, type-specific antibody screening has been evaluated in several studies, and currently such screening can not be recommended to prevent neonatal herpes [39,40].

Treatment

There is no cure for HSV infection, but the use of antiviral medications in nonpregnant women has been shown to reduce the frequency and duration of outbreaks, reduce the frequency of asymptomatic shedding, and reduce transmission [41]. Acyclovir has also been used extensively in pregnant women [31]. In a pharmacokinetics study of acyclovir and valacyclovir, acyclovir was concentrated in the amniotic fluid, but there was no evidence of preferential fetal drug accumulation [42].

The manufacturer of acyclovir and valacyclovir, in cooperation with the Centers for Disease Control and Prevention in Atlanta, Georgia, maintained a registry for exposure to these drugs during pregnancy through 1999. More than 700 infants reported were exposed to acyclovir during the first trimester, and there does not appear to be an increase in adverse fetal or neonatal effects [43]. One potential complication is fetal neutropenia, similar to that seen in infants who have HSV on long-term suppressive acyclovir therapy, although no cases have been reported in newborns to antepartum prophylaxis [44]. There are insufficient data on valacyclovir and famciclovir exposure in the pregnancy registry for analyses.

The current guidelines for antiviral treatment in nonpregnant women are listed below in Box 1. Antiviral treatment may be administered orally to pregnant women who have first-episode genital herpes or severe recurrent herpes. In patients who have severe disease, oral treatment can be extended for more than 10 days if lesions are incompletely healed after that time [10]. Acyclovir should be administered IV to pregnant women who have severe HSV infection or disseminated herpetic infections.

In nonpregnant women, episodic therapy with acyclovir, famciclovir, or valacyclovir has been shown to decrease the proportion of patients who have outbreaks, reduce the duration of symptoms, and shorten the duration of viral shedding [45]. Suppressive therapy reduces the frequency of genital herpes recurrences by 70% to 80% among patients who have frequent recurrences (ie, ≥6 recurrences per year), and many patients report no symptomatic outbreaks [10]. Patients on suppressive therapy must be counseled that although recurrences are less frequent, viral shedding still occurs, so they are still capable of

Box 1. Antiviral treatment guidelines for nonpregnant women

First clinical episode—recommended regimens

Acyclovir, 400 mg orally three times a day for 7–10 days; or
Acyclovir 200 mg orally 5 times a day for 7–10 days; or
Famciclovir, 250 mg orally three times a day for 7–10 days; or
Valacyclovir, 1 g orally twice a day for 7–10 days

Recurrent episodes—recommended episodic regimens

Acyclovir, 400 mg orally three times a day for 5 days; or
Acyclovir, 200 mg orally 5 times a day for 5 days; or
Acyclovir, 800 mg orally twice a day for 5 days; or
Acyclovir, 800 mg orally 3 times a day for 2 days; or
Famciclovir, 125 mg orally twice a day for 5 days; or
Valacyclovir, 500 mg orally twice a day for 3–5 days; or
Valacyclovir, 1 g orally once daily for 5 days

Severe primary infection or disseminated infection

Acyclovir, intravenous 5–10 mg/kg every 8 hours for 2–7 days or until clinical improvement, followed by oral antiviral therapy to complete at least 10 days total therapy [10]

transmitting the disease. In a large clinical trial, individuals taking valacyclovir once daily for prophylaxis had a decreased rate of transmission to their sexual partners compared with those individuals randomized to placebo [41].

The efficacy of suppressive therapy during pregnancy to prevent recurrences near term has been evaluated in several studies [46–52]. A recent meta-analysis of randomized controlled trials [53] was performed to assess the effectiveness of acyclovir suppressive therapy given after 36 weeks on the risk of a clinical recurrence at delivery, cesarean delivery for recurrent genital herpes, and the detection of HSV at delivery among women with a history of recurrent genital herpes. The risk of recurrence at delivery was significantly reduced (odds ratio [OR] 0.25, 95% confidence interval [CI] 0.15–0.40), as was the rate of Cesarean delivery (OR 0.61, 95% CI 0.43–0.86) for women who received suppression. The odds of viral detection at delivery using culture were reduced (OR 0.11, 95% CI 0.04–0.31) among treated women; however, in one trial, virus was detected in one woman receiving acyclovir [52]. The use of acyclovir suppression in late pregnancy has also been evaluated in economic analyses, and suppression was found to be cost-effective [54]. The doses of antiviral medication used in the randomized trials in pregnancy were higher than the corresponding doses in nonpregnant women. Possible regimens for suppression include: acyclovir 400 mg orally three times a day and valacyclovir 500 mg orally twice a day. No clinical trials have been conducted using famciclovir. Valacyclovir results in higher plasma acyclovir levels than acyclovir when given in late pregnancy; however, no clinical studies have compared acyclovir to valacyclovir in pregnancy [42].

Because of the severity of neonatal infection, cesarean delivery has been used widely in instances when active genital herpetic recurrences are suspected. According to the American College of Obstetricians and Gynecologists [55], cesarean delivery is indicated in women who have an active genital lesion or in those who have a typical prodrome of an impending outbreak. Thus, cesarean delivery is performed only if primary or recurrent lesions are visualized near the time of labor or when the membranes are ruptured. In a very large retrospective study [56], there was an 85% reduction in the risk of neonatal HSV with cesarean delivery (7.7% versus 1.2%) among women who had HSV shedding at delivery.

Neonatal issues

An exposed infant of a mother known or suspected of having genital herpes initially should be isolated and cultures taken for herpes. It is not necessary to separate baby and mother when the mother has genital herpetic lesions; instead, she is instructed in hand washing and to avoid any contact between her lesions, her hands, and the baby. Breast feeding is allowed under these conditions. Maternal antiviral therapy should not deter breast feeding, because acyclovir does not reach appreciable levels in breast milk with valacyclovir treatment [57]. Family members who have oral herpetic lesions should avoid kissing the newborn and should use careful hand-washing techniques.

Chancroid

Haemophilus ducreyi can cause painful, nonindurated genital ulcers, often accompanied by painful inguinal lymphadenopathy. Although common in some developing countries, it has become rare in the United States. Importantly, the infection is a high-risk cofactor for HIV and syphilis transmission [10]. There have been no reported adverse effects of chancroid on pregnancy outcomes.

Diagnosis by culture is difficult because appropriate media are not widely available from commercial sources. Instead, a probable clinical diagnosis is made when dark-field examination or syphilis serologic tests are negative and herpesvirus tests on the ulcer are negative. Recommended treatment options in pregnancy are azithromycin, 1 g orally as a single dose; erythromycin base, 500 mg orally three times daily for 7 days; or ceftriaxone, 250 mg in a single intramuscular dose [10]. The efficacy of azithromycin for the treatment of chancroid in pregnant women has not been established, however.

Gonorrhea

The incidence of gonorrhea in the United States has decreased 75% since 1975. The incidence rate for 2003 was 116.2 cases per 100,000 population, which is the lowest rate ever reported for this disease [7]. The prevalence of gonorrhea during pregnancy in selected US prenatal clinics in 2003 was 0.9%, and varied from 0.19% to 4.0%. Risk factors for infection in pregnancy include being single, adolescence, poverty, drug abuse, prostitution, other sexually transmitted diseases, and lack of prenatal care [58]. Concomitant chlamydial infection is present in about 40% of pregnant women infected with gonorrhea [58].

In most pregnant women, gonococcal infection is limited to the lower genital tract, including the cervix, urethra, and periurethral and vestibular glands. Adverse pregnancy outcomes have been associated with infection. Untreated gonococcal cervicitis is associated with septic spontaneous abortion and infection after induced abortion [59]. Preterm delivery, premature rupture of membranes, chorioamnionitis, and postpartum infection are more common in women who have *Neisseria gonorrhoeae* detected at delivery [60]. Neonatal infections are manifest most commonly as ophthalmia neonatorum, scalp abscess, or disseminated disease.

Diagnosis

The diagnosis of gonorrhea is best made either with culture or with nucleic acid amplification tests (NAATs). If culture is done, modified Thayer-Martin media should be used and the specimen should not be refrigerated. For either culture or NAAT testing, an endocervical specimen should be obtained. The use of nucleic acid amplification tests for rectal and oropharyngeal specimens has had limited evaluation in published studies [10].

Because of the complications associated with gonococcal infection in pregnancy, a screening test is recommended at the first prenatal visit or before an induced abortion. A repeat culture after 28 weeks is recommended in high-risk populations, including those infected early in pregnancy [10,61]. Postpartum screening has been recommended in the at-risk teenage population [62,63].

Treatment

Antimicrobial-resistant *N gonorrhoeae* have rendered most β-lactam drugs ineffective for therapy [64]. In a study of 62 pregnant women who had probable endocervical gonorrhea [65], intramuscular ceftriaxone (125 mg) and oral cefixime (400 mg) resulted in a cure rate of 95% and 96%, respectively. Ceftriaxone and cefixime are recommended for uncomplicated gonococcal infection during pregnancy, although cefixime has limited availability at present [66]. Spectinomycin, 2 g IM in a single dose is an alternative for pregnant women allergic to penicillin or β-lactam antibiotics. Azithromycin at a 2-g dose is efficacious, but it is associated with gastrointestinal (GI) symptoms. At an oral dose of 1 g, azithromycin is insufficiently effective and is not recommended for gonococcal therapy [10]. Screening for syphilis and *Chlamydia trachomatis* should precede treatment, if possible. If chlamydial testing is unavailable, presumptive therapy is given. Treatment is recommended for sexual contacts, but a test-of-cure is unnecessary if symptoms resolve.

Recommended regimens are: (1) 400 mg cefixime orally in a single dose (note, however, that the manufacturer has discontinued production for the US market); or (2) 125 mg ceftriaxone IM in a single dose. Treatment for chlamydia should be included with either.

Disseminated gonococcal infections

Gonococcal bacteremia may lead to petechial or pustular skin lesions, arthralgias, septic arthritis, or tenosynovitis. Pregnant women may account for a disproportionate amount of disseminated gonococcal infection in women [67]. Endocarditis rarely complicates pregnancy, but it may be fatal [68]. Because of the rarity of this condition, consultation with experts in treatment of sexually transmitted infections should be considered. The Centers for Disease Control and Prevention recommend ceftriaxone, 1000 mg IM or IV every 24 hours [10]. Treatment for disseminated GC should be continued for 24 to 48 hours after improvement, and then therapy should be changed to an oral agent to complete at least 1 week of therapy. For gonococcal endocarditis, therapy should be continued for at least 4 weeks.

Chlamydial infections

C trachomatis is an obligate intracellular bacterium that has several serotypes, including those that cause lymphogranuloma venereum. *C trachomatis* genital infection remains the most common infectious disease reported to state health departments and to the Centers for Disease Control and Prevention, especially among sexually active adolescents and young adults [7]. The national rate of reported chlamydia in 2003 was 304.3 cases per 100,000 population. The continuing increase in reported cases likely represents expansion of screening, more sensitive screening tests, and more complete national reporting. *C trachomatis* infection is also common in pregnant women, and its incidence depends on the demographic makeup of the population. In 2003, the median chlamydia test positivity rate among young women screened at selected prenatal clinics in 27 states, Puerto Rico, and the Virgin Islands was 7.4%, with a range of 2.4% to 19.7% [7]. Risk factors for chlamydial infection include age less than 25 years, presence or history of other sexually transmitted disease, multiple sexual partners, and a new sexual partner within 3 months [10].

The effect of asymptomatic chlamydial infection on pregnancy outcome remains controversial. The risk of spontaneous abortion does not appear to be increased [69]; however, untreated maternal cervical chlamydial infection increases the risk for preterm delivery, premature rupture of the membranes, and perinatal mortality [70–72]. Infection with chlamydia does not appear to be associated with an increased risk of chorioamnionitis or with pelvic infection after cesarean delivery [73,74].

There is vertical transmission to 30% to 50% of infants delivered vaginally to infected women, and *C trachomatis* is the most common identifiable infectious cause of ophthalmia neonatorum. Although neonatal eye prophylaxis for gonococcal infection with silver nitrate, erythromycin, or tetracycline is effective, none of these prevent chlamydial conjunctivitis or pneumonia [10,75].

Diagnosis

Important advances for the detection of chlamydia have been associated with a rise in the reporting of this common infection. NAATs, including polymerase chain reaction (PCR), ligase chain reaction (LCR), transcription-mediated amplification (TMA), and strand displacement amplification (SDA), are highly sensitive compared with culture and maintain high specificity [76].

Routine screening for *C trachomatis* during pregnancy is a complex issue [77]. The Centers for Disease Control and Prevention recommends screening at the first prenatal visit and again in the third trimester for women less than 25 years old or those who have new or multiple sex partners [10].

Recurrent chlamydial colonization after treatment has been found in as many as 17% of women treated in pregnancy [78]. This high rate of recurrent colonization may be related to the reduced efficacy of amoxicillin or erythromycin, or to failure to complete recommended therapy (see treatment section below).

Because of the high risk of recurrence, repeat screening in the third trimester seems reasonable in women who have positive initial cultures or for those at high risk.

Treatment

The recommended regimens for the treatment of chlamydia during pregnancy are either azithromycin, 1 g orally in a single dose or amoxicillin 500 mg three times daily for 7 days. Erythromycin base, 500 mg orally four times a day for 7 days is an alternative regimen. There have been several clinical trials evaluating the efficacy of azithromycin for therapy in pregnancy. Trials in women report efficacy rates ranging from 64% to 95% [79–82]. Side effects are less common with azithromycin compared with erythromycin. Only 7% of women receiving azithromycin had significant side effects, compared with 39% of those given erythromycin. Amoxicillin and erythromycin are equally effective for treatment during pregnancy—reported cure rates are approximately 82% for amoxicillin and 85% for erythromycin [83,84]. These cure rates are lower than in nonpregnant adults. This may be explained in part by reduced efficacies in pregnancy, and by the failure to complete treatment due to the adverse side effect profile of these therapies during pregnancy. Amoxicillin is better tolerated than erythromycin, and fewer patients may discontinue therapy before completion [83]. Repeat testing for chlamydia, preferably by NAAT, 3 weeks after completion of therapy is recommended for all pregnant women to ensure therapeutic cure because of the sequelae that may occur in the mother or neonate if the infection persists.

There are several reports that antenatal and postnatal exposure to macrolide antibiotics increases the risk of hypertrophic pyrolic stenosis in infants of treated mothers [85–88]. Neither erythromycin estolate nor tetracyclines should be used during pregnancy.

Lymphogranuloma venereum

There are several serovars of *C trachomatis* that cause lymphogranuloma venereum (LGV). The primary genital infection may be transient and seldom recognized. For treatment during pregnancy, erythromycin, 500 mg four times daily, is given for at least 21 days [10]. Although data regarding efficacy are scarce, some authorities recommend azithromycin given in multiple doses over 3 weeks [10].

Human papillomavirus

Genital papillomavirus infection, either symptomatic or asymptomatic, is common. Of 2597 high-risk pregnant women enrolled in one center of the Vaginal Infections and Prematurity Study, 28% were seropositive for HPV-16 capsid antibodies [89]. The most important sequela is development of cervical, vaginal, vulvar, and anal neoplasia and cancer [90]. Mucocutaneous external genital warts are usually caused by HPV types 6 and 11, but may also be caused by intermediate- and high-oncogenic risk HPV [91,92].

External genital warts

Genital warts frequently increase in number and size during pregnancy, sometimes filling the vagina or covering the perineum. When large or diffuse, they can complicate vaginal delivery and episiotomy. The relationship of HPV to episiotomy breakdown is controversial [93,94]. Because papillomavirus infection can be subclinical and multifocal, women who have vulvar lesions may also have cervical infection, and vice versa [90,95].

Maternal infection may be associated with juvenile onset recurrent respiratory papillomatosis, a rare, benign neoplasm of the larynx. It can cause hoarseness and respiratory distress in children, and is due often to HPV types 6 or 11. A Danish population-based study estimated a very low risk of transmission (7 in 1000) from infected women [96]. Recently, HPV PCR and DNA sequencing techniques were used to examine parental and newborn samples [97]. They found infection in only 9 of 574 (1.6%) of newborn samples, and they found no HPV DNA in any of the infants who returned for follow-up. Importantly, there was concordance of HPV type in only one mother–infant pair, and the transmission rate was only 3.7% among HPV-positive women. These data support the rarity of perinatal HPV transmission and suggest other potential sources of exposure or contamination.

Diagnosis

Diagnosis is most often made by visualization of the lesions. If doubt exists, a biopsy should be performed. Because of variations in inter- and intraobserver interpretation, Pap smears are not a reliable method for diagnosis. Although there are genetic probes available to identify HPV subtypes, the clinical utility of these tests in the management of external condyloma has not been determined.

Treatment

In pregnancy, some specialists reserve treatment of genital warts to those situations in which intervention is necessary to relieve significant obstruction of the birth canal that may otherwise complicate vaginal delivery. Others recommend intervention because of the risk of enlargement during the gestation. Choice of therapy is directed toward minimizing toxicity to the mother and fetus. Although there are several agents available for use in adult women, pregnancy limits their use.

Podophyllin resin, podofilox 0.5% solution or gel, 5-fluorouracil cream, imiquimod 5% cream, and interferon therapy should not be used in pregnancy because of concerns about maternal and fetal safety [10]. The podophyllin derivatives are associated with inhibition of cell mitosis, 5-fluorouracil is associated with dysmorphogenesis, and the effect of the immunomodulators (imiquimod and interferon) on pregnancy is unknown [98,99].

Trichloroacetic or bichloracetic acid in concentrations up to 85% in alcohol is an effective treatment for small lesions and can be used safely in pregnancy. The solution can be applied to external lesions with a swab weekly for up to 4 weeks. Some clinicians prefer cryotherapy or laser ablation of lesions in pregnancy. Successful results with the CO_2 have been reported in several series [100,101]. Occasionally, warts attain enormous size, and these may even necessitate cesarean delivery. If the woman is seen several weeks before delivery, the large lesions sometimes can be removed by excision, electrocautery, cryosurgery, or laser ablation. CO_2 laser has been used during pregnancy to remove large Büschke-Lowenstein tumors under anesthesia [102].

Pregnant women who have external genital warts should be informed that the risk of respiratory papillomatosis is low (0.7%) [96], and there is no evidence that cesarean delivery reduces the risk of neonatal disease. No current evidence indicates that the reduction in viral DNA that results from antepartum treatment impacts any risk of peripartum transmission.

Trichomonas infections

The protozoan *Trichomonas vaginalis* is the etiologic agent of trichomoniasis, one of the most common sexually transmitted infections in the world [103]. In the United States, it is responsible for an estimated 7 million new infections annually [1]. The prevalence in pregnancy is approximately 7% to 13% [104–106]. The race-specific prevalence was 23% for blacks, 6.6% for Hispanics, and 6.1% for white women. Trichomonas infection in pregnancy has been associated with preterm premature rupture of membranes, preterm delivery, and low birthweight infants [107].

Diagnosis

Trichomonads are demonstrated readily in a wet mount of vaginal secretions as flagellated, ovoid, motile organisms that are somewhat larger than leukocytes. The sensitivity of this technique depends on a number of factors, including the concentration of organisms, the degree of dilution, and the experience of the examiner, but is generally considered to be 60% to 85% [108]. Trichomonads are identified most accurately by culture, traditionally using Diamond's medium; however, a new commercially available culture method composed of liquid medium in a clear pouch has been shown to have equivalent sensitivity to the traditional method (InPouch TV by BioMed Diagnostics, San Jose, California) [109]. This method has been used successfully with both clinician-obtained and self-obtained specimens [110]. Recent studies have evaluated the test characteristics of a rapid point-of-care test for *T vaginalis*, XenoStrip-Tv (Genzyme, Cambridge, Massachusetts) [111,112]. The sensitivity of the XenoStrip-Tv when compared with culture was 74% to 79%, and the specificity was 99%; however, the rapid test had a higher sensitivity than wet mount. Another point-of-care test for the diagnosis of trichomoniasis in women has also been licensed by the FDA: the OSOM Trichomonas Rapid Test (Genzyme). The FDA has also approved a DNA probe-based test for *T vaginalis* (Affirm VPIII, Becton Dickinson, Franklin Lakes, New Jersey) that has a sensitivity of 90% to 100% compared with traditional culture [113]. PCR techniques are also under development [114,115].

Treatment

Metronidazole is likely to provide parasitological cure for trichomoniasis [116]. Cure rates generally exceed 90%. Both single-dose and long-term courses of treatment appear to be equally effective [117,118]. Oral treatment may be more effective than intravaginal treatment alone in achieving parasitological cure [119].

Unfortunately, there are few data regarding efficacy of any regimen in pregnancy. According to the Centers for Disease Control and Prevention, pregnant women can be treated with a 2-g single dose of oral metronidazole or 500 mg twice a day for 7 days [64]. Many studies of metronidazole use in pregnancy have failed to detect an association with teratogenic or mutagenic effects in infants, even when it is used in the first trimester [120–122].

Tinidazole, a 5-nitroimidazole compound, is chemically related to metronidazole. This drug has been used widely outside the United States for treatment of trichomoniasis and has recently been licensed for use in this country. A 2-g oral dose of tinidazole has overall clinical efficacy equal to metronidazole (90% to 100%) [123]. Tinidazole is considered FDA pregnancy category C, and its use in the first trimester is not recommended [124,125].

An increased rate of adverse outcomes among treated women was found in two randomized trials [126,127] that evaluated the effect of screening and treatment for trichomonas. The Maternal-Fetal Medicine Units Network enrolled asymptomatic women in a randomized, placebo-controlled trial to test the efficacy of treatment for trichomoniasis on preterm birth reduction [126]. The second study [127] was a subanalysis of data collected as part of a community-randomized trial of presumptive sexually transmitted infection treatment during pregnancy in Uganda. Although rates of preterm birth were similar, there was an increased rate of low birthweight in women treated for trichomonas in a maternal cohort from Rakai.

In both studies, it appears that treatment of trichomoniasis is associated with increased risks of adverse outcomes. The explanation for this finding is unclear. Because of the risks, universal screening of asymptomatic women and subsequent treatment of trichomoniasis to prevent preterm birth is not recommended. All symptomatic women should be evaluated and treated if trichomoniasis is diagnosed. Because of a higher relapse rates in women whose partners were not treated, the Centers for Disease Control recommends that all partners be treated [10].

Bacterial vaginosis

Bacterial vaginosis (BV) is a clinical syndrome resulting from replacement of the normal H_2O_2-producing *Lactobacillus* species in the vagina with high concentrations of anaerobic bacteria (eg, *Prevotella* spp and *Mobiluncus* spp), along with *Gardnerella vaginalis*, and *Mycoplasma hominis*. BV is strikingly common among women of reproductive age, and an estimated 3 million cases occur annually in the United States. Although BV is a common cause of vaginal discharge or malodor, up to 50% of women who have BV are asymptomatic. The pathophysiology of the microbial alteration is not fully understood, particularly in pregnancy [128]. BV during pregnancy may be associated with adverse pregnancy outcomes, including premature rupture of the membranes, preterm labor, preterm birth, chorioamnionitis, postabortion endometritis, and postpartum endometritis [129,130].

Diagnosis

BV can be diagnosed by the use of clinical or Gram's-stain criteria. Clinical diagnosis with Amsel's criteria requires three of the following symptoms or signs:

- A homogeneous, white, noninflammatory discharge that smoothly coats the vaginal walls
- The presence of clue cells on microscopic examination
- A pH of vaginal fluid >4.5
- A fishy odor of vaginal discharge before or after addition of 10% potassium hydroxide (KOH) (ie, the whiff test)

When a Gram's stain is used, determining the relative concentration of the bacterial morphotypes characteristic of the altered flora of BV is an acceptable laboratory method (Nugent criteria) for diagnosing BV.

Treatment

All symptomatic pregnant women should be tested and treated. The main benefit of therapy for clinical BV in pregnant women is to relieve vaginal symptoms and signs of infection. Because of the potential risk for postoperative infectious complications associated with BV, some providers screen and treat women who have BV in addition to providing routine antimicrobial prophylaxis before abortions. More information is needed before recommending treatment of asymptomatic BV before these procedures, however, particularly cesarean delivery.

There is some debate about the optimal regimen for treating clinical infection in pregnancy, but therapeutic cure rates are about 70% [131]. For women at high risk for preterm delivery based on their history, and who have BV during the index pregnancy, evidence from three trials [132–134] has demonstrated that oral therapy with metronidazole (one trial combined metronidazole and oral erythromycin) reduced the risk of premature delivery by 25% to 75%. Two trials used 7 to 14 days of systemic therapy, which would treat possible upper tract infection [132–134].

Three trials of oral treatment for bacterial vaginosis to reduce preterm birth among mixed patient populations have been conducted [134–136]. Two of these trials [134,135] found no reduction in preterm birth among treated women. One large trial [135] randomized a total of 1953 asymptomatic women of high-and low risk to treatment with a dose of metronidazole, 2 g orally, which was repeated 48 hours later, or to placebo. The first treatment occurred between 16 and 24 weeks, and the treatment/placebo regimen was repeated once between 24 and 30 weeks. There were no significant differences in the rate of birth at less than 37 weeks (12.2% versus 12.5%; RR 1, 95% CI 0.8–1.2), less than 35 weeks, or less than 32 weeks. The groups also did not differ significantly with regard to neonatal death during the stay in the nursery, admission to the neonatal intensive care unit, or the presence of neonatal sepsis.

An earlier, smaller trial [134] randomized asymptomatic women who had BV (diagnosed by culture at 24 weeks gestation) to a short regimen of metronidazole, 400 mg 2 times a day for 2 days (repeated at 29 weeks for those who had recurrent BV), or to placebo. The rate of prematurity was 4.5% in the treatment group and 6.3% in the control group (*P* not significant) and the predetermined sample size was not reached.

The one positive trial [137] used oral clindamycin, 300 mg twice daily for 5 days to treat bacterial vaginosis detected between 16 and 22 weeks. Women receiving clindamycin had significantly fewer deliveries at less than 37 weeks (5% versus 12%, $P<.001$) than did those who received placebo. There were no differences, however, in neonatal outcomes.

Seven trials have evaluated the use of 2% intravaginal clindamycin treatment of bacterial vaginosis to prevent prematurity [137–143]. In six trials, 2% intravaginal clindamycin cream was given between 10 and 27 weeks' gestation to women who had BV, and all but one showed an increase in the rate of prematurity [137–142]. The seventh study evaluated a program of screening and treatment compared with routine prenatal care [143]. Women in the intervention group who were found to have a pathological vaginal flora or microscopically diagnosed infection received treatment. Bacterial vaginosis was treated for 6 days with clindamycin 2% vaginal cream. Persistent or recurrent disease was treated with oral clindamycin, 300 mg twice daily for 7 days. Candidiasis and trichomoniasis were also treated. The majority of infections were due to bacterial vaginosis (169 in treatment versus 166 in placebo women). The difference in the rates of spontaneous preterm birth between the intervention group and the control group was significant (3.0% versus 5.3%, $P<.01$). The groups did not differ significantly with regard to necrotizing enterocolitis, neonatal sepsis, and neonatal death during hospitalization.

In summary, asymptomatic low-risk women should not be screened and treated for bacterial vaginosis to reduce preterm birth. Screening and treatment of high-risk women may be performed. Treatment of symptomatic women with oral metronidazole is appropriate. Many studies of metronidazole use in pregnancy have failed to detect an association with teratogenic or mutagenic effects in infants, even when it is used in the first trimester [120–122]. Clinical trials do not indicate that a woman's response to therapy and the likelihood of relapse are affected by the treatment of her sexual partner; therefore, routine treatment of sex partners is not recommended [144,145].

Vulvovaginal candidiasis

The etiologic agent of vulvovaginal candidiasis (VVC) is typically *Candida albicans*, but infections with other *Candida* spp can occur. Symptoms of VVC include local pruritis and burning, vaginal discharge, vaginal soreness, dyspareunia and dysuria [146]. The disease is very common—an estimated 75% of women will have at least one episode of infection. With the advent of over-the-counter preparations and self-initiated therapy, a classification system for VVC can be helpful to guide therapeutic choices (Box 2) [10].

The diagnosis of VVC is often made clinically by the presence of typical symptoms and signs, supplemented by the identification of yeast on a wet preparation or using culture [146]. Ten to 20% of women can have asymptomatic colonization, so treatment should be reserved to those women who have symptoms.

Box 2. Characteristics of uncomplicated and complicated vulvovaginal candidiasis

Uncomplicated VVC
- Sporadic or infrequent VVC
- Mild-to-moderate VVC
- Likely to be *C albicans*
- Non–immune compromised women

Complicated VVC
- Recurrent VVC
- Severe VVC
- Non-albicans candidiasis
- Uncontrolled diabetes, debilitation or immune suppression, or pregnancy

Treatment

In nonpregnant women, uncomplicated VVC is effectively treated with the short-course topical or oral preparations. A recent meta-analysis [147] evaluated ten randomized trials of treatments for symptomatic VVC in pregnancy. Based on five trials, imidazole drugs were more effective than nystatin when treating vaginal candidiasis in pregnancy (OR 0.21, 95% CI 0.16–0.29) [148–152]. Single-dose treatment was no more or less effective than 3 or 4 days treatment; however, two trials involving 81 women showed that treatment lasting for 4 days was less effective than treatment for 7 days (OR 11.7, 95% CI 4.2–29.2). Based on two trials, treatment for 7 days was no more or less effective than treatment for 14 days (OR 0.41, 95% CI 0.16–1.05). In summary, topical imidazole appears to be more effective than nystatin. Treatments for 7 days may be necessary in pregnancy rather than the shorter courses more commonly used in nonpregnant women [147]. Intravaginal agents should be used as listed below; clotrimazole cream and miconazole cream and suppositories are available over the counter:

- Clotrimazole 1% cream, 5 g intravaginally for 7–14 days; or
- Clotrimazole 100 mg vaginal tablet for 7 days; or
- Miconazole 2% cream, 5 g intravaginally for 7 days; or
- Miconazole 100 mg vaginal suppository, one suppository for 7 days; or
- Terconazole 0.4% cream, 5 g intravaginally for 7 days

Recurrent VVC is usually defined as four or more episodes of symptomatic VVC each year. Women who have recurrent VVC should have vaginal cultures performed to confirm the diagnosis, and to identify unusual species such as *Candida glabrata* [153]. Options for initial therapy would include 7 to 14 days of topical azole therapy [10]. Recommended regimens for maintenance include clotrimazole (500 mg dose vaginal suppositories once weekly) and itraconazole (400 mg dose vaginally once monthly or 100 mg dose vaginally once daily).

The optimal treatment of non-albicans VVC remains unknown. Longer duration of therapy (7–14 days) with a non-fluconazole azole drug is recommended as first-line therapy. Women who have severe VVC or those who have debilitating medical conditions also benefit from longer courses (7–14 days) of conventional therapy [10].

Fluconazole, 150 mg orally in a single dose, is often used to treat VVC in nonpregnant patients. A large Scandinavian cohort study [154] compared birth outcomes (malformations, low birthweight, and preterm delivery) of women exposed to fluconazole to the outcomes among 13,327 women who did not receive any prescriptions during their pregnancies. The prevalence of malformations was similar (3.3% versus 5.2% for women who had used fluconazole in the first trimester and controls). Additionally, there were no differences in the risk of preterm delivery (OR 1.17, 95% CI 0.63–2.17) or low birthweight (OR 1.19, 95% CI 0.37–3.79). At the present time, use of fluconazole is not recommended in pregnancy [10].

Molluscum contagiosum

Molluscum contagiosum is a dome-shaped lesion with central umbilication. The lesions are found on epithelial surfaces, but not mucosal membranes. Sometimes a curdlike, milky core can be expressed. Lesions are slow-growing and usually multiple. The etiologic agent is a member of the pox virus family, and infection is usually self-limiting, lasting 6 to 9 months on average. There are two forms of infection. One is seen in young children, resulting from skin-to-skin contact or fomite transmission. The other occurs in adolescents and adults, and results from sexual transmission [155]. Diagnosis of this lesion is primarily made by gross appearance, or a skin biopsy may be performed. Skin biopsy is usually only performed when the diagnosis is in question.

Effective treatment can be achieved with skin curettage, cryotherapy, expression of the umbilicated core, or excision. The latter will cause scarring, so it is not routinely recommended. The use of tri-chloracetic acid is also effective.

Scabies

Scabies is a highly contagious infection caused by *Sarcoptes scabiei*, also known as the itch mite. It is an obligate parasite that burrows into, resides in, and reproduces in human skin. It is worldwide in its distribution and occurs in all races and socioeconomic classes. It is not a vector for other infectious diseases. It is transmitted by intimate contact, often sexual, but casual contact may incur transmission as well. Fomites may also be an important means of transmission.

Most people who have scabies complain of intense pruritus that is worse at night. Areas prone to infection include interdigital spaces, wrists, axillary folds, the peri-umbilical area, pelvic area, and ankles. Infection is usually erythematous and papules or vesicles may be present, with excoriations often seen. The classic linear burrows (short, wavy lines that cross skin lines) should be sought to assist in the diagnosis. Formal diagnosis is made by microscopically examining skin scrapings of suspected sites for the organism, eggs, or feces.

Treatment

The drug of choice for treatment is permethrin cream, which has a higher cure rate than lindane [156]. Permethrin is safe for use in pregnancy and is considered category B. Lindane is also in pregnancy category B, but is not recommended for treatment of pregnant women. Household contacts should also be treated, and recently worn clothes and linens should be washed in hot soapy water and placed in a hot dryer. Fingernails should be trimmed as part of the treatment, and patients should be counseled that the itching may persist for up to 2 weeks after therapy.

Recommended regimen in pregnancy

Permethrin (5% cream): applied to all areas of the body from the neck down and washed off after 8 to 14 hours.

Pediculosis pubis

Pediculosis pubis is also known as the crab louse. An estimated 3 million cases occur each year in the United States. It may be spread through fomites, although the usual acquisition is through sexual contact. This the most contagious of the sexually transmitted infections—the risk of acquiring pediculosis is 95% with a single sexual encounter. Most patients complain of intense pruritus or irritation in the pubic hair area. The diagnosis is made by visualizing the lice, larvae, or nits with a magnifying glass.

Treatment

All sexual contacts, family members, and close contacts should be treated, even if they are asymptomatic. Recently worn clothing or linens should be washed in hot, soapy water and dried in a hot dryer. Dry cleaning is also acceptable. Petrolatum jelly should be applied to infested eyelashes. After therapy, a fine-tooth comb should be used to remove any remaining lice or nits. If lice or eggs are found 5 to 7 days after therapy, the treatment should be repeated.

Recommended regimens for pregnancy

Permethrin (1% cream) should be applied to affected areas and washed off after 10 minutes; or pyrethrin with piperonyl butoxide should be applied to the affected area and washed off after 10 minutes.

Summary

Sexually transmitted infections remain a major public health concern in the United States. Unfortunately, these infections are relatively common during pregnancy, and many are associated with an increase in adverse outcomes among infected women and their infants. Education, screening, treatment, and prevention are important components of prenatal care for women at risk. Because the management of sexually transmitted infections is often altered in the pregnant patient, it is important for all care providers to familiarize themselves with the guidelines for pregnant patients. Optimal treatment and prevention of these sexually transmitted infections is associated with improved pregnancy outcomes.

References

[1] Weinstock H, Berman S, Cates W. Sexually transmitted diseases among American youth: incidence and prevalence estimates, 2000. Perspect Sex Reprod Health 2004;36(1):6–10.

[2] Chesson HW, Blandford JM, Gift TL, et al. The estimated direct medical cost of sexually transmitted diseases among American youth, 2000. Perspect Sex Reprod Health 2004; 36(1):11–9.

[3] Gray RH, Wabwire-Mangen F, Kigozi G, et al. Randomized trial of presumptive sexually transmitted disease therapy during pregnancy in Rakai, Uganda. Am J Obstet Gynecol 2001; 185(5):1209–17.

[4] Goldenberg RL, Thompson C. The infectious origins of stillbirth. Am J Obstet Gynecol 2003;189(3):861–73.

[5] Goldenberg RL, Andrews WW, Yuan AC, et al. Sexually transmitted disease and adverse outcomes of pregnancy. Clin Perinatol 1997;24:23–41.

[6] Centers for Disease Control and Prevention. Sexually transmitted disease surveillance 2002 supplement, syphilis surveillance report. Atlanta (GA): US Department of Health and Human Services, Centers for Disease Control and Prevention; 2004.

[7] Centers for Disease Control and Prevention. Sexually transmitted disease surveillance report 2003. Atlanta (GA): US Department of Health and Human Services, Centers for Disease Control and Prevention; 2004.

[8] Genc M, Ledger WJ. Syphilis in pregnancy. Sex Transm Infect 2000;76:73–9.

[9] Watson-Jones D, Changalucha J, Gumodoka B, et al. Syphilis in pregnancy in Tanzania. I. Impact of maternal syphilis on outcome of pregnancy. J Infect Dis 2002;186(7):940–7.

[10] Centers for Disease Control and Prevention. Sexually transmitted disease treatment guidelines 2002. MMWR Recomm Rep 2002;51(RR-6):1–78.

[11] Hollier LM, Hill J, Sheffield JS, et al. State laws regarding prenatal syphilis screening in the United States. Am J Obstet Gynecol 2003;189(4):1178–83.

[12] Lumbiganon P, Piaggio G, Villar J, et al. The epidemiology of syphilis in pregnancy. Int J STD AIDS 2002;13(7):486–94.

[13] Wendel GD. Gestational and congenital syphilis. Clin Perinatol 1988;15(2):287–303.

[14] Augenbraun M, Workowski K. Ceftriaxone therapy for syphilis: report from the emerging infections network. Clin Infect Dis 1999;29(5):1337–8.

[15] Augenbraun MH. Treatment of syphilis 2001: nonpregnant adults. Clin Infect Dis 2002; 35(Suppl 2):S187–90.

[16] Wendel Jr GD, Sheffield JS, Hollier LM, et al. Treatment of syphilis in pregnancy and prevention of congenital syphilis. Clin Infect Dis 2002;35(Suppl 2):S200–9.

[17] Centers for Disease Control and Prevention. Azithromycin treatment failures in syphilis infections—San Francisco, California, 2002–2003. MMWR Morb Mortal Wkly Rep 2004; 53:197–8.

[18] Wendel Jr GD, Stark BJ, Jamison RB, et al. Penicillin allergy and desensitization in serious infections during pregnancy. N Engl J Med 1985;312:1229–32.

[19] Alexander JM, Sheffield JS, Sanchez PJ, et al. Efficacy of treatment for syphilis in pregnancy. Obstet Gynecol 1999;93:5–8.

[20] Myles TD, Elam G, Park-Hwang E, et al. The Jarisch-Herxheimer reaction and fetal monitoring changes in pregnant women treated for syphilis. Obstet Gynecol 1998;92:859–64.

[21] Nathan L, Twickler DM, Peters MT, et al. Fetal syphilis: correlation of sonographic findings and rabbit infectivity testing of amniotic fluid. J Ultrasound Med 1993;12:97–101.

[22] Hollier LM, Harstad TW, Sanchez PJ, et al. Fetal syphilis: clinical and laboratory characteristics. Obstet Gynecol 2001;97:947–53.

[23] Barton JR, Thorpe Jr EM, Shaver DC, et al. Nonimmune hydrops fetalis associated with maternal infection with syphilis. Am J Obstet Gynecol 1992;167:56–8.

[24] Sheffield JS, Sanchez PJ, Morris G, et al. Congenital syphilis after maternal treatment for syphilis during pregnancy. Am J Obstet Gynecol 2002;186:569–73.

[25] Fleming DT, McQuillian GM, Johnson RE, et al. Herpes simplex virus type 2 in the United States, 1976 to 1994. N Engl J Med 1997;337:1105–11.
[26] Mertz GJ, Rosenthal SL, Stanberry LR. Is herpes simplex virus type 1 (HSV-1) now more common than HSV-2 in first episodes of genital herpes? Sex Transm Dis 2003;30:801–2.
[27] Brown ZA, Selke S, Zeh J, et al. The acquisition of herpes simplex virus during pregnancy. N Engl J Med 1997;337:509–15.
[28] Frenkel LM, Garratty EM, Shen JP, et al. Clinical reactivation of herpes simplex virus type 2 infection in seropositive pregnant women with no history of genital herpes. Ann Intern Med 1993;118:414–8.
[29] Harger JH, Amortegui AJ, Meyer MP, et al. Characteristics of recurrent genital herpes simplex infections in pregnant women. Obstet Gynecol 1989;73:367–72.
[30] Hutto C, Arvin A, Jacobs R, et al. Intrauterine herpes simplex virus infections. J Pediatr 1987;110:97–101.
[31] Ratanajamit C, Vinther Skriver M, Jepsen P, et al. Adverse pregnancy outcomes in women exposed to acyclovir during pregnancy: a population-based observational study. Scand J Infect Dis 2003;35:255–9.
[32] Brown ZA, Benedetti J, Ashley R, et al. Neonatal herpes simplex virus infection in relation to asymptomatic maternal infection at the time of labor. N Engl J Med 1991;324:1247–52.
[33] Koelle DM, Benedetti J, Langenberg A, et al. Asymptomatic reactivation of herpes simplex virus in women after the first episode of genital herpes. Ann Intern Med 1992;116:433.
[34] Wald A, Ericsson M, Krantz E, et al. Oral shedding of herpes simplex virus type 2. Sex Transm Infect 2004;80:272–6.
[35] Brown ZA. HSV-2 specific serology should be offered routinely to antenatal patients. Rev Med Virol 2000;10:141–4.
[36] Wald A, Ashley-Morrow R. Serological testing for herpes simplex virus (HSV)-1 and HSV-2 infection. Clin Infect Dis 2002;35:S173–82.
[37] Scoular A. Using the evidence base on genital herpes: optimizing the use of diagnostic tests and information provision. Sex Transm Infect 2002;78:160–5.
[38] Wilkinson D, Barton S, Cowan F. HSV-2 specific serology should not be offered routinely to antenatal patients. Rev Med Virol 2000;10:145–53.
[39] Rouse DJ, Stringer JS. An appraisal of screening for maternal type-specific herpes simplex virus antibodies to prevent neonatal herpes. Am J Obstet Gynecol 2000;183:400–6.
[40] Barnabas RV, Carabin H, Garnett GP. The potential role of suppressive therapy for sex partners in the prevention of neonatal herpes: a health economic analysis. Sex Transm Infect 2002;78:425–9.
[41] Corey L, Wald A, Patel R, et al. Once-daily valacyclovir to reduce the risk of transmission of genital herpes. N Engl J Med 2004;350:11–20.
[42] Kimberlin DF, Weller S, Whitley RJ, et al. Pharmacokinetics of oral valacyclovir and acyclovir in late pregnancy. Am J Obstet Gynecol 1998;179:846–51.
[43] Stone KM, Reiff-Eldridge R, White AD, et al. Pregnancy outcomes following systemic prenatal acyclovir exposure: conclusions from the international acyclovir pregnancy registry, 1984–1999. Birth Defects Res A Clin Mol Teratol 2004;70:201–7.
[44] Kimberlin DW. Neonatal herpes simplex infection. Clin Microbiol Rev 2004;17:1–13.
[45] Spruance SL, Tyring SK, DeGregorio B, et al. A large-scale placebo-controlled, dose-ranging trial of peroral valaciclovir for episodic treatment of recurrent herpes genitalis. Arch Intern Med 1996;156:1729–35.
[46] Braig S, Luton D, Sibony O, et al. Acyclovir prophylaxis in late pregnancy prevents recurrent genital herpes and viral shedding. Eur J Obstet Gynecol Reprod Biol 2001;96:55–8.
[47] Brocklehurst P, Kinghorn G, Carney O, et al. A randomized placebo controlled trial of suppressive acyclovir in late pregnancy in women with recurrent genital herpes infection. Br J Obstet Gynaecol 1998;105:275–80.

[48] Scott LL, Sanchez PJ, Jackson GL, et al. Acyclovir suppression to prevent cesarean section after first episode genital herpes in pregnancy. Obstet Gynecol 1996;87:69–73.
[49] Scott LL, Hollier LM, McIntire D, et al. Acyclovir suppression to prevent clinical recurrences at delivery after first episode genital herpes in pregnancy: an open-label trial. Infect Dis Obstet Gynecol 2001;9:75–80.
[50] Scott LL, Hollier LM, McIntire D, et al. Acyclovir suppression to prevent recurrent genital herpes at delivery. Infect Dis Obstet Gynecol 2002;10:71–7.
[51] Stray-Pederson B. Acyclovir in late pregnancy to prevent neonatal herpes simples [letter]. Lancet 1990;336:756.
[52] Watts DH, Brown ZA, Money D, et al. A double-blind randomized, placebo-controlled trial of acyclovir in late pregnancy for the reduction of herpes simplex virus shedding and cesarean delivery. Am J Obstet Gynecol 2003;188:836–43.
[53] Sheffield JS, Hollier LM, Hill JB, et al. Acyclovir prophylaxis to prevent herpes simplex virus recurrence at delivery: a systematic review. Obstet Gynecol 2003;102:1396–403.
[54] Scott LL, Alexander J. Cost-effectiveness of acyclovir suppression to prevent recurrent genital herpes in term pregnancy. Am J Perinatol 1998;15:57–62.
[55] American College of Obstetricians and Gynecologists. Management of herpes in pregnancy. Practice Bulletin No. 8, October, 1999.
[56] Brown ZA, Wald A, Ashley-Morrow RA, et al. Effect of serologic status and cesarean delivery on transmission rates of herpes simplex virus from mother to infant. JAMA 2003;289:203–9.
[57] Sheffield JS, Fish DN, Hollier LM, et al. Acyclovir concentrations in human breast milk after valacyclovir administration. Am J Obstet Gynecol 2002;186:100–2.
[58] Christmas JT, Wendel GD, Bawdon RE, et al. Concomitant infection with *Neisseria gonorrhoeae* and *Chlamydia trachomatis* in pregnancy. Obstet Gynecol 1989;74:295–8.
[59] Burkman RT, Tonascia JA, Atienza MF, et al. Untreated endocervical gonorrhea and endometritis following elective abortion. Am J Obstet Gynecol 1976;126:648–51.
[60] Alger LS, Lovchik JC, Hebel JR, et al. The association of *Chlamydia trachomatis*, *Neisseria gonorrhoeae*, and group B streptococci with preterm rupture of the membranes and pregnancy outcome. Am J Obstet Gynecol 1988;159:397–404.
[61] Miller Jr JM, Maupin RT, Mestad RE, et al. Initial and repeated screening for gonorrhea during pregnancy. Sex Transm Dis 2003;30:728–30.
[62] Ickovics JR, Niccolai LM, Lewis JB, et al. High postpartum rates of sexually transmitted infections among teens: pregnancy as a window of opportunity for prevention. Sex Transm Infect 2003;79:469–73.
[63] Mahon BE, Rosenman MB, Graham MF, et al. Postpartum *Chlamydia trachomatis* and *Neisseria gonorrhoeae* infections. Am J Obstet Gynecol 2002;186:1320–5.
[64] Centers for Disease Control and Prevention. Sexually transmitted diseases treatment guidelines 2002. MMWR Recomm Rep 2002;51(RR-6):1–78.
[65] Ramus R, Sheffield JS, Mayfield JA, et al. A randomized trial that compared oral cefixime and intramuscular ceftriaxone for the treatment of gonorrhea in pregnancy. Am J Obstet Gynecol 2001;185:629–32.
[66] Brocklehurst P. Antibiotics for gonorrhoea in pregnancy. Cochrane Database Syst Rev 2002; 2:CD000098.
[67] Ross JD. Systemic gonococcal infection. Genitourin Med 1996;72:404–7.
[68] Bataskov KL, Hariharan S, Horowitz MD, et al. Gonococcal endocarditis complicating pregnancy: a case report and literature review. Obstet Gynecol 1991;78:494–6.
[69] Sozio J, Ness RB. Chlamydial lower genital tract infection and spontaneous abortion. Infect Dis Obstet Gynecol 1998;6:8–12.
[70] Martius J, Krohn MA, Hillier SL, et al. Relationships of vaginal lactobacillus species, cervical *Chlamydia trachomatis*, and bacterial vaginosis to predict preterm birth. Obstet Gynecol 1988;71:89–95.
[71] Gravett MG, Nelson HP, DeRouen T, et al. Independent associations of bacterial vaginosis and *Chlamydia trachomatis* infection with adverse pregnancy outcome. JAMA 1986; 236:1899–903.

[72] Andrews WW, Goldenberg RL, Mercer B, et al. The Preterm Prediction Study: association of second-trimester genitourinary chlamydia infection with subsequent spontaneous preterm birth. Am J Obstet Gynecol 2000;183:662–8.
[73] Blanco JD, Diaz KC, Lipscomb KA, et al. *Chlamydia trachomatis* isolation in patients with endometritis after cesarean section. Am J Obstet Gynecol 1985;152:278–9.
[74] Gibbs RS, Schachter J. Chlamydial serology in patients with intra-amniotic infection and controls. Sex Transm Dis 1987;14:213–5.
[75] Isenberg SJ, Apt L, Wood M. A controlled trial of povidone-iodine as prophylaxis against ophthalmia neonatorum. N Engl J Med 1995;332:562–6.
[76] Black CM. Current methods of laboratory diagnosis of *Chlamydia trachomatis* infections. Clin Microbiol Rev 1997;10:160–84.
[77] Kohl KS, Markowitz LE, Koumans EH. Developments in the screening for *Chlamydia trachomatis*: a review. Obstet Gynecol Clin North Am 2003;30:637–58.
[78] Miller Jr JM. Recurrent chlamydial colonization during pregnancy. Am J Perinatol 1998; 15:307–9.
[79] Adair CD, Gunter M, Stovall TG, et al. Chlamydia in pregnancy: a randomized trial of azithromycin and erythromycin. Obstet Gynecol 1998;91:165–8.
[80] Jacobson GF, Autry AM, Kirby RS, et al. A randomized controlled trial comparing amoxicillin and azithromycin for the treatment of *Chlamydia trachomatis* in pregnancy. Am J Obstet Gynecol 2001;184:1352–4.
[81] Kacmar J, Cheh E, Montagno A, et al. A randomized trial of azithromycin versus amoxicillin for the treatment of *Chlamydia trachomatis* in pregnancy. Infect Dis Obstet Gynecol 2001;9:197–202.
[82] Wehbeh HA, Ruggeirio RM, Shahem SR, et al. Single-dose azithromycin for chlamydia in pregnant women. J Reprod Med 1998;43:509–14.
[83] Silverman NS, Sullivan M, Hochman M, et al. A randomized, prospective trial comparing amoxicillin and erythromycin for the treatment of *Chlamydia trachomatis* in pregnancy. Am J Obstet Gynecol 1994;170:829–32.
[84] Brocklehurst P, Rooney G. Interventions for treating genital *Chlamydia trachomatis* infection in pregnancy. Cochrane Database Syst Rev 2000;(2):CD000054.
[85] Cooper WO, Ray WA, Griffin MR. Prenatal prescription of macrolide antibiotics and infantile hypertrophic pyloric stenosis. Obstet Gynecol 2002;100:101–6.
[86] Cooper WO, Griffin MR, Arbogast P, et al. Very early exposure to erythromycin and infantile hypertrophic pyloric stenosis. Arch Pediatr Adolesc Med 2002;156:647–50.
[87] Sorensen HT, Skriver MV, Pedersen L, et al. Risk of infantile hypertrophic pyloric stenosis after maternal postnatal use of macrolides. Scand J Infect Dis 2003;35:104–6.
[88] Adimora AA. Treatment of uncomplicated genital *Chlamydia trachomatis* infections in adults. Clin Infect Dis 2002;35:S183–6.
[89] Hagensee ME, Slavinsky 3rd J, Gaffga CM, et al. Seroprevalence of human papillomavirus type 16 in pregnant women. Obstet Gynecol 1999;94:653–8.
[90] Ault K. Human papillomavirus infections: diagnosis, treatment and hope for a vaccine. Obstet Gynecol Clin North Am 2003;30:809–17.
[91] Division of STD Prevention. Prevention of genital HPV infection and sequelae: report of an external consultants' meeting. Atlanta (GA): Department of Health and Human Services: Centers for Disease Control and Prevention; 1999.
[92] Wiley DJ, Douglas J, Beutner K, et al. External genital warts: diagnosis, treatment and prevention. Clin Infect Dis 2002;35(Suppl 2):S210–24.
[93] Snyder RR, Hammond TL, Hankins GDV. Human papillomavirus associated with poor healing of episiotomy repairs. Obstet Gynecol 1990;76:664–7.
[94] Goldaber KG, Wendel PJ, McIntire DD, et al. Postpartum perineal morbidity after fourth degree perineal repair. Am J Obstet Gynecol 1993;168:489–93.
[95] Spitzer M, Krumholz BA, Seltzer VL. The multicentric nature of disease related to human papillomavirus infection of the female lower genital tract. Obstet Gynecol 1989;73:303–7.

[96] Silverberg MJ, Thorsen P, Lindeberg H, et al. Condyloma in pregnancy is strongly predictive of juvenile-onset recurrent respiratory papillomatosis. Obstet Gynecol 2003;101:645–52.

[97] Smith EM, Ritchie JM, Yankowitz J, et al. Human papillomavirus prevalence and types in newborns and parents. Sex Transm Dis 2004;31(1):57–62.

[98] Miller RA. Podophyllin. Int J Dermatol 1985;24:491–8.

[99] Shuey DL, Buckalew AR, Wilke TS, et al. Early events following maternal exposure to 5-fluorouracil lead to dysmorphology in cultured embryonic tissues. Teratology 1994;50: 379–86.

[100] Arena S, Marconi M, Frega A, et al. Pregnancy and condyloma. Evaluation about therapeutic effectiveness of laser CO_2 on 115 pregnant women. Minerva Ginecol 2001;53:389–96.

[101] Schwartz DB, Greenberg MD, Daoud Y, et al. Genital condylomas in pregnancy: use of trichloroacetic acid and laser therapy. Am J Obstet Gynecol 1988;158:1407–16.

[102] Garozzo G, Nuciforo G, Rocchi CM, et al. Buschke-Lowenstein tumour in pregnancy. Eur J Obstet Gynecol Reprod Biol 2003;111:88–90.

[103] World Health Organization. Global prevalence and incidence of selected curable sexually transmitted infections. Geneva (Switzerland): World Health Organization; 2001. p. 27.

[104] Klebanoff MA, Carey JC, Hauth JC, et al. Failure of metronidazole to prevent preterm delivery among pregnant women with asymptomatic *Trichomonas vaginalis* infection. N Engl J Med 2001;345:487–93.

[105] Cotch MF, Pastorek II JG, Nugent RP, et al. Demographic and behavioral predictors of *Trichomonas vaginalis* infection among pregnant women. Obstet Gynecol 1991;78:1087–92.

[106] Witkin SS, Inglis SR, Polaneczky M. Detection of *Chlamydia trachomatis* and *Trichomonas vaginalis* by polymerase chain reaction in introital specimens from pregnant women. Am J Obstet Gynecol 1996;175:165–7.

[107] Cotch MF, Pastorek II JG, Nugent RP, et al. *Trichomonas vaginalis* associated with low birth weight and preterm delivery. Sex Transm Dis 1997;24:353–60.

[108] Krieger JN, Tam MR, Stevens CE, et al. Diagnosis of trichomoniasis. JAMA 1988;259: 1223–7.

[109] Draper D, Parker R, Patterson E, et al. Detection of *Trichomonas vaginalis* in pregnant women with the InPouch TV system. J Clin Microbiol 1993;31:1016–8.

[110] Schwebke JR, Morgan SC, Pinson GB. Validity of self obtained vaginal specimens for diagnosis of trichomoniasis. J Clin Microbiol 1997;35:1618–9.

[111] Kurth A, Whittington WLH, Golden MR, et al. Performance of a new, rapid assay for detection of *Trichomonas vaginalis*. J Clin Microbiol 2004;42:2940–3.

[112] Pillay A, Lewis J, Ballard RC. Evaluation of Xenostrip-Tv, a rapid diagnostic test for *Trichomonas vaginalis* infection. J Clin Microbiol 2004;42:3853–6.

[113] Brown HL, Fuller DA, Davis TE, et al. Evaluation of the Affirm Ambient Temperature Transport System for the detection and identification of *Trichomonas vaginalis*, *Gardnerella vaginalis*, and *Candida* species from vaginal fluid specimens. J Clin Microbiol 2001;39: 3197–9.

[114] Lawing L, Hedges S, Schwebke J. Detection of trichomonosis in vaginal and urine specimens from women by culture and PCR. J Clin Microbiol 2000;38:3585–8.

[115] Madico G, Quinn TC, Rompalo A, et al. Diagnosis of *Trichomonas vaginalis* infection by PCR using vaginal swab samples. J Clin Microbiol 1998;36:3205–10.

[116] Gulmezoglu AM. Interventions for trichomoniasis in pregnancy. Cochrane Database Syst Rev 2002;(3):CD000220.

[117] Thin RN, Symonds MAE, Booker R, et al. Double-blind comparison of a single dose and a five-day course of metronidazole in the treatment of trichomoniasis. Br J Vener Dis 1979; 55:354–6.

[118] Hager WD, Brown ST, Kraus SJ, et al. Metronidazole for vaginal trichomoniasis. JAMA 1980;244:1219–20.

[119] Forna F, Gulmezoglu AM. Interventions for treating trichomoniasis in women. Cochrane Database Syst Rev 2003;2:CD000218.

[120] Roe F. Safety of nitroimidazoles. Scand J Infect Dis 1985;46(Suppl):72–8.

[121] Caro-Paton T, Carvajal A, Martin de Diego I, et al. Is metronidazole teratogenic? A meta-analysis. Br J Clin Pharmacol 1997;44:179–82.
[122] Sorensen HT, Larsen H, Jensen ES, et al. Safety of metronidazole during pregnancy: a cohort study of risk of congenital abnormalities, preterm delivery and low birth weight in 124 women. J Antimicrob Chemother 1999;44:854–6.
[123] Gulmezoglu AM, Garner P. Trichomoniasis treatment in women: a systematic review. Trop Med Int Health 1998;3:553–8.
[124] Karhunan M. Placental transfer of metronidazole and tinidazole in early human pregnancy after a single infusion. Br J Clin Pharmacol 1984;18:254–7.
[125] Czeizel AE, Kazy Z, Vargha P. Oral tinidazole treatment during pregnancy and teratogenesis. Int J Gynaecol Obstet 2003;83:305–6.
[126] Klebanoff MA, Carey JC, Hauth JC, et al. Failure of metronidazole to prevent preterm delivery among pregnant women with asymptomatic *Trichomonas vaginalis* infection. N Engl J Med 2001;345:487–93.
[127] Kigozi GG, Brahmbhatt H, Wabwire-Mangen F, et al. Treatment of trichomonas in pregnancy and adverse outcomes of pregnancy: a subanalysis of a radomized trial in Rakai, Uganda. Am J Obstet Gynecol 2003;189:1398–400.
[128] Nelson DB, Macones G. Bacterial vaginosis in pregnancy: current findings and future directions. Epidemiol Rev 2002;24:102–8.
[129] Crowley T, Low N, Turner A, et al. Antibiotic prophylaxis to prevent post-abortal upper genital tract infection in women bacterial vaginosis: randomised controlled trial. BJOG 2001; 108:396–402.
[130] Watts DH, Krohn MA, Hillier SL, et al. Bacterial vaginosis as a risk factor for post-cesarean endometritis. Obstet Gynecol 1990;75:52–8.
[131] Koumans EH, Markowitz LE, Hogan V for the CDC BV Working Group. Indications for therapy and treatment recommendations for bacterial vaginosis in nonpregnant and pregnant women: a synthesis of data. Clin Infect Dis 2002;35:S152.
[132] Hauth JC, Goldenberg RL, Andrews WW, et al. Reduced incidence of preterm delivery with metronidazole and erythromycin in women with bacterial vaginosis. N Engl J Med 1995; 333:1732–6.
[133] Morales WJ, Schorr S, Albritton J. Effect of metronidazole in patients with preterm birth in preceding pregnancy and bacterial vaginosis: a placebo-controlled, double-blind study. Am J Obstet Gynecol 1994;171:345–9.
[134] McDonald HM, O'Loughlin JA, Vigneswaran R, et al. Impact of metronidazole therapy on preterm birth in women with bacterial vaginosis flora (*Gardnerella vaginalis*): a randomised, placebo controlled trial. Br J Obstet Gynaecol 1997;104:1391–7.
[135] Carey JC, Klebanoff MA, Hauth JC, et al. Metronidazole to prevent preterm delivery in pregnant women with asymptomatic bacterial vaginosis. National Institute of Child Health and Human Development Network of Maternal-Fetal Medicine Units. N Engl J Med 2000; 342:534–40.
[136] Ugwumadu A, Manyonda I, Reid F, et al. Effect of early oral clindamycin on late miscarriage and preterm delivery in asymptomatic women with abnormal vaginal flora and bacterial vaginosis: a randomised controlled trial. Lancet 2003;361:983–8.
[137] McGregor JA, French JI, Jones W, et al. Bacterial vaginosis is associated with prematurity and vaginal fluid mucinase and sialidase: results of a controlled trial of topical clindamycin cream. Am J Obstet Gynecol 1994;170:1048–59.
[138] Joesoef MR, Hillier SL, Wiknjosastro G, et al. Intravaginal clindamycin treatment for bacterial vaginosis: effects on preterm delivery and low birth weight. Am J Obstet Gynecol 1995; 173:1527–31.
[139] Rosenstein IJ, Morgan DJ, Lamont RF, et al. Effect of intravaginal clindamycin cream on pregnancy outcome and on abnormal vaginal microbial flora of pregnant women. Infect Dis Obstet Gynecol 2000;8:158–65.
[140] Vermeulen GM, Bruinse HW. Prophylactic administration of clindamycin 2% vaginal cream to reduce the incidence of spontaneous preterm birth in women with an increased recur-

rence risk: a randomised placebo-controlled double-blind trial. Br J Obstet Gynaecol 1999;106: 652–7.
[141] Kurkinen-Raty M, Vuopala S, Koskela M, et al. A randomized controlled trial of vaginal clindamycin for early pregnancy bacterial vaginosis. Br J Obstet Gynaecol 2000;107: 1427–32.
[142] Kekki M, Kurki T, Pelkonen J, et al. Vaginal clindamycin in preventing preterm birth and peripartum infections in asymptomatic women with bacterial vaginosis: a randomized, controlled trial. Obstet Gynecol 2001;97:643–8.
[143] Kiss H, Petricevic L, Husslein P. Prospective randomised controlled trial of an infection screening programme to reduce the rate of preterm delivery. BMJ 2004;329:371–6.
[144] Colli E, Landoni M, Parazzini F. Treatment of male partners and recurrence of bacterial vaginosis: a randomized trial. Genitourin Med 1997;73:267–70.
[145] Vejtorp M, Bollerup AC, Vejtorp L, et al. Bacterial vaginosis: a double-blind randomized trial of the effect of treatment of the sexual partner. Br J Obstet Gynaecol 1988;95:920–6.
[146] Vazquez JA, Sobel JD. Mucosal candidiasis. Infect Dis Clin North Am 2002;16:793–820.
[147] Young GL, Jewell D. Topical treatment for vaginal candidiasis (thrush) in pregnancy. Cochrane Database Syst Rev 2001;(4):CD000225.
[148] Davis JE, Frudenfeld JH, Goddard JL. Comparative evaluation of monistat and mycostatin in the treatment of vulvovaginal candidiasis. Obstet Gynecol 1974;44:403–6.
[149] McNellis D, McLeod M, Lawson J, et al. Treatment of vulvovaginal candidiasis in pregnancy. A comparative study. Obstet Gynecol 1977;50:674–8.
[150] Qualey JR, Cooper C. Monistat cream (miconazole nitrate) a new agent for the treatment of vulvovaginal candidiasis. J Reprod Med 1975;15:123–5.
[151] Ruiz-Velasco V, Rosas-Arceo J. Prophylactic clotrimazole treatment to prevent mycoses contamination of the newborn. Int J Gynaecol Obstet 1978;16:70–1.
[152] Tan CG, Good CS, Milne LJ, et al. A comparative trial of six day therapy with clotrimazole and nystatin in pregnant patients with vaginal candidiasis. Postgrad Med J 1974; 50(Suppl 1):102–5.
[153] Sobel J. Management of patients with recurrent vulvovaginal candidiasis. Drugs 2003; 63:1059–66.
[154] Sorensen HT, Nielsen GL, Olesen C, et al. Risk of malformations and other outcomes in children exposed to fluconazole in utero. Br J Clin Pharmacol 1999;48:234–8.
[155] Felman YM, Nikitas JA. Sexually transmitted molluscum contagiosum. Dermatologic Clinics 1983;1:103–11.
[156] Amer M, El-Garib I. Permethrin vs. crotamiton and lindane in the treatment of scabies. Int J Dermatol 1992;31:357–8.

ELSEVIER
SAUNDERS

Clin Perinatol 32 (2005) 657–670

CLINICS IN
PERINATOLOGY

Herpes Simplex Virus in Pregnancy: New Concepts in Prevention and Management

James Hill, MD[a,*], Scott Roberts, MD[b]

[a]Department of Obstetrics and Gynecology, Department of the Army, Womack Army Medical Center, 2817 Reilly Road MCXC, Fort Bragg, NC 28310-730, USA
[b]Division of Maternal-Fetal Medicine, Department of Obstetrics and Gynecology, University of Texas Southwestern Medical Center, 5323 Harry Hines Boulevard, Dallas, TX 75390-9032, USA

Genital herpes simplex virus (HSV) infection is one of the most common viral sexually transmitted diseases in the United States [1,2]. Based on the findings of the National Health and Nutrition Examination Surveys (NHANES III), it is estimated that 45 million adolescents and adults are infected with genital HSV [1,3]. Most genital herpes infections in the United States are caused by HSV type 2 (HSV-2), and 25% to 30% of women of reproductive age have HSV-2 antibodies [1,4–6]. What is more striking is that genital herpes is frequently under-recognized, and that only 5% to 10% of these women have a history of genital herpes [1,4–6]. Because such a small percentage of women are aware of being infected with HSV, the risk of maternal transmission of this virus to the fetus or newborn is a significant health issue.

Transmission

Genital herpes can be caused by either HSV-1 or HSV-2, and is transmitted through direct sexual contact. Transmission requires physical contact of the susceptible mucosal surfaces or small cracks in the skin of the genital tract with the virus. The virus replicates at these sites and spreads through sensory nerve fibers to the sacral dorsal root ganglia. The risk of acquiring HSV infections

* Corresponding author.
E-mail address: james.b.hill@us.army.mil (J. Hill).

0095-5108/05/$ – see front matter. Published by Elsevier Inc.
doi:10.1016/j.clp.2005.05.008

is related to a number of factors: age of the patient, number of lifetime sexual partners, duration and frequency of sexual intercourse, race, and family income [7]. Women have a higher risk of acquiring HSV-2 from an infected male compared with the acquisition of HSV-2 from female to male, and this is probably related to anatomic differences that lead to greater mucosal surface area exposure [8].

Men and women may intermittently shed HSV virus from the genital tract in the absence of visible lesions or prodromal symptoms. Therefore, transmission of genital herpes can occur as a consequence of close contact with a person who is undergoing asymptomatic viral shedding of HSV [9]. Mertz and colleagues [7] examined asymptomatic shedding, and estimated that 70% of HSV transmission occurs during times when the infected partner is asymptomatic. Because viral shedding is usually asymptomatic, there often is no way to predict when it will occur. A number of recent studies have reported that most cases of neonatal herpes occur in women who asymptomatically shed virus near delivery [5,10–12].

Approximately 1500 to 2000 newborns contract neonatal herpes each year [13]. The overall incidence of neonatal HSV infection was recently described as 1 in 1900 among women who had no HSV antibodies, and 1 in 8000 among women who were seropositive for HSV-1 and HSV-2 [14]. Perinatal transmission is usually the result of contact with the maternal genital tract when it is shedding virus. The frequency of vertical transmission at term is higher among women who acquire HSV near-term (25% to 50%) than among those who have past HSV-2 and reactivated HSV infection at delivery (<1%) [14]. HSV-2 seropositive women asymptomatically shed HSV-2 in their cervical secretions about 2% of the time at delivery [14,15]. Only 1% of exposed infants develop neonatal HSV, presumably due to the protective effects of maternally transferred antibodies. Even though the transmission rate is low, the high seroprevalence of HSV-2 in the general population (30% to 60%) results in over half of the cases of neonatal HSV coming from HSV-2 seropositive mothers [14,16].

Transmission of HSV at the time of delivery can occur when the newborn comes into contact with the virus, as the infant passes through the birth canal. The risk of transmission during this time is dependent upon whether the disease is primary, nonprimary first episode, or recurrent (see the section below on the clinical spectrum of HSV infection). The risk of neonatal transmission is greatest when the mother acquires HSV-1 or HSV-2 infection close to the time of labor, with a 50% risk when the infection is primary ,and a 33% risks when the infection is a nonprimary first episode.

The risk of neonatal transmission is much less, between 1% and 5%, when the mother acquires genital herpes during the first half of pregnancy or prepregnancy and experiences a symptomatic activation at the time of delivery. The risk of acquisition increases when the mother is seronegative for HSV-1 and HSV-2 and her partner is HSV-2 seropositive. Eighty-five percent of neonatal herpes result from viral transmission near delivery. It has also been reported that the fetus may acquire the virus while in utero, due to an ascending cervical infection or transplacental passage of the virus [17,18]. These infections are more likely to occur during a primary outbreak, because of the higher viral load [19].

Diagnosis

It is sometimes very difficult to clinically distinguish between genital herpes infection and other genital ulcerative diseases, and thus the diagnosis of HSV is often missed. The diagnosis of HSV is also frequently missed because the clinical presentation of genital herpes is often atypical. A primary HSV infection may present with multiple grouped vesicles within 2 weeks of exposure to an infectious virus. These vesicles are usually very painful, and can often present with tender lymphadenopathy; however, an atypical HSV outbreak may present as a small fissure, an erythematous region, or raw area in the absence of visible lesions. A strong level of clinical suspicion is important in securing an accurate and prompt diagnosis.

Laboratory confirmation of genital herpes can be performed in several ways. The most widely used test for detecting HSV from clinical specimens is viral isolation by cell culture, which can usually be type-specific (HSV-1 or HSV-2). Although the gold standard for diagnosing HSV infection is isolation of the virus by cell culture, its sensitivity is limited by duration of viral shedding [20,21]. When sampling lesions that are not in the ulcerated state, these lesions should be unroofed and the fluid sampled; however, the sensitivity of this technique is prone to sampling and transport errors.

The presence of intranuclear inclusion and multinuclear giant cells on the Papanicolaou and Tzanck preparation supports the diagnosis of herpes simplex. These tests, however, are not very reliable screening tests, and have a specificity of approximately 65% [9,22,23]. The diagnosis should be confirmed by other tests, such as a viral culture or polymerase chain reaction (PCR).

A more sensitive technique that is readily available in detecting genital HSV is the virus type-specific DNA PCR method [24,25]. Herpes simplex virus DNA detection by PCR is more sensitive in detecting HSV DNA in genital lesions than in viral cultures. Ulcers from recurrent infections are less likely to be culture positive. The DNA PCR is more sensitive than viral isolation by cell culture in detecting asymptomatic genital herpes simple virus [26,27].

Type-specific serologic testing is an adjunct for defining the clinical stage of HSV infection, and the availability of these assays has increased in recent years. These type-specific antibody tests differentiate HSV-1 from HSV-2 by measuring the type-specific glycoproteins (g) G1 and G2 (gG1 for HSV-1 and gG2 for HSV-2), structural proteins that elicit HSV-antibody production from the HSV virion.

Enzyme-linked immunosorbent assay (ELISA)and HSV antigen determination are also very useful assays. The Herpes simplex virus Type I IgG ELISA kit provides a fast and easy method for the detection of antibodies to herpes simplex virus. Diagnosis of HSV-1 or HSV-2 can be confirmed by a significant rise of the

IgG titer within a few days. Focus Technologies (Cypress, California) provides an HSV-1 and HSV-2 ELISA, and an immunoblot test for herpes antibody detection. An additional ELISA, Captia ELISA, is provided by Trinity Biotech (Bray, Ireland). Recently, the Food and Drug Administration (FDA) approved the rapid test formerly known as the POCkit test. It is being marketed as the BiokitHSV-2 Rapid Test (Biokit USA, Lexington, Massachusetts, 800-926-3353) and as the Sure-Vue HSV-2 (Fisher Scientific, Pittsburgh, Pennsylvania). The ELISA assay has a sensitivity of 96% to 100%, and the rapid tests have a sensitivity of 93% to 100%.

Clinical spectrum of herpes simplex virus infection

Genital herpes can be classified into one of three categories: primary, nonprimary first episode, or recurrent infection. Primary genital herpes is defined as the first episode of genital herpes, when the patient has no pre-existing antibodies against HSV-1 or HSV-2.

In the presence of antibodies against HSV-1, first episodes of genital HSV-2 infection are defined as nonprimary first episode, and the symptoms are milder. Recurrent genital herpes simplex infection is characterized by intermittent episodes of viral reactivation with associated pain, burning, and swelling. The duration of symptoms is variable, but may be up to one week. The average number of recurrences for HSV-2 infections is four to six per year.

Herpes in pregnancy

The rate of recurrence for genital herpes is higher in pregnant compared with nonpregnant women, and is more common with HSV-2 than HSV-1 [8,12,28,29]. In a study of 137 patients who had a primary genital herpes infection [29], the likelihood of HSV-2 infections was 60%, compared with 14% who had HSV-1 infection. A patient who has a first symptomatic episode of genital herpes during pregnancy has a risk of an outbreak at delivery of 36% [30,31]. In a study of 457 patients who had HSV-2 isolated from a genital lesion and positive HSV-2 serology [32], 38% of patients had as many as six recurrences, and 20% had more than ten.

The most significant risk of genital herpes infection during pregnancy is transmission of the virus to the fetus or newborn. This transmission occurs more commonly during delivery as the fetus comes into contact with infected vaginal secretions. In-utero transmission occurs less frequently. The rates of neonatal infection were evaluated in a recent study of 40,023 pregnant women who were classified as having primary, nonprimary and reactivation disease with serologic testing and PCR techniques [14]. In this cohort of women, there were 10 cases of neonatal HSV-2 infection and 8 cases of HSV-1 infection. The majority of neonatal infections occurred in women who have first-episode disease (7 of 20 infants), compared with 1 in 46 infants born to mothers who had reactivation infection. Other risk factors for neonatal HSV included younger maternal age, delivery before 38 weeks, HSV isolated from the cervix, and HSV-1 at the time of labor. For all women who were seropositive for HSV, the overall transmission rate was 22 per 100,000 live births.

Some studies, primarily case reports [33–35], have suggested an increased risk of microcephaly, microophthalmia, intracranial calcifications, and chorioretinitis with in-utero infection during the first trimester. There is also an increased risk of spontaneous abortion associated with primary infection in the first trimester; primary infection later in pregnancy has been associated with preterm labor and intrauterine growth restriction.

Because 85% of neonatal herpes cases result from viral transmission near delivery, the American College of Obstetrics and Gynecology [36] currently recommends a cesarean delivery for all women who have an active lesion or prodromal symptoms at delivery. Although the risk of transmission to the newborn is low in mothers who have recurrent infections, cesarean delivery is warranted because of the significant consequences of neonatal herpes infection. It is also important to note that 70% of neonatal herpes cases occur in women who asymptomatically shed virus near delivery [5,10–12]. The risk of transmission to the neonate from asymptomatic shedding in women who have recurrent HSV is estimated to be approximately 1 in 10,000 [14].

In women who have preterm premature rupture of membranes and active genital lesions, there are published case reports supporting conservative management in the setting of recurrent HSV infection. It is important to note that in this setting, administration of antiviral therapy has not been proven to shorten the duration of active lesions [36].

Invasive procedures, such as amniocentesis, percutaneous umbilical-cord blood sampling, and transabdominal chorionic villus sampling, are safe in patients who have recurrent HSV infection. In patients who have primary infection, these procedures should be avoided until after symptoms of lesions resolve. Fetal scalp monitoring may be used in women who have recurrent HSV, as long as no lesions are present and the woman does not have prodromal symptoms. Breastfeeding is only contraindicated in the presence of an active lesion on the breast.

Neonatal herpes

The neonate acquires herpes infections transplacentally, intrapartum, and postpartum. Ninety percent of neonatal herpes is perinatally acquired. More than 70% of infants who have neonatal HSV infection are born to mothers who lack symptoms or signs of HSV lesions at delivery [37]. Transplacental infection is rare and occurs in only up to 5% of newborn herpes cases [38]. These infants are almost invariably born to mothers who have acquired primary HSV infection during pregnancy. The gravid patient should be counseled that congenital herpes infection from recurrent disease is an extremely rare event, if it ever happens at all. Transplacental infection is devastating to the newborn. Hutto and coworkers [38] summarized 13 culture-proven cases in which 92% of newborns presented with skin lesions within 7 days of life. Central nervous system (CNS) lesions were present in 92%, microcephaly in 54%, hydranencephaly in 38%, and microphthalmia in 15%. Overall 31% of newborns who had transplacental infection died. Neurologic sequelae were present in nearly all survivors.

Seventy percent of neonatal HSV infections are caused by HSV-2. Most of the neonatal infections caused by HSV-1 are associated with the acquisition of primary HSV-1 late in pregnancy, and subsequent exposure of the fetus to secretions in the genital tract at time of delivery [39]. HSV-1 infection can be acquired from maternal or paternal oral-labial infection or from a hospital worker.

There are three major categories of neonatal HSV infection: (1) localized infection (skin, eye, and mouth only), (2) CNS involvement (with or without SEM), and (3) disseminated disease (which also includes signs of the first two categories). Neonatal HSV becomes symptomatic in the first 4 weeks of life, with two thirds of the cases having onset in the first week, and 25% to 33% on the first day of life [40,41]. Disseminated disease has the highest mortality and morbidity and presents at mean day 11 of life. CNS infection has a lower mortality but still a high morbidity, and presents at mean day 17 of life. Skin, eye, or mouth (SEM) only infection has both low morbidity when antiviral agents (eg, acyclovir) are used, and presents at mean day 11 of life [37,40]. The discrepancy between the timing of presentation of CNS versus SEM and disseminated disease may be due to later CNS reactivation of asymptomatic disease [42]. In general, CNS morbidity is less severe with HSV-1 than HSV-2 infection [39].

Evidence for improved ascertainment and treatment of disease comes from the National Institutes of Health (NIH) Collaborative Antiviral Study Group [43]. Comparing the frequency of differing presentations of neonatal herpes from 1973 to 1981 with 1982 to 1987, the frequency of disseminated disease decreased from 51% to 23%, and the frequency of SEM increased from 18 to 44%. CNS infection remained stable: 32% to 34%. It may be that improved diagnosis of SEM only and antiviral treatment now prevents some disseminated disease.

Management of genital herpes in pregnancy

Until 1988, a weekly viral culture to detect asymptomatic shedding in late pregnancy was the recommended policy. This was difficult from an administrative standpoint, and increased cesarean rates, much of the time due to inadequate culture surveillance, with results being unavailable before labor and delivery. In the presence of a positive culture, cesarean delivery was recommended. Several cases of neonatal herpes were reported despite the use of weekly surveillance cultures and cesarean delivery [17,44]. Other criticism of this policy came from cost-effectiveness analysis, which estimated a cost of $37 million dollars per case of neonatal herpes averted with the policy of weekly cultures. Most convincing were data from a study by Arvin and colleagues [45] that demonstrated the poor predictive value of antepartum cultures for cervical shedding before labor and delivery.

In 1988, the American College of Obstetricians and Gynecologists (ACOG) [46] recommended that in the absence of visible lesions or prodromal symptoms at the onset of labor, vaginal delivery was acceptable. Furthermore, even in the presence of membrane rupture for more than 4 hours, cesarean delivery was still appropriate in the presence of active genital herpes lesions. Although this policy resulted in a decrease in the number of cesarean deliveries performed for historical maternal genital herpes, there was continued concern that excess cesarean deliveries were being performed in the face of a very low-incidence disease [47]. Randolph and coworkers [48] provided data from a decision analysis reporting 1580 excess cesarean deliveries for every one poor neonatal outcome prevented, and a cost of $2.5 million per case of neonatal HSV averted. They also estimated that four mothers would die from complications of cesarean for every seven babies saved from HSV related deaths.

Several trials have been performed to evaluate the efficacy of acyclovir prophylaxis in decreasing cesarean delivery for genital herpes [49–53]. In general, a reduction in the occurrence of herpes lesions in HSV seropositive gravidas at the time of labor has been demonstrated. This has led to a decrease in the number of cesarean deliveries performed for maternal genital herpes.

Given the new paradigm of acyclovir prophylaxis during the last several weeks of pregnancy to decrease active lesions at the time of delivery, Randolph and colleagues [54] again presented data from a cost-effectiveness analysis. This decision analysis estimated considerable savings with the use of acyclovir prophylaxis followed by cesarean deliveries for genital lesions ($493,641 cost per case of neonatal HSV averted) when compared with the no prophylaxis, cesarean for genital lesions policy ($1,319,457 cost per case). Neither would be considered a bargain in light of the unknown efficacy of cesarean delivery to prevent vertical transmission of herpes in gravidas with recurrent disease. The expense is highlighted with the knowledge that more than 70% of neonates who have herpes infection are born to asymptomatic women [17,37].

In 1999, ACOG reaffirmed the 1988 recommendations concerning performing cesarean section for women who have genital herpes lesions (or prodromal symptoms in the case of recurrent herpes) at the time of labor and delivery. Acyclovir prophyalxis should be considered for women at or beyond 36 weeks who had a first episode of HSV occurring during the current pregnancy, and could be considered for women at risk for recurrent disease [36]. Currently the Centers for Disease Control (CDC) does not recommend use of prophylactic antiviral therapy in gravidas with recurrent genital herpes. There remain concerns about neonatal safety [55,56]. Acyclovir may be administered orally to pregnant women who have first episode genital herpes or severe recurrent herpes, and should be administered intravenously (IV) to pregnant women who have severe HSV infection [55]. It is important to recognize that primary HSV cannot be distinguished from nonprimary first-episode disease unless serology is performed [57].

Important data have come from Brown and coworkers [14], who established very important features of HSV infection. First, there are clear differences between neonatal infection rates in HSV seropositive and seronegative gravidas; the highest rates being in HSV seronegative women who acquired primary HSV-1 and HSV-2 during pregnancy, and whose infants lacked type-specific transplacental antibodies. Second, there was a reduced risk of transmitting HSV-2 and virtually no risk of transmitting HSV-1 infection vertically if women had previous HSV-2 infection. Third, cesarean delivery was found to be protective against the acquisition of neonatal HSV, previously only an assumption. The use of direct fetal monitors was found to increase the risk of neonatal HSV infection in the presence of active cervical shedding [14].

The more recent trials on acyclovir [10,52] found not only reduction in cesarean deliveries for genital lesions present at delivery, but also significant decreases in asymptomatic cervical shedding at the time of delivery. Meta-analysis of five randomized trials (including the two aforementioned) supports this finding [53]. Demonstrating the superior sensitivity of PCR, Watts and coworkers [52] detected asymptomatic cervical shedding in 22% of placebo treated and 0% of acyclovir treated patients within 2 days of delivery ($P = 0.001$). When contrasted with a 2% and a 0% rate of culture positivity in the same patients, one wonders if earlier failed attempts at demonstrating reduced cervical shedding in asymptomatic patients were due to the lack of sensitivity of culture techniques rather than lack of effect of the nucleoside analog [50,51].

Valacyclovir, an acyclovir prodrug, has been evaluated in women who have a history of herpes during pregnancy. One study using 500 mg orally once per day was unable to demonstrate reductions in cervical shedding, lesions at delivery, or cesarean sections [58]; however at 500 mg orally twice per day, reductions in all three were seen [59]. A reduced frequency of dosing compared with acyclovir may increase patient compliance and efficacy.

In December 2004, a cost-effectiveness analysis [60] estimated reasonable incremental costs for screening women universally during pregnancy for HSV-2. Reduced rates of neonatal infection and cesarean deliveries are estimated from identifying and prophylaxing women seropositive for HSV-2. Acceptable costs were also identified for screening partners of seronegative women and treating HSV-2 seropositive partners. The additional benefits of this strategy are small.

Importantly, recurrent lesions remote from the vulva, vagina, and cervix are not indications for cesarean delivery. Cervical shedding occurs no more often than in pregnant gravidas without genital lesions, approximately 2%. These lesions should be covered at the time of labor and delivery to avoid incidental neonatal contact [61].

Antiviral use in pregnancy

The safety of systemic acyclovir, valacyclovir, and famciclovir in pregnant women has not been established. Prospective pregnancy registries established by Glaxo Wellcome (Triangle Park, North Carolina) indicate no increase in teratogenicity to gravidas exposed to acyclovir in the first trimester [62]. Extremely high doses do not result in gene damage to mammalian embryos in culture [63]. There are as yet too few data concerning valacyclovir and famciclovir to make similar claims. A study of the pharmacokinetics of oral acyclovir in pregnancy indicates that acyclovir is well-tolerated, is concentrated in the amniotic fluid, and does not accumulate in the fetus [64]. It passes through the placenta to the fetal circulation by passive diffusion [65]. Concerns over the use of these agents as prophylaxis against cervical shedding and reactivation of disease center around the potential of antivirals to blunt neonatal response to infection, and theoretically to increase the rate of disseminated disease, or to delay diagnosis of infection to a point where neonatal herpes is not high on the differential list (eg, after 1 month of age) [5,56]. Acyclovir is associated with a delayed and decreased antibody response to HSV [66,67]. This may be due to decreased viral load and antigenic stimulation rather than to direct stimulation of the immune system. Reversible nephrotoxicity has been reported in fewer than 5% of patients given acyclovir [68]. Renal toxicity may become apparent in newborns exposed to maternal prophylaxis if they are born having sepsis or have compromised renal function [5].

Acyclovir, valacyclovir, and famciclovir have all been recommended for use to treat first-episode and recurrent HSV infections, as well as for suppression in the nonpregnant individual [55,69]. Acyclovir is an acyclic nucleoside analog that is substrate for HSV-specified thymidine kinase. It concentrates in HSV-infected cells and is converted to the active derivative acyclovir triphosphate. It is not concentrated in uninfected cells. The active form is a competitive inhibitor of viral DNA polymerase and inhibits viral DNA synthesis. Its safety lies in its selectivity for HSV-infected cells [70,71]. Acyclovir has a category C pregnancy classification.

Valacyclovir is the valine ester prodrug of acyclovir, and has a category B pregnancy classification. The ester side chain increases bioavailability in the gut. The ester is removed and more than 99% of the valacyclovir is converted back to acyclovir. The benefit is that the frequency of dosing can be reduced while maintaining therapeutic concentrations of the drug. Valacylovir has been evaluated in pregnancy [58,59]. In a study using valacyclovir at 500 mg once daily for maternal prophylaxis in women at term with recurrent genital herpes Andrews and coworkers [58] evaluated neonatal renal function extensively. There was no evidence of elevated creatinine, blood urea nitrogen, decreased urine output, or decreased glomerular filtration rate. Famciclovir is a prodrug of penciclovir, another antiviral agent in the nucleoside analog family. Penciclovir is not currently available in the United States. Famciclovir is currently being evaluated for its use in pregnancy, and has a category B pregnancy classification [72].

Vaccines

Vaccine trials have attempted to find a vaccine that was not only immunogenic against HSV, but also reduced acquisition of HSV infection and recurrence. Results have been disappointing, but efforts continue toward incorporating vaccines into an overall strategy to battle the current herpes epidemic.

Two study groups [73,74] have looked at the preparation of vaccines that would prevent or control HSV-2 infection. In the first group, two well-executed, placebo-controlled, randomized controlled trials (RCTs) were effected by the Chiron HSV Vaccine Study Group and reported by Corey and colleagues [73] in 1999. In each, a vaccine containing HSV-2 glycoproteins B_2 (gB_2) and D_2 (gD_2) in combination with the adjuvant MF59 were used in the treatment group. All subjects were HIV negative. The first looked specifically at HSV-2 seronegative partners of HSV-2 infected patients. The second looked at HSV-2 seronegative persons attending a sexually transmitted diseases (STDs) clinic who reported a history of STDs and four or more sexual partners within the year before enrollment.

The vaccine was administered at 0, 1, and 6 months, and study participants were followed for 12 months after the last vaccine dose. Although there was induction of high titers of neutralizing antibody, the vaccine proved ineffective in reducing HSV-2 acquisition rate in both men and women, regardless of baseline HSV-1 serostatus. Further, there was no vaccine effect noted on disease modification (eg, asymptomatic cervical shedding).

The GlaxoSmithKline Herpes Vaccine Efficacy Study Group presented findings of two Phase III, placebo-controlled RCTs in 2002 [74]. Again, HSV-2 glycoprotein D was used, but this time alum-3-de-0-acetylated monophosphoyl lipid A (MPL) was used as an adjuvant. All subjects were HIV-negative. The primary group in the first study was HSV-1 and HSV-2 seronegative individuals (268/847 were women). The second study was performed to evaluate safety of the vaccine in subjects of any HSV serologic status. In this second Phase III trial, 710 out of 2491 subjects were HSV-2 seronegative women. Two hundred of these women were also seronegative for HSV-1. Results of both trials indicated significant vaccine efficacy against HSV-2 disease in women who were HSV-1 and HSV-2 seronegative at baseline (73% and 74%, respectively). The researchers also found a nonsignificant trend toward protection from infection in this same group.

This raises an important point both for vaccines and nucleoside analog treatment/suppression. Protection against infection, not just the inhibition of symptoms, is necessary to inhibit the spread of disease [75,76]. There was apparent lack of protection from disease among HSV-1 positive, HSV-2 seronegative women in the second study. This lack of conferred immunity may be explained by partial protection from HSV-2 infection provided by previous HSV-1 infection [73,76].

The difference in success achieved by the D_2-MPL vaccine versus the B_2_D_2-MF59 vaccine may have to do with the enhancement of type 1 helper T cells

(Th-1)by the MPL adjuvant and type 2 helper T cells (Th-2) by MF59. The Th-1 response seen with the MPL adjuvant may be more important for the control of HSV infection at the mucosal level [77,78].

Based upon the later trials presented by Stanberry and colleagues [74], Garnett and coworkers [79] proposed that a vaccine that had efficacy in HSV-1/HSV-2 seronegative women could have a substantial impact on genital herpes epidemiology. The magnitude of the impact extends from women to men, but depends on whether the vaccine prevents asymptomatic viral shedding. This can occur in two ways: (1) prevention of disease is likely to correlate with prevention of asymptomatic shedding; and (2) prevention of infection implicitly prevents asymptomatic shedding [79].

The major adverse consequences of genital herpes are the risk of neonatal infection and the increased susceptibility and transmissibility of HIV. Clearly, trials performed to date are a beginning to our understanding of how we might control the current herpes epidemic. The optimal way to control HSV-2 epidemics potentially involves several approaches, including pre-exposure vaccines, postexposure vaccines, and antiviral therapy [80].

References

[1] Fleming DT, McQuillan GM, Johnson RE, et al (Center for Disease Control and Prevention, Atlanta, Gerorgia; Emory University; Atlanta, Georgia). Herpes simplex virus type 2 in the United States, 1976 to 1994. N Engl J Med 1997;337:1105–11.

[2] Corey L, Handsfield HH. Genital herpes and public health: addressing a global problem. JAMA 2000;283:791–4.

[3] Xu F, Schillinger JA, Sternberg MR, et al. Seroprevalence and coinfection with herpes simplex virus type 1 and type 2 in the United States, 1988–1994. J Infect Dis 2002;185: 1019–24.

[4] Brown ZA, Benedetti JK, Watts DH. A comparison between detailed and simple histories in the diagnosis of genital herpes complicating pregnancy. Am J Obstet Gynecol 1995;172: 1299–303.

[5] Prober CG, Corey L, Brown ZA, et al. The management of pregnancies complicated by genital infections with herpes simplex virus. Clin Infect Dis 1992;15:1031–8.

[6] Armstrong GL, Schillinger J, Markowitz L, et al. Incidence of herpes simplex virus type 2 infection in the United states. Am J Epidemiol 2001;153:912–20.

[7] Mertz GJ, Benedetti J, Selke SA, et al. Risk factors for the sexual transmission of genital herpes. Ann Intern Med 1992;116:197–202.

[8] Wald A, Zeh J, Selke S, et al. Virologic characteristics of subclinical and symptomatic genital herpes infection. N Engl J Med 1995;333:770–5.

[9] Hensleigh PA. Undocumented history of maternal genital herpes followed by neonatal herpes meningitis. J Perinatol 1994;14:216.

[10] Braig S, Luton D, Sibony O, et al. Acyclovir prophylaxis in late pregnancy prevents recurrent genital herpes and viral shedding. Eur J Obstet Gynecol Reprod Biol 2001;96:55–8.

[11] Brown ZA, Selke S, Zeh J, et al. The acquisition of herpes simplex virus during pregnancy. N Engl J Med 1997;337:509–15.

[12] Brown ZA, Benedetti J, Ashley R, et al. Neonatal herpes simplex virus infection in relation to asymptomatic maternal infection at the time of labor. N Engl J Med 1991;324:1247–52.

[13] Whitley RJ, Hutto C. Neonatal herpes simplex virus infections. Pediatr Rev 1985;7:119–26.

[14] Brown ZA, Wald A, Morrow RA, et al. Effect of serologic status and cesarean delivery on transmission rates of herpes simplex virus from mother to infant. JAMA 2003;289:203–9.
[15] Garland SM, Lee TN, Sacks S. Do antepartum herpes simplex virus cultures predict intrapartum shedding for pregnant women with recurrent disease? Infect Dis Obstet Gynecol 1999;7:230.
[16] Nahmias AJ, Lee FK, Beckman-Nahmias S. Sero-epidemiological and -sociological patterns of herpes simplex virus infection in the world. Scand J Infect Dis Suppl 1990;69:19–36.
[17] Stone KM, Brooks CA, Guinan ME, et al. National surveillance for neonatal herpes simplex virus infections. Sex Transm Dis 1989;16:152.
[18] Sweet RL, Gibbs RS. Herpes simplex virus infection. In: Infectious diseases of the female genital tract. 2nd edition. Baltimore (MD): Williams & Wilkins; 1990. p. 144–57.
[19] Maccato M. Herpes in pregnancy. Clin Obstet Gynecol 1993;36:869.
[20] Straus SE, Seidlen M, Takeff H. Effect of oral acyclovir treatment on symptomatic and asymptomatic virus shedding in recurrent genital herpes. Sex Transm Dis 1989;16:107.
[21] Kroon S. Management strategies in herpes: limiting the continued spread of genital herpes. Worthing (UK): PPS Europe Ltd; 1994. p. 17–22.
[22] Nahass GT, Goldstein BA, Zhu WY, et al. Comparison of Tzanck smear, viral culture, and DNA methods in detection of herpes simplex and varicella-zoster infection. JAMA 1992;2268:2541.
[23] Nahmias AJ, Roizman B. Infection with herpes-simplex viruses 1 and 2 (third of three parts). N Engl J Med 1973;289:781.
[24] Cone RW, Hobson AC, Huang MLW. Co-amplified positive control detects inhibition of polymerase chain reactions. J Clin Microbiol 1992;30:3185–9.
[25] Cone RW, Swenson P, Hobson AC, et al. Herpes simplex virus detection from genital lesions: a comparative study using antigen detection (HerpCheck) and culture. J Clin Microbiol 1993;31:1774–6.
[26] Hardy DA, Arvin AM, Yasukawa LL, et al. Use of polymerase chain reaction for successful identification of asymptomatic genital infection with herpes simplex virus in pregnant women at delivery. J Infect Dis 1990;162:1031–5.
[27] Boggess KA, Watts DH, Hobson AC, et al. Herpes simplex virus type 2 detection by culture polymerase chain reaction and relationship to genital symptoms and cervical antibody status during the third trimester of pregnancy. Am J Obstet Gynecol 1997;176:443–51.
[28] Brown ZA, Vontver LA, Benedetti J, et al. Genital herpes in pregnancy: risk factors associated with recurrences and asymptomatic viral shedding. Am J Obstet Gynecol 1985;24:153.
[29] Reeves WC, Corely L, Adams HG, et al. Risk of recurrence after first episode of genital herpes. Relation to HSV type and antibody response. N Engl J Med 1981;305:315.
[30] Frenkel LM, Garatty EM, Shen JP, et al. Clinical reactivation of herpes simplex virus type 2 infection in seropositive women with no history of genital herpes. Ann Intern Med 1993;118:414.
[31] Adler-Storthz K, Dreesman GR, Kaufman RH. A prospective study of herpes simplex virus infection in a defined population in Houston, Texas. Am J Obstet Gynecol 1985;151:582.
[32] Benedetti J, Corey L, Ashley R. Recurrence rates in genital herpes after symptomatic first-episode infection. Ann Intern Med 1994;121:847–54.
[33] Altshuler G. Pathogenesis of congenital herpesvirus infection: case report including a description of the placenta. Am J Dis Child 1974;127:427–9.
[34] Chalhub EF, Baenziger J, Feigen RD, et al. Congenital herpes simplex type II infection with extensive hepatic calcification bone lesions and cataracts: complete postmortem examination. Dev Med Child Neurol 1977;19:527–34.
[35] Monif GR, Kellner KR, Donnelly Jr WH. Congenital herpes simplex type II infection. Am J Obstet Gynecol 1985;152:1000–2.
[36] American College of Obstetricians and Gynecologists. Management of herpes in pregnancy. ACOG practice bulletin Number 8. Washington (DC): American College of Obstetricians and Gynecologists; 1999.
[37] Whitley RJ, Corey L, Arvin A, et al. Changing presentation of herpes simplex virus infection in neonates. J Infect Dis 1988;158:109–16.

[38] Hutto C, Arvin A, Jacobs R, et al. Intrauterine herpes simplex virus infection. J Pediatr 1987; 110:97–101.
[39] Corey L, Whitley RJ, Stone EF, et al. Difference in neurologic outcome after antiviral therapy of neonatal central nervous system herpes simplex virus type 1 versus herpes simplex virus type 2 infection. Lancet 1988;1:1–4.
[40] Koskiniemi M, Happonen JM, Jarvenapaa AI, et al. Neonatal herpes simplex virus infection: a report of 43 patients. Pediatr Infect Dis J 1989;8:30–5.
[41] Sullivan-Bolyai JZ, Hull HF, Wilson C, et al. Presentation of neonatal herpes simplex virus infections: implications for a change in therapeutic strategy. Pediatr Infect Dis J 1986;5:309–14.
[42] Kohl S. A hypothesis on the pathophysiology of neonatal herpes simplex encephalitis: clinical recurrence after asymptomatic primary infection. Pediatr Infect Dis J 1990;9:307–8.
[43] Whitley R, Arvin A, Prober C, et al. A controlled trial comparing vidaribine with acyclovir in neonatal herpes simplex virus infection. N Engl J Med 1991;324:444–9.
[44] Growdon WA, Apodaca L, Cragun J, et al. Neonatal herpes simplex virus infection occurring in second twin of an asymptomatic mother. Failure of a modern protocol. JAMA 1987;257: 508–11.
[45] Arvin AM, Hensleigh PA, Prober CG, et al. Failure of antepartum maternal cultures to predict the infant's risk of exposure to herpes simplex virus at delivery. N Engl J Med 1987;316:240–4.
[46] American College of Obstetricians and Gynecologists. Perinatal herpes simplex virus infections. ACOG technical bulletin 122. Washington (DC): American College of Obstetricians and Gynecologists; 1988.
[47] Roberts SW, Cox SM, Dash J, et al. Genital herpes during pregnancy: no lesions, no cesarean. Obstet Gynecol 1995;85:261–4.
[48] Randolph AG, Washington E, Prober CG. Cesarean delivery for women presenting with genital herpes lesions. Efficacy, risks, and costs [decision analysis]. JAMA 1993;270:77–82.
[49] Stray-Pederson B. Acyclovir in late pregnancy to prevent neonatal herpes simplex. Lancet 1990;336:1594–5.
[50] Scott LL, Sanchez PJ, Jackson GL, et al. Acyclovir suppression to prevent cesarean delivery after first-episode genital herpes. Obstet Gynecol 1996;87:69–73.
[51] Brockelhurst P, Kinghorn G, Carney O, et al. A randomized placebo controlled trial of suppressive acyclovir in late pregnancy in women with recurrent genital herpes infection. Br J Obstet Gynaecol 1998;105:275–80.
[52] Watts DH, Brown ZA, Money D, et al. A double-blind, randomized, placebo-controlled trial of acyclovir in late pregnancy for the reduction of herpes simplex virus shedding and cesarean delivery. Am J Obstet Gynecol 2003;188:836–43.
[53] Sheffield JS, Hollier LM, Hill JB, et al. Acyclovir prophylaxis to prevent herpes simplex virus recurrence at delivery: a symptomatic review. Obstet Gynecol 2003;102:1396–403.
[54] Randolph AG, Hartshorn RM, Washington AE. Acyclovir prophyalxis in late pregnancy to prevent neonatal herpes: a cost-effectiveness analysis. Obstet Gynecol 1996;88:603–10.
[55] Centers for Disease Control and Prevention. Sexually transmitted diseases guidelines. MMWR Morb Mortal Wkly Rep 2002;51(RR06):1–80.
[56] Prober CG. Management of the neonate whose mother received suppressive acyclovir therapy during late pregnancy. Pediatr Infect Dis J 2001;20(1):90–1.
[57] Mertz GL. Epidemiology of genital herpes infections. Infect Dis Clin North Am 1993;7:825–39.
[58] Andrews W, Kimberlin D, Whitley RJ, et al. Valaciclovir suppressive therapy in pregnant women reduces recurrent genital herpes (HSV): results of a randomized trial. Presented at the 23rd annual meeting of the Society for Maternal-Fetal Medicine. San Francisco, February 3–8, 2003.
[59] Sheffield JS, Hill J, Laibl V, et al. Valacyclovir suppression to prevent recurrent herpes at delivery: a randomized controlled trial. Obstet Gynecol 2005;105(Supplement):5s.
[60] Baker D, Brown Z, Hollier LM, et al. Cost-effectiveness of herpes simplex virus type 2 serologic testing and antiviral therapy in pregnancy. Am J Obstet Gynecol 2004;191:2074–84.
[61] Wittek AE, Yeager AS, Au DS, et al. Asymptomatic shedding of herpes simplex virus from the cervix and lesion site during pregnancy. Correlation of antepartum shedding with shedding at delivery. Am J Dis Child 1984;138:439–42.

[62] Reiff-Eldridge R, Heffner CR, Ephross SA, et al. Monitoring pregnancy outcomes after prenatal drug exposure through prospective pregnancy registries: a pharmaceutical company commitment. Am J Obstet Gynecol 2000;182:159–63.
[63] Klug S, Lewandowski C, Blankenbur G, et al. Effect of acyclovir of mammalian embryonic development in culture. Arch Toxicol 1985;58:89–96.
[64] Frenkel LM, Brown ZA, Bryson YJ, et al. Pharmacokinetics of acyclovir in the term human pregnancy and neonate. Am J Obstet Gynecol 1991;164:569–76.
[65] Gilstrap LC, Bawdon RE, Roberts SW, et al. The transfer of the nucleoside analog ganciclovir across the perfused human placenta. Am J Obstet Gynecol 1994;170:967–72 [discussion: 972–3].
[66] Sullender WM, Miller JL, Yasukawa LL, et al. Humoral and cell-mediated immunity in neonates with herpes simplex virus infection. J Infect Dis 1987;155:28–37.
[67] Bernstein DI, Lovett MA, Bryson YJ. The effects of acyclovir on antibody response to herpes simplex virus in primary genital herpetic infections. J Infect Dis 1984;150:7–13.
[68] Balfour HH, Rotbart HA, Feldman S, et al. Acyclovir treatment of varicella in otherwise healthy adolescents. J Pediatr 1992;120:627–30.
[69] American College of Obstetricians and Gynecologists. Gynecologic herpes simplex virus infections. ACOG practice bulletin number 57. Washington (DC): American College of Obstetricians and Gynecologists; 2004.
[70] Elion G, Furman PA, Fyfe JA, et al. Selectivity of action of an antiherpetic agent, 9-(2-hydroxyethoxymethyl) guanine. Proc Natl Acad Sci U S A 1977;79:5716–20.
[71] Brigden D, Whitman P. The clinical pharmacology of acyclovir and its prodrug. Scand J Infect Dis 1985;47(Suppl):33–9.
[72] Leung DT, Sacks SL. Current treatment options to prevent perinatal transmission of herpes simplex virus [review]. Expert Opin Pharmacother 2003;4(10):1809–19.
[73] Corey L, Langenberg AG, Ashley R, et al. Recombinant glycoprotein vaccine for the prevention of genital HSV-2 infection: two randomized controlled trials. JAMA 1999;282:331–40.
[74] Stanberry LR, Spruance SL, Cunningham AL, et al. Glycoprotein-D-adjuvant vaccine to prevent genital herpes. N Engl J Med 2002;347:1652–61.
[75] White PJ, Garnett GP. Use of antiviral treatment and prophylaxis is unlikely to have a major impact on the prevalence of herpes simplex virus type 2. Sex Transm Infect 1999;75(1):49–54.
[76] Langenberg AG, Corey L, Ashley RL, et al. A prospective study of new infections with herpes simplex virus type 1 and type 2. N Engl J Med 1999;341:1432–8.
[77] Stanberry LR, Cunningham AL, Mindel A, et al. Prospects for control of herpes simplex virus disease through immunization. Clin Infect Dis 2000;30:549–66.
[78] Deshpande SP, Kumaraguru U, Rouse BT. Why do we lack an effective vaccine against herpes simplex virus infections? Microbes Infect 2000;2:973–8.
[79] Garnett GP, Dubin G, Slaoui M, et al. The potential epidemiological impact of a genital herpes vaccine for women. Sex Transm Infect 2004;80:24–9.
[80] Schwartz EJ, Blower S. Predicting the potential of individual- and population- level effects of imperfect herpes simplex virus type 2 vaccines. J Infect Dis 2005;191:1734–46.

ELSEVIER
SAUNDERS

Clin Perinatol 32 (2005) 671–696

CLINICS IN
PERINATOLOGY

Human Herpes Viruses in Pregnancy: Cytomegalovirus, Epstein-Barr Virus, and Varicella Zoster Virus

Lisa M. Hollier, MD, MPH*, Heidi Grissom, MD, RPh

Division of Maternal-Fetal Medicine, Department of Obstetrics, Gynecology and Reproductive Sciences, University of Texas Houston Medical School Houston, Lyndon B. Johnson General Hospital, 5656 Kelley Street, Houston, TX 77026, USA

The human herpesvirus family is composed of large, enveloped DNA viruses that have close structural similarity [1]. The family includes the herpes simplex viruses types 1 and 2, varicella zoster virus (VZV), Epstein-Barr virus (EBV), cytomegalovirus (CMV), and human herpes viruses types 6, 7, and 8. These viruses all share the ability to establish latency and reactivate at a later time. Primary maternal infection with CMV and varicella during pregnancy has been associated with fetal abnormalities and neonatal disease.

Cytomegalovirus

CMV (human herpes virus-5) is a double-stranded DNA virus. There are several different types of CMVs, but humans and higher primates are the only known reservoirs for the human subtype of CMV. For the remainder of this discussion, CMV will be used to represent human CMV. Infection with CMV is endemic, and the virus infects individuals worldwide across all social and demographic groups. It is the most common cause of congenital viral infection, affecting approximately 0.2% to 2% of the 4 million infants born in the United States each year, resulting in 10,000 to 80,000 congenitally infected children.

* Corresponding author.
E-mail address: lisa.m.hollier@uth.tmc.edu (L.M. Hollier).

0095-5108/05/$ – see front matter
doi:10.1016/j.clp.2005.05.003 *perinatology.theclinics.com*

Due to the virus's ubiquitous nature, ideal methods for diagnosing, treating, and preventing infection remain elusive.

The cytomegalovirus is the largest member of the herpesvirus family. Similar to the other herpes viruses, the virus consists of a core enclosed by a capsid. The capsid is surrounded by an amorphous tegument, which itself is surrounded by the lipid-containing envelope. The envelope contains numerous immunogenic proteins, the most numerous of which is glycoprotein B [1]. There appears to be genetic heterogeneity within the CMV genotype, and individual strains have been characterized by restriction fragment-length polymorphisms [2–4].

Clinical presentation

Transmission among healthy individuals requires repeated or prolonged intimate contact. In sexually active adolescents and adults, the virus is often transmitted sexually. Among sex workers, the seroprevalence of CMV approximates 100% [5,6]. The incubation period ranges from 20 to 60 days. Infection is mainly asymptomatic in healthy individuals, but immunocompromised individuals may suffer from serious infections [7]. If symptoms are present, typically they include fever, malaise, headache, and myalgia [8,9]. Lymphadenopathy may be present. Laboratory findings may include a relative lymphocytosis, with increased numbers of atypical lymphocytes and thrombocytopenia. The total white blood cell count can be low, normal, or elevated. Moderate elevation of liver enzymes often occurs.

During the initial viral infection, viremia occurs. Not only can the virus be detected in the blood, but tests are also available to detect antigen, viral DNA, and RNA. The body combats the primary infection with a vigorous T lymphocyte response. The appearance of atypical lymphocytes is a hallmark of this infection, and they are predominantly activated CD8+ T lymphocytes. Peak titers of IgM antibody can usually be detected during the first 1 to 3 months after the onset of infection; thereafter the titers decline. In immunocompetent adults, the IgM should be virtually undetectable within 12 months [9]. Although some authors report that CMV IgM can also be produced by the immunocompetent host during nonprimary infections, others disagree [9,10]. The difference in clinical studies may reflect the differing specificity of the antibody assays. The detection of IgM antibodies may not always indicate primary infection, because it can persist for up to 18 months, and 10% of women who have recurrent infection have IgM antibodies [11].

Following resolution of the initial infection, the virus establishes latency within the host tissues. The exact sites of latency are unclear, but are likely diverse. CMV has been isolated in oropharyngeal secretions, urine, feces, semen, vaginal secretions, breast milk, blood, and tears [12]. The excretion of virus after the initial infection may persist for years. Reactivation of latent virus can also occur and lead to recurrent, symptomatic infection.

Most infections resolve spontaneously within a period of 2 to 6 weeks, but complications include heterophil antibody-negative mononucleosis syndrome, hepatitis, and pneumonia. Rare complications can include myocarditis, pleuritis, arthritis, encephalitis, and Guillain-Barrè syndrome [13]. The body's immune response may contribute to the development of a mono syndrome similar to that following EBV.

Diagnosis

Acute infection in immunocompetent adults is often difficult to detect, because the infection is frequently asymptomatic. Primary infection during pregnancy would be optimally diagnosed by the detection of CMV-specific IgG antibodies in a previously seronegative woman; however, although this approach provides a definitive diagnosis, it would require a screening program to evaluate for the presence (or absence) of CMV antibodies in early pregnancy. Because such a screening program is not currently practical, alternative strategies using a combination of tests are described in Fig. 1. Assays for the presence of CMV IgM and IgG should be performed. The identification of significant titers of CMV-specific IgM antibody is suggestive of a primary infection, though caution should be exercised when interpreting positive results. Some assays have reduced specificity, and the false-positive results are an important limitation of IgM detection. The specificity of the antibody detection is higher with assays using multiple CMV antigens. For example, the AxSYM CMV IgM (Abbott Laboratories, Abbott Park, Illinois) uses four different protein antigens and has a specificity of greater than 95% [14]. The detection of CMV-specific IgM in a pregnant woman may be related to a primary infection when a high titer of antibody falls sharply in sequential blood samples. Alternatively, low levels that decline slowly may be related to a primary infection with onset some months earlier, and possibly before pregnancy [9]. Finally, IgM levels may be persistent in a small proportion of women.

When CMV IgM antibodies are detected, testing of the avidity of anti-CMV IgG antibodies can be useful to distinguish primary from nonprimary infection. When antibodies to a particular antigen are initially produced, the antibodies have low avidity for the antigen. As the antibody response matures, the avidity of the antibody for the antigen becomes progressively higher. This test is expressed in terms of the avidity index, which is the percentage of the antibody bound to antigen following a denaturing procedure. The utility of IgG avidity testing in the confirmation of primary CMV infection has been demonstrated [15,16]. In one study of 78 women who had detectable IgM [15], high or intermediate CMV-IgG avidity indexes during the first trimester of pregnancy were not associated with congenital infection; however, one case of congenital CMV infection was observed despite a high avidity index in the second trimester of the pregnancy.

Because of limitations with the serologic diagnosis of primary infections, additional testing of women determined to be at risk is appropriate. The presence of CMV in the blood can be evaluated by detection of the virus itself (in tissue culture), CMV antigens, viral DNA, and viral RNA. There are several qualitative

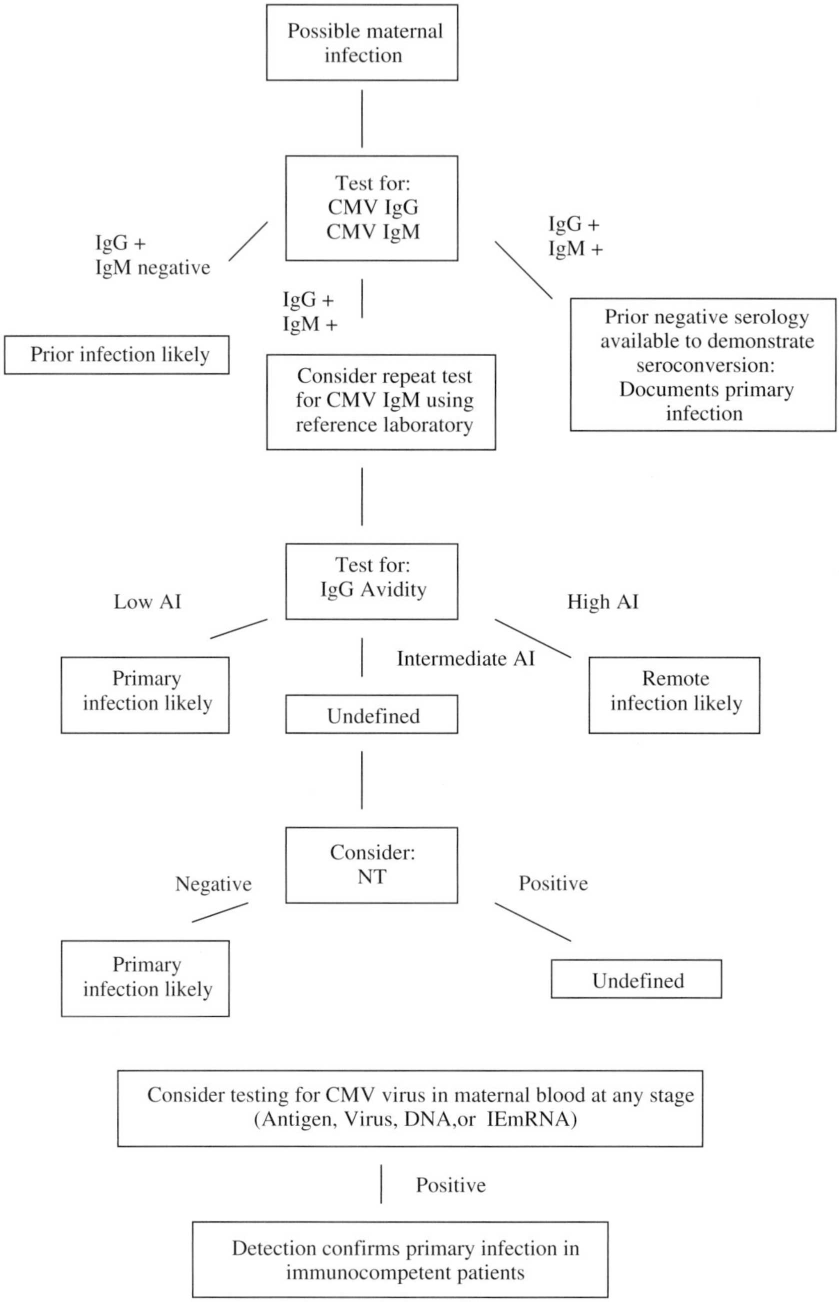

Fig. 1. Diagnosis of maternal CMV infection. AI, avidity index; NT, neutralization test. (*From* Revello M, Gerna G. Diagnosis of congenital HCMV infection. Clin Microbiol Rev 2002;15(4): 680–715; with permission.)

and quantitative polymerase chain reaction tests to detect CMV DNA in blood (eg, COBAS AMPLICOR CMV MONITOR test; Roche Molecular systems, Branchburg, New Jersey) or white blood cells (eg, Digene Hybrid Capture System CMV DNA Assay, Abbott Laboratories, Abbott Park, Illinois). Presence of the virus in the blood of an immunocompetent host may be diagnostic of primary infection, but data are currently limited [17].

Findings suggestive of recurrent infection include the isolation of virus, viral DNA, or viral antigen in clinical samples from a patient having no serologic evidence of primary disease.

Transmission

A number of studies have shown that approximately 50% of pregnant patients are seropositive for CMV antibodies [18–20]. In general, factors associated with higher rates of seropositivity include lower socioeconomic status, maternal age more than 30, nonwhite race, less than college education, and close contact with young children [21].

The incidence of primary infection during pregnancy ranges from 1% to 4%, depending on the characteristics of the population. Risk factors for a primary infection include young age, and the presence of young children in the home [20,22]. The prevalence of symptoms in women who have primary infection during pregnancy ranges from 5% to 68%, and symptoms experienced are similar to nonpregnant patients [9,23].

Congenital CMV infection is acquired by vertical transmission. The incidence ranges from 0.5% to 2% of all live births [24]. Hematogenous spread appears to be the most likely pathway for transmission to the fetus. Studies in animal models suggest that placental infection occurs first, followed by replication of the virus and then transfer to the fetus [25]. Once fetal infection occurs, the virus replicates in the renal tubular epithelium. Virus is excreted into the amniotic fluid and the cycle can repeat. Neonates can also acquire infection from maternal breast milk.

Perhaps in part because maternal viremia tends to occur only with primary infections, women who have evidence of immunity are less likely to exhibit symptomatic vertical transmission. In a large population-based study of 16,218 women [20], a 30% to 40% intrauterine transmission risk with primary CMV infection during pregnancy was reported. In contrast, the risk of transmission with recurrent maternal infection is between 0.2% and 1.8% [26]. Naturally acquired immunity results in a 69% reduction in the risk of congenital CMV infection in future pregnancies [27]. Due to the high prevalence of maternal seropositivity, there are a substantial number of congenitally infected infants born to mothers who have recurrent infection. In women who are seropositive for CMV, reinfection with a different strain of CMV can lead to intrauterine transmission and symptomatic congenital infection [28].

Only 10% to 15% of the congenitally infected infants are symptomatic at birth; however, more severe sequelae are seen in children whose mothers had

Table 1
Abnormalities associated with congenital cytomegalovirus infection

Antenatal ultrasound findings	Early postnatal findings	Late findings
Microcephaly	Microcephaly	Developmental delay
Periventricular calcifications	Periventricular calcifications	Mental retardation
Intracranial hemorrhage	Ventriculomegaly	Seizures
Ventriculomegaly	Chorioretinitis	Visual impairment
Echogenic bowel	Hyperbilirubinemia	Sensorineural hearing loss
Hepatosplenomegaly	Hepatosplenomegaly	
	Hepatitis	
Fetal growth restriction	Growth delay	

Data from Refs. [30–36].

primary infection during pregnancy [29]. Classic abnormalities seen with symptomatic CMV infection are detailed in Table 1 [30–36], and include fetal growth restriction, microcephaly, hepatosplenomegaly, ventriculomegaly, periventricular calcifications, pneumonia, hyperbilirubinemia, and choiroretinitis (Figs. 2, 3). There is a 20% to 30% mortality rate among these symptomatic infants, and 90% of the survivors have serious neurologic sequelae [30]. Most of the deaths result from disseminated intravascular coagulation, hepatic dysfunction, or bacterial superinfection. Mental retardation, hearing loss, visual impairment, seizures, and developmental delay have all been described. In addition, 5% to 15% of the asymptomatic infected infants can exhibit these sequelae, especially sensorineural hearing loss, later in life [31]. In approximately 40%, the bilateral hearing impairment is so severe (50–100 dB) that communication and learning are disturbed [32].

The symptoms of congenital CMV infection appear to be related to the timing of maternal infection. Infection with CMV in the first half of pregnancy is fre-

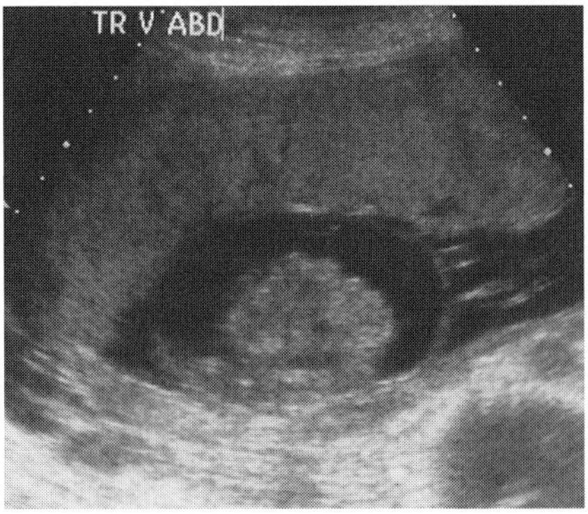

Fig. 2. Ultrasound image of transverse view through the fetal abdomen, demonstrating significant fetal ascites. The fetus was diagnosed with congenital CMV. (Image courtesy of Dr. Joan M. Mastrobattista.)

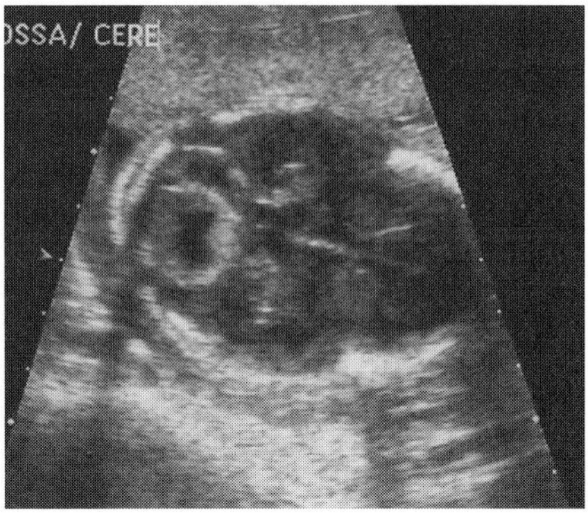

Fig. 3. Ultrasound image of the posterior fossa, demonstrating a hemorrhagic lesion of the cerebellum. The fetus was diagnosed with congenital CMV. (Image courtesy of Dr. Joan M. Mastrobattista.)

quently associated with symptomatic disease, whereas maternal infection in the second half is more commonly associated with initially asymptomatic infections.

Diagnosis of congenital infection

Despite extensive investigation, prenatal diagnosis of CMV remains a complicated and difficult issue. One algorithm for prenatal diagnosis is outlined in Fig. 4. Clinical samples can be obtained with amniocentesis or percutaneous umbilical blood sampling (PUBS). Amniotic fluid can also be removed at the time of blood sampling. Both procedures carry risks of pregnancy loss: approximately 0.5% for amniocentesis and 1% for PUBS. Among infected women, invasive diagnosis carries the risk of iatrogenic fetal infection, though this risk may be more theoretical than actual [37].

In 1971, Davis and colleagues [38] reported making the diagnosis of congenital CMV antenatally by isolating the virus from the amniotic fluid of a symptomatic patient. Because CMV replicates in the renal tubular epithelium and viruria is a consistent finding in infected neonates, detection of virus in amniotic fluid became the gold standard for diagnosis [19,39–43]. The sensitivity of viral culture on amniotic fluid ranges from 77% to 100%, and specificity ranges from 96% to 100% [44,45]. Polymerase chain reaction (PCR) has improved sensitivity compared with culture-based techniques (93% versus 82% in one study of 86 women who had primary CMV) [9]. Both techniques are unlikely to achieve a sensitivity of 100% when used in the clinical arena, because there is a delay between the primary maternal infection and the transmission of quantifiable virus in the fetal compartment. In addition to imperfect sensitivity, the specificity may also be limited. False-positive results from PCR analyses on amniotic fluid have been reported [46,47].

The quantity of cytomegalovirus detected in the amniotic fluid may be related to the presence or absence of abnormalities. Using quantitative PCR techniques, higher quantities of viral DNA were identified in the amniotic fluid of symp-

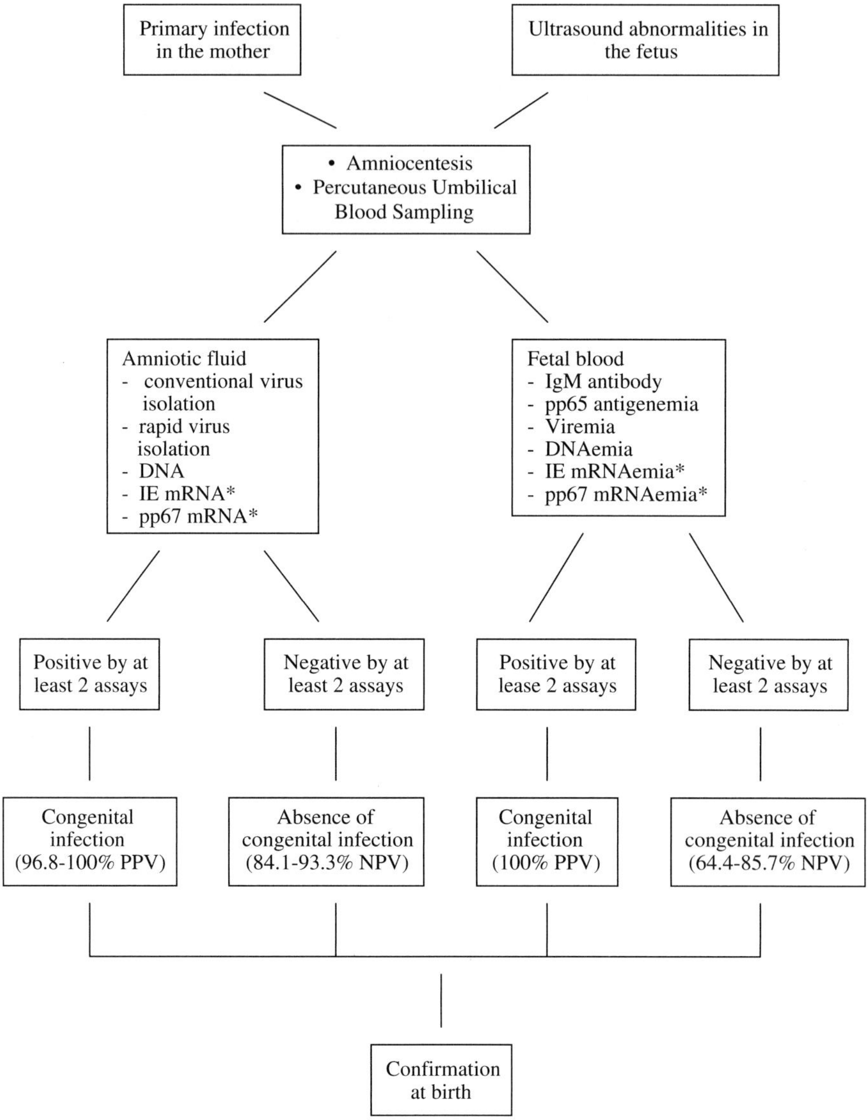

Fig. 4. Diagnosis of fetal CMV infection. NPV, negative predictive value; PPV, positive predictive value. (*From* Revello MG, Gerna G. Pathogenesis and prenatal diagnosis of human cytomegalovirus infection. J Clin Virol 2004;29:81; with permission.)

tomatic fetuses and newborns compared with fetuses and newborns who had no symptoms [9]. Using similar PCR techniques, higher quantities of viral DNA were associated with a higher probability of symptomatic infection [47].

Gestational age also plays an important role in the ability to diagnose CMV prenatally. In a prospective study of 237 women who had suspected primary

CMV infection, repeated samples were obtained from a subset of women [37]. In 24 infected pregnancies with multiple samples, antenatal diagnosis was possible in 96%. The findings were negative in 75% of the samples taken before 21 weeks. Other authors also report diminished sensitivity before 21 weeks [39,43,48]. The time from initial maternal infection to fetal testing is also an important factor. Because of the necessary time interval from maternal infection through transmission, fetal infection, and viral shedding, the amniotic fluid is most likely to be positive if tested 7 weeks or more after the maternal infection [37].

The detection of antiCMV IgM antibodies in fetal blood is believed to be diagnostic of infection, although one false-positive case has been described [40]. As with fetuses infected with syphilis, the presence of fetal IgM is associated with symptomatic infection [49]. One limiting aspect of IgM testing is the high false-negative rate reported by numerous authors [39,42,43]. In addition, fetal IgM is not detectable in the first half of pregnancy, probably because of the immaturity of the fetal immune system.

Fetal blood cultures are rarely positive, even in severely affected cases. It is possible that other hematologic parameters may be useful for determining severity of disease, although they are not diagnostic of CMV. Checking for fetal thrombocytopenia or abnormal liver function tests, as well as determining viral load, has been suggested [41].

Management in pregnancy

Unfortunately, the improvements in the diagnosis of maternal primary CMV infection and the detection of fetal infection have outpaced any improvement in the treatment of infected infants. There are currently no well-studied, effective therapies for CMV in pregnancy. Ganciclovir is a nucleoside analog that is used to treat CMV infection in immunocompromised hosts. The drug has significant hematologic toxicity and, therefore a narrow therapeutic index. Using the ex-vivo human placenta model, ganciclovir was found to cross the placenta by diffusion [50]. Attempts to treat fetuses who have symptomatic infection have not been effective in preventing congenital infection. Intravascular injection of ganciclovir to a 29-week fetus who had significant biochemical abnormalities was associated with a drop in detectable virus in the amniotic fluid; however, the fetus was stillborn at 32 weeks [43]. Treatment of an infected fetus who had intra-amniotic injection of ganciclovir was attempted beginning at 25 weeks gestation. Although a decrease in detectable virus was demonstrated during the pregnancy, the fetus had symptomatic CMV disease at birth [51]. There are reports [52,53] on the use of ganciclovir in neonates, though the findings are not terribly encouraging. In a multicenter clinical trial of ganciclovir for congenital CMV infection, detection of viral excretion in the urine resolved during treatment; however, excretion recurred after therapy was completed. Improvement or stabilization of hearing loss occurred in only 16% of symptomatic infants after 6 months [52].

Foscarnet is a DNA polymerase inhibitor that has been used to treat CMV in AIDS patients and transplant recipients. It also has a narrow therapeutic index, and most treated patients develop some degree of renal impairment. There are currently no reports on its safety or efficacy in pregnancy. There are concerns about its use in neonates because it is deposited in bone, teeth, and cartilage [54].

Prevention

Diagnosis of maternal infection is possible, as is detection of congenital infection; however, beyond therapeutic termination of pregnancy, intervention to prevent adverse neonatal consequences is not possible. Thus, neither the American Academy of Pediatrics [55] nor the American College of Obstetricians and Gynecologists [56] recommends routine serologic screening for CMV immunity.

Because there are no effective therapies for congenital CMV infection, prevention is the ideal solution. Several vaccines have been developed, including a live-attenuated vaccine, a recombinant virus vaccine, and several subunit vaccines. DNA vaccines have been investigated in animals. The live-attenuated vaccine using the Towne strain was tested in clinical trials enrolling renal transplant recipients [57–60]. The vaccine induced both a humoral and cell-mediated immune response. Although there was no difference in the rate of CMV infection among vaccinated individuals, those who received the vaccine had a significant reduction in disease severity. In an older economic analysis published 15 years ago [61], vaccination of seronegative women was determined to be economically beneficial. Despite this finding, there is a reluctance to immunize women of childbearing age, because there are many unanswered questions, including the ability of the vaccine strain to reactivate and infect, the possibility that the vaccine strain may be shed from the cervix and in breast milk, and the possible oncogenic potential of CMV. Additionally, reports of new infections in previously immune individuals raise questions about the efficacy of vaccination in general.

Additional efforts involve the development of vaccines against subunits of the viral genome. Promising subunits include gB (one of the most prevalent envelope glycoproteins), gH (a target of the neutralizing antibody response), and pp65 (a viral phosphoprotein). Animal models showed that immunity induced by the gB subunit vaccine reduced the incidence and severity of congenital CMV disease [62]. Subunit vaccines eliminate the concerns of viral reactivation and oncogenicity.

Women of childbearing age should be educated about CMV and its transmission. This education should include counseling about the careful handling of potentially soiled articles such as diapers, and thorough hand washing when around young children or immunocompromised hosts. Careful attention to hygiene may be effective in helping to prevent transmission. Women could be counseled regarding the utility of serologic screening, and such screening offered to women before pregnancy.

Despite hundreds of publications regarding the effects of CMV infection during pregnancy, it remains the most common cause of congenital viral infection, affecting approximately 10,000 to 80,000 infants born in the United States each year. Ideal methods for diagnosing, treating, and preventing infection remain elusive.

Epstein-Barr virus infections

Epstein-Barr virus (human herpesvirus-6) is a double-stranded DNA virus that is familiar as the cause of infectious mononucleosis. Infection with EBV is common, and most women of reproductive age have been infected in childhood [63]. Whether infection during pregnancy increases the risks of abortion or prematurity remains unclear. Similarly, although congenital abnormalities have been associated with EBV infection, the data do not demonstrate a causal relationship.

Epstein-Barr virus is commonly transmitted through contact with infected oral secretions. The incubation period is about 4 to 6 weeks. Typical signs and symptoms of infectious mononucleosis include fever, sore throat, significant fatigue, and posterior cervical or auricular adenopathy [64]. Other findings can include splenomegaly, hepatomegaly, and a morbilliform or papular rash. Fatigue, myalgias, and malaise may persist for several months after the acute infection has resolved. Liver function tests are elevated in approximately 90% of cases. Serious complications involving the pulmonary, ophthalmologic, neurologic, and hematologic systems can develop. Primary infection is always followed by the establishment of a permanent viral carrier state [65]. In a large prospective study of healthy seropositive adults [66], 90% shed EBV at some point as detected by the standard lymphocyte transformation assay, with 25% shedding virus on every testing occasion.

The virus has a DNA core surrounded by an icosahedral nucleocapsid and by the viral envelope, which contains glycoproteins. Acute infection with EBV is accompanied by activation of B cells, resulting in the production of IgM and IgG antibodies to viral capsid antigens (VCA) soon after infection [67]. Many infected individuals also develop antibodies to early antigens (EA) which usually fall to undetectable levels by 6 months after infection. Antibodies to EBV-associated nuclear antigen (EBNA) develop 3 to 4 weeks after primary infection and probably persist for life [68].

About 1 week after the onset of the disease, many patients develop heterophile antibodies. These are IgM antibodies that do not bind EBV proteins, and are identified using the heterophile test (Monospot). Their production likely results from the polyclonal activation of B cells [65].These antibodies peak at weeks 2 to 5, and are usually present for 3 months after the onset of illness. In some patients, they may persist for up to 1 year. A small proportion of patients who have mononucleosis (10% to 20%) may never develop heterophile antibodies.

In addition to the humoral immune response, early in the course of infection the body mounts a mononuclear lymphocytosis composed primarily of natural killer and T cells specific for EBV [63].The importance of the T cell response is apparent by the severity of the infection in persons who have suppression of cellular immunity. The cytotoxic T cells persist for the life of the host.

Infectious mononucleosis is considered a self-limited illness. Treatment is generally symptomatic, and includes hydration, analgesics, antipyretics, and rest. Corticosteroids, acyclovir, and antihistamines are not routinely recommended [69]. In circumstances of complicated disease, antiviral agents have been used, and corticosteroids may benefit patients who have autoimmune hemolytic anemia, severe thrombocytopenia, and respiratory compromise or severe pharyngeal edema.

The virus cannot be isolated directly in tissue culture, so other methods are required to make a diagnosis. The presence of an atypical lymphocytosis of at least 20%, or atypical lymphocytosis of at least 10% plus lymphocytosis of at least 50% provides support for the diagnosis. The heterophile antibody test (Monospot) has been used frequently for the diagnosis of infectious mononucleosis. This test detects heterophile antibodies, which are typically IgM antibodies that nonspecifically react against different proteins. Monospot tests are positive in approximately 85% of patients who have infectious mononucleosis. Because of the time delay between infection and production of antibodies, the test can be falsely negative early in the illness [70]. A Monospot may remain positive for as long as 12 to 18 months after acute infection with EBV. False-positive and false-negative results may occur. The commercially available Monospot test is somewhat more sensitive than the classic hetrophile test.

Specific serologic tests are helpful in patients who have symptoms and who lack heterophile antibodies, and for individuals who have atypical presentations. Additionally, they provide an advantage over the heterophile test for the diagnosis of recent primary infection. Because antibodies to VCA are produced earlier than those to EBV-associated nuclear antigens, the diagnosis of recent primary infection can be established by the presence of VCA IgM antibodies in the absence of antibodies to EBNA-1 [71]. Three to 6 weeks later, seroconversion to EBNA-1 positivity can also be demonstrated. Unfortunately, serology is complicated by the fact that some individuals do not produce antibodies in the patterns noted, and in some, antibodies persist for prolonged periods. Therefore, a patient who has a primary infection may exhibit the same serologic profile as a patient who had a past infection, and vice versa [71].

A PCR assay has been developed and tested in a population with known EBV status based on serologic testing [72]. Twenty-one (75%) of the patients in the primary EBV infection group, one (4%) of the seronegatives and none of the seropositives had detectable EBV DNA. PCR has also been used to detect EBV DNA in the cerebrospinal fluid of AIDS patients who have lymphoma, and to monitor the amount of EBV DNA in the blood of patients who have lymphoproliferative disease.

Because immunity to EBV typically exceeds 95% of the reproductive population, primary infection during pregnancy is uncommon [73,74]. Evidence regarding the association of congenital abnormalities and EBV infection is limited to small series and case reports. Six cases of primary infection during pregnancy were reported, and those pregnancies ended with spontaneous abortion, preterm delivery, and a variety of congenital abnormalities. The fetuses/neonates were not studied for evidence of infection [75]. Other reported cases of primary infection during pregnancy have resulted in normal outcomes [76,77].

Studies of neonates also do not support a pattern of abnormalities associated with EBV infection. EBV has rarely been identified in the neonate; it was found in none of over 2000 infants screened by detection of spontaneous transformation of lymphocytes, and in only 2 of 67 infants by the detection of virus by PCR.

Varicella

Varicella zoster is a DNA virus in the herpes family. Primary infection with the virus causes chickenpox, one of the contagious childhood exanthems. After resolution of the primary infection, the virus enters the latent phase and remains in the sensory ganglia until reactivation characterized by a rash that occurs along a dermatome distribution—termed herpes zoster (shingles).

Before licensure of the varicella vaccine in 1995, varicella infected approximately 3 million individuals each year [78]. Fewer than 5% of the cases occur in patients 20 years of age or older, but 55% of fatal cases are in this age group [79]. Fortunately, varicella in pregnancy is relatively rare. A large prospective study [80] documented maternal chickenpox in only 5 per 10,000 pregnancies in the United States. The disease is important, however, because complications can be severe. These complications include maternal pneumonia, fetal malformations, and life-threatening neonatal infection. Additionally, recent epidemiologic evidence suggests a recent upward shift in the age distribution of primary infections in the United States, which may reflect the increased use of the vaccine in younger age groups [81].

Clinical presentation

Varicella virus is transmitted by the respiratory route through droplets, and is highly contagious. Approximately 90% of persons without antibodies develop disease after exposure [82]. Varicella enters through the respiratory tract and the conjunctiva. The virus is believed to replicate at the site of entry in the nasopharynx and in regional lymph nodes. Primary viremia occurs 4 to 6 days later, and this stage disseminates the virus to other organs, such as the liver, spleen, and sensory ganglia. Further replication occurs in the vicera, followed by a secondary viremia, with viral infection of the skin [83]. Infected patients are contagious from 1 or 2 days before the lesions develop until all lesions are covered with scabs.

After an incubation period of 10 to 21 days, a prodrome develops that consists of systemic symptoms such as headache, fever, and malaise. One or 2 days later, lesions begin on the face or trunk as small pruritic macules and progress to papules and vesicles. The rash follows a classic course, with several waves of lesions cropping up every 2 to 3 days. The entire course of the disease lasts 6 to 10 days.

The body combats the primary infection with a cell-mediated antibody response. IgG, IgM, and IgA are produced within 2 to 5 days after infection, and reach a maximum after 2 to 3 weeks [84]. The IgG crosses the placenta to provide passive immunity to the fetus. Although there can be significant variation in the number of lesions, all primary infections are believed to confer immunity. Rare reports exist in the literature regarding the development of recurrent clinical chickenpox [85].

Most childhood infections are benign; however, the disease may have serious sequelae in adults. In children, the most common complication of varicella is bacterial superinfection of skin lesions, caused most often by *Staphylococcus aureus* or *Streptococcus pyogenes* [86]. In adults, pneumonia can complicate up to 20% of cases, which may necessitate hospitalization and even mechanical ventilation [78]. Encephalitis is the most serious CNS complication of varicella, and has an incidence of one or two episodes per 10,000 varicella cases, with the highest incidence in adults and infants [87,88]. Other complications include myocarditis, pericarditis, adrenal insufficiency, glomerulonephritis, hepatic dysfunction, and thrombocytopenic purpura [89].

Diagnosis

Both chickenpox and herpes zoster are usually diagnosed clinically by the characteristic presentation of the diseases, and laboratory testing is rarely necessary. Two situations in which diagnosis can provide helpful information are to confirm the diagnosis of varicella before initiation of antiviral therapy in a patient who presents with unusual symptoms, and confirmation of susceptibility or immunity in exposed pregnant women.

Viral culture has been considered the gold standard for diagnosis; however, culturing virus from the fluid in unruptured vesicles is cumbersome. Rapid virus identification techniques are indicated for cases having severe or unusual disease to initiate antiviral therapy [83]. The direct fluorescent antibody test is the method of choice for rapid clinical diagnosis. Specimens should be obtained by unroofing a vesicle and then rubbing the base of the lesion with a polyester swab. Results are generally available in several hours [83]. PCR for varicella DNA has been used for the diagnosis of herpes zoster. In one study [90], PCR results confirmed the clinical diagnosis of zoster in 95% of individuals tested. Primers selected from VZV gene 28 proved to be most sensitive.

Multiple antibody detection assays exist, including enzyme linked immunosorbent assay (ELISA), fluorescent antimembrane antibody (FAMA), latex agglutination (LA), and complement fixation tests. The complement fixation tests are insensitive, and have identified previously infected individuals as susceptible. Although the FAMA test is generally considered more sensitive and specific than the others, the sensitivity of this technique has been questioned. In a recent series [91], the FAMA was negative in 25.7% of patients who had clinical symptoms consistent with varicella. The study cited a prolonged time period between rash onset and maternal blood sampling, particularly in the early years of the study. False-positive results from these tests are rare, but have been reported [92]. Knowledge of the specific type of test performed at each laboratory is important, because of the variability in time necessary to obtain results.

Confirmation of immunity to varicella is the most important step after maternal exposure. Although a positive history of chickenpox is a good indicator of immunity, a negative history of clinical disease is unreliable. One study of pregnant women exposed to varicella used the fluorescent membrane antibody test to screen for immunity [93]. Over 80% of women who had a negative or indeterminate history of prior varicella had antibodies indicative of previous infection. All exposed pregnant women not having a history of varicella should be tested for antibody, although most are immune.

Post-exposure prophylaxis

Administration of varicella zoster immunoglobulin (VZIG) is recommended within 96 hours of exposure of a pregnant woman who is nonimmune to VZV. VZIG is also recommended if it is not possible to obtain antibody test results within this time period. Passive immunity is not effective if VZIG is given more than 5 days after exposure. A preparation of VZIG used in Germany was reported to be 90% effective in preventing severe varicella infection in exposed pregnant women [94]. There have been no prospective studies evaluating the efficacy of VZIG for the prevention of congenital varicella.

The dose recommended by the manufacturer is 125 U (1 vial) per 10 kg, with a maximum of 625 U. This injection volume can exceed 12 mL, so some authorities recommend 4 vials [92]. One vial can be given in each buttock and one in each thigh. This slightly decreased dose does not appear to decrease efficacy. The cost of the immunoglobulin ranges from $105 to $125 per vial in addition to hospital charges. Because of this significant expense, screening for immunity is cost effective [95].

One untested option may be the use of acyclovir for prophylaxis. In a small, randomized trial of prophylaxis of family contacts [96], the severity of the disease was reduced among treated children and infants. Among the 25 who received acyclovir, 4 (16%) developed the disease and 1 (4%) had a fever. On the other hand, all of 25 control subjects developed the disease and 17 (68%) had a fever. Despite the absence of clinical disease, seroconversion was observed in 84% of subjects who received acyclovir. Subsequent studies indicate that oral acyclovir more effectively inhibits replication of VZV in secondary viremia than that of the primary viremia [97].

Treatment

Pregnant patients who develop varicella should be kept isolated from other potentially nonimmune gravidas. Hospitalization is not necessary for all infected women; however, supportive care with fluids, analgesic agents, and antipruritic agents is important. The patient should report to her physician any pulmonary symptoms and any worsening of her skin lesions. Acyclovir is a synthetic nucleoside analog that inhibits replication of human herpes viruses and is currently classified by the Food and Drug Administration (FDA) as a pregnancy Category C drug. Early therapy with oral acyclovir (administered at <24 hours after rash onset) decreases the time to healing of skin lesions in adult varicella, decreases the duration of fever, and lessens symptoms [98,99]. The recommended dose of acyclovir is 800 mg orally five times per day for 7 days. Early acyclovir has been used to limit the course of illness during pregnancy. Some experts have recommended its use [100], whereas others suggest caution in use during pregnancy [99]. Importantly, initiation of oral therapy after the first day of illness is of no value in uncomplicated cases of adult varicella. Finally, as with varicella zoster immune globulin, treatment with acyclovir has not been shown to prevent the effects of congenital varicella syndrome (see below).

Hospitalization and intravenous acyclovir are recommended for any patient who has evidence of disseminated disease or symptoms suspicious for pneumonia (see below) [89]. Currently, no randomized clinical trials have evaluated acyclovir for varicella pneumonia; however, numerous case reports document its use [78,101–103]. Acyclovir has less intrinsic activity in vitro against varicella zoster than against herpes simplex, so larger doses are generally required for clinical varicella zoster infection [104].

Complications

Varicella pneumonia

Pulmonary symptoms typically manifest approximately 4 days after the development of the varicella rash. Typical clinical symptoms include tachypnea, dyspnea, cough, hemoptysis, chest pain, and cyanosis. The radiographic findings are classic: bilateral, diffuse, peribronchial nodular infiltrates. The correlation among the radiographic findings, the auscultatory findings, and the clinical signs and symptoms is poor. Often the auscultatory findings are minimal, whereas the chest radiograph is markedly abnormal. Although some cases can be severe, the disease is often self-limited, with the symptoms resolving within 7 days.

Through the years, controversy has existed regarding the frequency and severity of varicella in pregnant women compared with nonpregnant women. In a recent prospective study, 25% of women who had primary varicella noted dyspnea, but only 5.2% had evidence of varicella pneumonia on chest radiograph [91]. Over time, the mortality rate for varicella pneumonia has decreased dramatically—early reviews reported mortality rates in pregnancy (41%) greatly exceeded rates in nonpregnant women (17%) [105]. Reviews after the advent of acyclovir found a decreased mortality rate of 14% in pregnant women. Recently, a case-control study [106] reported 18 women who had varicella pneumonia with no maternal mortality. The maternal outcome may be related to the gestational age when infected. Women who had varicella pneumonia were significantly more likely to have developed varicella at a later gestational age [106]. Additionally, women developing pneumonia during the third trimester were more likely to die than women infected in the second trimester [78]. Pregnant women who had varicella pneumonia were also significantly more likely to be current smokers.

Intravenous acyclovir at a dose of 7.5 mg/kg every 8 hours has been recommended for the treatment of varicella pneumonia [99]. It has become standard therapy for patients having or at risk of developing complications of varicella infection, despite the fact that there have been no randomized controlled trials for its use in the treatment of varicella pneumonia.

Even in patients who are aggressively treated with antiviral agents, pulmonary failure can occur. In one series of varicella pneumonia in pregnancy at an indigent care facility [102], 40% of patients required intubation with mechanical ventilation. Extracorporeal membrane oxygenation (ECMO) has been used in patients who developed respiratory failure despite treatment with acyclovir [101,107].

Complications of varicella pneumonia include premature delivery, which has been reported in nearly 40% of gravidas having varicella pneumonia in an older series [78]. In a more recent report, 1 out of 18 women delivered early (a preterm stillbirth at 25 weeks within 1 week of the onset of illness) [106]. Other complications associated with hypoxemia include transient heart rate decelerations, which may resolve with improvements in ventilatory status [108].

Fetal effects

In 1947, Laforet and Lynch [109] reported a constellation of findings after maternal varicella infection. The most commonly associated anomalies were central nervous system lesions, limb hypoplasia, and skin scarring. It has been postulated that the manifestations of congenital varicella are the complications of recurrent zoster infections in the fetus [110]. Table 2 outlines many of the abnormalities that have been associated with intrauterine varicella.

The fetal effects of varicella depend largely on the gestational age at infection. Infection in the first trimester does not appear to increase the risk for spontaneous abortion [111]; however, viral infection in the first half of pregnancy can cause a wide variety of malformations that have been associated with infection as late

Table 2
Abnormalities associated with congenital varicella

Neural	Skeletal	Ocular	Cutaneous	Miscellaneous
Microcephaly	Limb hypoplasia	Chorioretinitis	Extensive scarring	Hydronephrosis
Hydrocehalus	Joint contractures	Congenital cataract	Hypopigmentation	Intestinal fibrosis
Cortical atrophy		Hypoplasia of optic disc	Vesicular lesions	Neurogenic bladder
Horner's syndrome				Vocal cord paralysis
Bulbar palsy				Diaphragmatic paralysis

From Scott LL, Hollier LM, Dias K. Perinatal herpesvirus infections: herpes simplex, varicella, and cytomegalovirus. Infect Dis Clin North Am 1997;11(1):40; with permission.

as 24 weeks' gestation. In a compilation of four studies [112], the overall risk of congenital varicella was 2.3%. A recent study [91] followed a cohort of 231 infants born to women who had primary varicella during pregnancy, and found only 1 infant who had definite evidence of varicella and 2 infants (both having hydrops before 20 weeks gestation) who had probable congenital infection, for an overall incidence of 1.3% (95% confidence interval [CI] 0.3, 3.7). Some infants infected in utero are asymptomatic at birth but have delayed manifestations of the illness, including the development of herpes zoster during infancy or early childhood. Rates of 0.8% of infants exposed to VZV during 13 to 24 weeks' gestation and 1.7% of infants exposed during 25 to 36 weeks' gestation have been reported [113].

Prenatal diagnosis

Antenatal diagnosis of congenital varicella syndrome is difficult for several reasons. First, a broad spectrum of abnormalities can result from varicella infection in utero. In addition, attempts at recovering virus from the affected fetus or neonate have been unsuccessful. Immunologic data also have been difficult to obtain. Fetal IgM has been detected in blood samples obtained by cordocentesis. Varicella-specific IgM is present early in the course of fetal infection and may disappear by delivery [114]. This early production with subsequent disappearance of IgM may explain negative IgM results commonly seen in infected infants at delivery. Varicella zoster virus DNA has been identified in the amniotic fluid and in fetal tissue using PCR techniques [115,116].

There is, however, limited enthusiasm for invasive prenatal diagnosis. The risk of congenital varicella syndrome in exposed pregnancies is roughly equivalent to the rates of pregnancy loss associated with the performance of invasive testing. Additionally, identification of the virus in chorionic villi, amniotic fluid, or fetal blood does not predict the severity and effect of fetal infection [115,117].

Noninvasive diagnosis with ultrasound has been investigated. Ultrasound findings that have been associated with congenital varicella include intracranial calcifications, porencephalic cysts, hepatic calcifications (liver echogenicities), echogenic bowel, ascites, hydrops, and polyhydramnios [33,115,118,119]. MRI may prove a useful adjunct to the sonographic detection of fetal effects. Central nervous system abnormalities not visualized on ultrasound (including cerebellar hypoplasia) were identified with MRI [118].

Neonatal infection

Just as fetal effects depend on the gestational age at infection, the neonatal outcome depends on the timing of maternal chickenpox before delivery. Neonatal varicella is the result of transplacental viral infection. The infants most likely to exhibit clinical disease are those whose mothers develop the rash up to 5 days before delivery, or up to 2 days after delivery. This period of increased susceptibility is due to the time required for maternal IgG production and transplacental passage of antibody [120]. The neonatal illness typically develops within 5 to 10 days after delivery, and is of varying severity. Some infants develop a widespread skin rash and severe pneumonia, whereas other infants have only sparse skin lesions, without evidence of systemic disease.

Treatment with VZIG is recommended for all exposed neonates if the mother had chickenpox within 5 days before and up to 2 days after delivery. The appropriate dose is 125 U (1 vial). In addition, VZIG should be given to all exposed neonates who are delivered at or before 28 weeks' gestation, because of the poor antibody transfer at early gestational ages [121]. Unfortunately, VZIG does not prevent 100% of cases of neonatal varicella. In one series [122], half of the infants who received prophylaxis developed chickenpox, though the severity of the infection was reduced.

Herpes zoster

Herpes zoster, or shingles, represents reactivation of latent infection due to the VZV. Reactivation occurs in approximately 3% of infected patients; thus this complication is rare in pregnancy. The disease is characterized by eruption of vesicles on an erythematous base, similar to that seen with the initial infection. With reactivation, however, the lesions occupy a dermatome distribution. Fortunately, congenital varicella has not been reported after herpes zoster in pregnancy.

The new mother who has an outbreak of shingles can be allowed to breastfeed, provided that the skin lesions do not involve the breast. Viral cultures obtained on breast milk from women who had zoster and acute varicella have been negative.

Other considerations

If a child in the home has chickenpox, it is prudent to evaluate the maternal history. If the mother's history is positive for chickenpox or if immunity can be identified by antibody testing, it is reasonable to allow the mother and newborn to return home, because the newborn has transplacentally acquired antibody to varicella. If, however, the mother is not immune, it is reasonable to keep the mother and newborn isolated from the infected child. Another option is to give VZIG to mother and newborn [92].

Prevention

A live, attenuated varicella vaccine (Varivax, Merck, West Point, Pennsylvania) was approved by the FDA in 1995. Two doses of vaccine given 4 to 8 weeks apart are recommended for healthy adolescents and adults [123]. Among persons aged 13 or greater, 78% of vaccinees seroconverted after the first dose of varicella virus vaccine, and 99% seroconverted after a second dose administered 4 to 8 weeks later [123]. Varicella virus vaccine provides 70% to 90% protection against infection and 95% protection against severe disease for 7 to 10 years after vaccination.

Fever following vaccination may occur in up to 10% of vaccinees. The main adverse reactions to the vaccine are tenderness and erythema at the vaccine site and rash. The local symptoms (eg, soreness, swelling, erythema, rash, pruritus, hematoma, pyrexia, induration, and numbness) occur in about 25% of vaccine. In approximately 5%, a mild, varicella-like rash may develop, either at the site of injection or nonlocalized [123]. Transmission of the virus from a vaccine to persons without immunity is possible, particularly in individuals who develop a rash after vaccination. Herpes zoster has been reported among adult vaccinees, with an estimated incidence of 12.8 per 100,000 person years [124]. This risk after vaccination does not appear to be increased compared with individuals who have natural varicella infection.

The vaccine should be considered for susceptible nonpregnant women of child-bearing age. These should be women who are not pregnant, but who may become pregnant in the future [123]. The vaccine is not currently recommended for use in pregnancy. The Advisory Committee on Immunization Practices (ACIP) and the American Academy of Pediatrics (AAP) recommend that a woman not become pregnant for at least 1 month following each dose of the vaccine. This differs from the package insert, which recommends a 3-month delay. The risk of congenital anomalies following vaccination with attenuated varicella vaccine is likely to be very low or absent. Merck, in collaboration with the Centers for Disease Control and Prevention (CDC), has established a Varicella Vaccine in Pregnancy Registry. Women who are given varicella vaccine inadvertently during pregnancy can be enrolled in the registry by calling The Merck National Service Center at 1-800-986-8999 [125].

Summary

Viruses of the human herpesvirus family can have profound effects on pregnancy. Primary maternal infection with CMV or varicella during pregnancy has been associated with fetal abnormalities and neonatal disease. Public awareness of the role of cytomegalovirus in the etiology of developmental disorders and chronic disabilities needs to be increased. With time, we may see new interventions for treatment of infected pregnant women and the prevention of long-term effects. Attention must be focused on the development of a safe and effective vaccine. With the introduction of the varicella vaccine and its efficacy, the rate of varicella in pregnancy is expected to decrease dramatically. Physicians caring for women have the opportunity to prevent the complications of varicella by identifying and vaccinating susceptible women.

References

[1] Roizman B. Herpesviridae: a brief introduction. In: Fields BN, Knipe DM, Howley PM, et al, editors. Field virology. 3rd edition. Philadelphia: Lippincott-Raven; 1996. p. 2221–30.

[2] Chou S. Differentiation of cytomegalovirus strains by restriction analysis of DNA sequences amplified from clinical specimens. J Infect Dis 1990;162:738–42.

[3] Chou S, Dennison KM. Analysis of interstrain variation in cytomegalovirus glycoprotein B sequences encoding neutralization- related epitopes. J Infect Dis 1991;163:1229–34.

[4] de Albuquerque DM, Costa SC. Genotyping of human cytomegalovirus using non-radioactive single-strand conformation polymorphism (SSCP) analysis. J Virol Methods 2003;110(1):25–8.

[5] Karas Z, Blok R, Zabel J, et al. [Seroepidemiologic study of cytomegaly and rubella in pregnant women and prostitutes]. Przegl Epidemiol 1992;46(4):303–7 [Polish].

[6] Dannenmaier B, Alle W, Hoferer EW, et al. Incidences of antibodies to hepatitis B, herpes simplex and cytomegalovirus in prostitutes. Zentralbl Bakteriol Mikrobiol Hyg [A] 1985; 259(2):275–83.

[7] Peckham CS. Cytomegalovirus infection: congenital and neonatal disease. Scand J Infect Dis Suppl 1991;80:82–7.

[8] Klemola E, Kaarianinen L. Cytomegalovirus as a possible cause of a disease resembling infectious mononucleosis. BMJ 1965;2:1099.

[9] Revello MG, Gerna G. Diagnosis and management of human cytomegalovirus infection in the mother, fetus, and newborn infant. Clin Microbiol Rev 2002;15(4):680–715.

[10] Nielsen CM, Hansen K, Andersen HMK, et al. An enzyme labeled nuclear antigen immunoassay for detection of cytomegalovirus IgM antibodies in human serum: specific and nonspecific reactions. J Med Virol 1987;22:67–76.

[11] Maine GT, Lazzarotto T, Landini MP. New developments in the diagnosis of maternal and congenital CMV infection. Expert Rev Mol Diagn 2001;1:19–29.

[12] Britt WJ, Alford CA. Cytomegalovirus. In: Fields BV, Knipe DM, Howley PM, et al, editors. Fields virology. 3rd edition. Philadelphia: Lippincott-Raven; 1996. p. 2493.

[13] Freij BJ, Sever JL. Herpesvirus infections in pregnancy: risks to embryo, fetus, and neonate. Clin Perinatol 1988;15:203–31.

[14] Maine GT, Stricker R, Schuler M, et al. Development and clinical evaluation of a recombinant-antigen-based cytomegalovirus immunoglobulin M automated immunoassay using the Abbott AxSYM analyzer. J Clin Microbiol 2000;38:1476–81.

[15] Bodeus M, Goubau P. Predictive value of maternal-IgG avidity for congenital human cytomegalovirus infection. J Clin Virol 1999;12:3–8.

[16] Grangeot-Keros L, Mayaux MJ, Lebon P, et al. Value of cytomegalovirus (CMV) IgG avidity index for the diagnosis of primary CMV infection in pregnant women. J Infect Dis 1997;175: 944–6.

[17] Revello MG, Zavattoni M, Sarasini A, et al. Human cytomegalovirus in blood of immunocompetent persons during primary infection: prognostic implications for pregnancy. J Infect Dis 1998;177(5):1170–5.

[18] Griffiths PD, Baboonian C, Rutter D, et al. Congenital and maternal cytomegalovirus infection in a London population. Br J Obstet Gynaecol 1991;98(2):135–40.

[19] Lamy M, Mulongo K, Gadisseux J, et al. Prenatal diagnosis of fetal cytomegalovirus infection. Am J Obstet Gynecol 1992;166:91–4.

[20] Stagno S, Pass R, Cloud G, et al. Primary cytomegalovirus infection in pregnancy: incidence, transmission to fetus, and clinical outcome. JAMA 1986;256(14):1904–8.

[21] Griffiths P, Baboonian C, Ashby D. The demographic characteristics of pregnant women infected with cytomegalovirus. Int J Epidemiol 1985;14:447–52.

[22] Yow MD, Williamson DW, Leeds LJ, et al. Epidemiologic characteristics of cytomegalovirus infection in mothers and their infants. Am J Obstet Gynecol 1988;158:1189–95.

[23] Pass RF, Boppana S. Cytomegalovirus. In: Jeffries DJ, Hudson CE, editors. Viral infections in obstetrics and gynecology. New York: Arnold; 1999. p. 35–56.

[24] Yow MD. Congenital cytomegalovirus disease. A NOW problem. J Infect Dis 1989;159:163–7.
[25] Goff E, Griffith B, Booss J. Delayed amplification of cytomegalovirus infection in the placenta and maternal tissues during late gestation. Am J Obstet Gynecol 1987;156(5):1265–70.
[26] Demmler GJ. Infectious Diseases Society of America and Centers for Disease Control. Summary of a workshop on surveillance for congenital cytomegalovirus disease. Rev Infect Dis 1991;13:315–29.
[27] Fowler KB, Stagno S, Pass RF. Maternal immunity and prevention of congenital cytomegalovirus infection. JAMA 2003;289:1008–11.
[28] Boppana SB, Rivera LB, Fowler KB, et al. Intrauterine transmission of cytomegalovirus to infants of women with preconceptional immunity. N Engl J Med 2001;344:1366–71.
[29] Fowler KB, Stagno S, Pass RF, et al. The outcome of congenital cytomegalovirus infection in relation to maternal antibody status. N Engl J Med 1992;326:663–7.
[30] Stagno S, Whitley R. Herpesvirus infections of pregnancy. Part I. Cytomegalovirus and Epstein-Barr virus infections. N Engl J Med 1985;313:1270–4.
[31] Reynolds DW, Stagno S, Stubbs KG, et al. Inapparent congenital cytomegalovirus infection with elevated cord IgM levels: causal relationship with auditory and mental deficiency. N Engl J Med 1974;290(6):291–6.
[32] Gaytant MA, Steegers EAP, Semmekrot BA, et al. Congenital cytomegalovirus infection: review of the epidemiology and outcome. Obstet Gynecol Surv 2002;57:245–56.
[33] Yaron Y, Hassan S, Geva E, et al. Evaluation of fetal echogenic bowel in the second trimester. Fetal Diagn Ther 1999;14(3):176–80.
[34] Pass R, Stagno S, Myers GJ, et al. Outcome of symptomatic congenital cytomegalovirus infection. Results of long-term follow-up. Pediatrics 1980;66(5):758–62.
[35] Malinger G, Lev D, Sahalka N, et al. Fetal cytomegalovirus infection of the brain: the spectrum of sonographic findings. AJNR Am J Neuroradiol 2003;24:28–32.
[36] Noyola DE, Demmler GJ, Nelson CT, et al. Early predictors of neurodevelopmental outcome in symptomatic congenital cytomegalovirus infection. J Pediatr 2001;138(3):325–31.
[37] Liesnard C, Donner C, Brancart F, et al. Prenatal diagnosis of congenital cytomegalovirus infection: prospective study of 237 pregnancies at risk. Obstet Gynecol 2000;95:881–8.
[38] Davis LE, Tweed GV, Chin TD, et al. Intrauterine diagnosis of cytomegalovirus infection: viral recovery from amniocentesis fluid. Am J Obstet Gynecol 1971;109(8):1217–9.
[39] Donner C, Liesnard C, Content J, et al. Prenatal diagnosis of 52 pregnancies at risk for congenital cytomegalovirus infection. Obstet Gynecol 1993;82:481–6.
[40] Hogge WA, Buffone GJ, Hogge JS. Prenatal diagnosis of cytomegalovirus (CMV) infection: a preliminary report. Prenat Diagn 1993;13(2):121–6.
[41] Hohlfeld P, Vial Y, Maillard-Brignon C, et al. Cytomegalovirus fetal infection: prenatal diagnosis. Obstet Gynecol 1991;78(4):615–8.
[42] Lynch L, Daffos F, Emanuel D, et al. Prenatal diagnosis of fetal cytomegalovirus infection. Am J Obstet Gynecol 1991;165(3):714–8.
[43] Nicolini U, Kustermann A, Tassis B, et al. Prenatal diagnosis of congenital human cytomegalovirus infection. Prenat Diagn 1994;14(10):903–6.
[44] Enders G, Bader U, Lindemann L, et al. Prenatal diagnosis of congenital cytomegalovirus infection in 189 pregnancies with known outcome. Prenat Diagn 2001;21:362–77.
[45] Revelo MG, Lilleri D, Zavattoni M, et al. Prenatal diagnosis of congenital human cytomegalovirus infection in amniotic fluid by nucleic acid sequence-based amplification assay. J Clin Microbiol 2003;41:1772–4.
[46] Guerra B, Lazzarotto T, Quarta S, et al. Prenatal diagnosis of symptomatic congenital cytomegalovirus infection. Am J Obstet Gynecol 2000;183:476–82.
[47] Lazzarotto T, Ripalti A, Bergamini G, et al. Prenatal diagnosis of congenital cytomegalovirus infection. J Clin Microbiol 1998;36:3540–4.
[48] Catanzarite V, Dankner WM. Prenatal diagnosis of congenital cytomegalovirus infection: false negative amniocentesis at 20 weeks' gestation. Prenat Diagn 1993;13(11):1021–5.

[49] Revello MG, Zavattoni M, Sarasini A, et al. Prenatal diagnostic and prognostic value of human cytomegalovirus load and IgM antibody response in blood of congenitally infected fetuses. J Infect Dis 1999;180:1320–3.
[50] Gilstrap LC, Bawdon RE, Roberts SW, et al. The transfer of the nucleoside analog ganciclovir across the perfused human placenta. Am J Obstet Gynecol 1994;170(4):967–72.
[51] Revello MG, Gerna G. Diagnosis and implications of human cytomegalovirus infection in pregnancy. Fetal and Maternal Medicine Review 1999;11:117–34.
[52] Whitley RJ, Cloud G, Gruber W, et al. Ganciclovir treatment of symptomatic congenital cytomegalovirus infection: results of a phase II study. J Infect Dis 1997;175(5):1080–6.
[53] Hocker JR, Cook LN, Adams G, et al. Ganciclovir therapy of congenital cytomegalovirus pneumonia. Pediatr Infect Dis J 1990;9:743–5.
[54] Hanshaw JB. Cytomegalovirus infections. Pediatr Rev 1995;16:43–8.
[55] American Academy of Pediatrics. Cytomegalovirus infection. In: Pickering LK, editor. Red book: 2003 report of the Committee on Infectious Diseases. 26th edition. Elk Grove Village (IL): American Academy of Pediatrics; 2003. p. 259–62.
[56] American College of Obstetricians and Gynecologists. Perinatal viral and parasitic infections. ACOG practice bulletin 2000;20:1–13.
[57] Plotkin SA, Furukawa T, Zygraich N, et al. Candidate cytomegalovirus strain for human vaccination. Infect Immun 1975;12(3):521–7.
[58] Balfour HH, Velo PK, Saachs GW. Cytomegalovirus vaccine trial in 400 renal transplant candidates. Transplant Proc 1985;17:81–3.
[59] Plotkin SA, Starr SE, Friedman HM, et al. Effect of Towne live virus vaccine on cytomegalovirus disease after renal transplant. A controlled trial. Ann Intern Med 1991;114:525–31.
[60] Plotkin SA, Higgins R, Kurtz JB, et al. Multicenter trial of Towne strain attenuated virus vaccine in seronegative renal transplant recipients. Transplantation 1994;58:1176–8.
[61] Porath A, McNutt R, Smiley L, et al. Effectiveness and cost benefit of a proposed live cytomegalovirus vaccine in the prevention of congenital disease. Rev Infect Dis 1990;12(1):31–40.
[62] Harrison CJ, Britt WJ, Chapman NM, et al. Reduced congenital cytomegalovirus (CMV) infection after maternal immunization with a guinea pig CMV glycoprotein before gestational primary CMV infection in the guinea pig model. J Infect Dis 1995;172(5):1212–20.
[63] Rickinson AB, Kieff E. Epstein-Barr virus. In: Knipe DM, Howley PM, Griffin DE, editors. Fields virology. 4th edition. Philadelphia: Lippincott, Williams & Wilkins; 2001. p. 2575–627.
[64] Peter J, Ray CG. Infectious mononucleosis. Pediatr Rev 1998;19:276–9.
[65] Henle G, Henle W. The virus as etiologic agent of infectious mononucleosis. In: Epstein MA, Achong BG, editors. The Epstein-Barr virus. Berlin: Springer-Verlag; 1979. p. 297–320.
[66] Yao QY, Rickinson AB, Epstein MA. A reexamination of the Epstein-Barr virus carrier state in healthy seropositive individuals. Int J Cancer 1985;35(1):35–42.
[67] Henle W, Henle G, Horwitz CA. Epstein-Barr virus-specific diagnostic tests in infectious mononucleosis. Hum Pathol 1974;5(5):551–65.
[68] Arvin AM, Maldonado YA. Other viral infections of the fetus and newborn. In: Remington JS, Klein JO, editors. Infectious diseases of the fetus and newborn infant. 5th edition. Philadelphia: WB Saunders; 2001. p. 855–9.
[69] Ebell MH. Epstein-Barr virus infectious mononucleosis. Am Fam Physician 2004;70:1279–87.
[70] Lennette ET. Epstein-Barr virus (EBV). In: Lennette EH, Lennette DA, Lennette ET, editors. Diagnostic procedures for viral, rickettsial, and chlamydial infections. 7th edition. Washington (DC): American Public Health Association; 1995.
[71] Hess RD. Routine Epstein-Barr virus diagnostics from the laboratory perspective: still challenging after 35 years. J Clin Microbiol 2004;42:3381–7.
[72] Pitetti RD, Laus S, Wadowsky RM. Clinical evaluation of a quantitative real time polymerase chain reaction assay for diagnosis of primary Epstein-Barr virus infection in children. Pediatr Infect Dis J 2003;22:736–9.
[73] Le CT, Chang RS, Lipson MH. Epstein-Barr virus infections during pregnancy. A prospective study and review of the literature. Am J Dis Child 1983;137(5):466–8.

[74] Gervais F, Joncas JH. Seropeidemiology in various population groups of the greater Montreal area. Comp Immunol Microbiol Infect Dis 1979;2(2–3):207–12.
[75] Icart J, Didier J, Dalens M, et al. Prospective study of Epstein-Barr virus (EBV) infection during pregnancy. Biomedicine 1981;34(3):160–3.
[76] Fleisher G, Bolognese R. Epstein-Barr virus infections in pregnancy: a prospective study. J Pediatr 1984;104(3):374–9.
[77] Fleisher G, Bolognese R. Infectious mononucleosis during gestation: report of three women and their infants studied prospectively. Pediatr Infect Dis 1984;3(4):308–11.
[78] Smego RA, Asperilla MO. Use of acyclovir for varicella pneumonia during pregnancy. Obstet Gynecol 1991;78:1112–6.
[79] Anonymous. Varicella-related deaths among adults—United States, 1997. MMWR Morb Mortal Wkly Rep 1997;46:409–12.
[80] Sever JA, White LR. Intrauterine viral infections. Annu Rev Med 1969;19:471–86.
[81] Gray GC, Palinkas LA, Kelly PW. Increasing incidence of varicella hospitalizations in the United States Army and Navy personnel. Pediatrics 1990;86:867–73.
[82] Centers for Disease Control and Prevention. Recommendations of the immunization practices advisory committee: varicella-zoster immune globulin for the prevention of chicken pox. MMWR Morb Mortal Wkly Rep 1984;33:84–90.
[83] Centers for Disease Control and Prevention. Epidemiology and prevention of vaccine-preventable diseases. 8th edition. Atlanta (GA): National Immunization Program, Centers for Disease Control and Prevention, US Department of Health and Human Services; 2005.
[84] Cradock-Watson JE, Rideholgh MKS, Bourne MS. Specific immunoglobulin responses after varicella and herpes zoster. J Hyg (Lond) 1979;82:319–36.
[85] Martin KA, Junker AK, Thomas EE, et al. Occurrence of chicken pox during pregnancy in women seropositive for varicella-zoster virus. J Infect Dis 1994;170:991–5.
[86] Aebi C, Ahmed A, Ramilo O. Bacterial complications of primary varicella in children. Clin Infect Dis 1996;23:698–705.
[87] Choo PW, Donahue JG, Manson JE, et al. The epidemiology of varicella and its complications. J Infect Dis 1995;172:706–12.
[88] Preblud SR. Age-specific risks of varicella complications. Pediatrics 1981;68:14–7.
[89] Ramin SM, Gilstrap LC. Varicella zoster in pregnancy. In: Pastorek JG, editor. Obstetric and gynecologic infectious disease. New York: Raven Press; 1994. p. 343–51.
[90] Sauerbrei A, Eichhorn U, Schacke M, et al. Laboratory diagnosis of herpes zoster. J Clin Virol 1999;14(1):31–6.
[91] Harger JH, Ernest JM, Thurnau GR, et al. Frequency of congenital varicella syndrome in a prospective cohort of 347 pregnant women. Obstet Gynecol 2002;100:260–5.
[92] Prober CG, Gershon AA, Grose C, et al. Consensus: varicella-zoster infections in pregnancy and the perinatal period. Pediatr Infect Dis J 1990;9:865–9.
[93] McGregor JA, Mark S, Crawford GP, et al. Varicella zoster antibody testing in the care of pregnant woman exposed to varicella. Am J Obstet Gynecol 1987;157:281–9.
[94] Enders G. Management of varicella-zoster contact and infection in pregnancy using a standardized varicella-zoster ELISA test. Postgrad Med J 1985;61(S4):23.
[95] Rouse DJ, Gardner M, Allen SJ, et al. Management of the presumed susceptible varicella (chickenpox)-exposed gravida: a cost-effectiveness/cost-benefit analysis. Obstet Gynecol 1996; 87:932–6.
[96] Asano Y, Yoshikawa T, Suga S, et al. Postexposure prophylaxis of varicella in family contact by oral acyclovir. Pediatrics 1993;92(2):219–22.
[97] Suga S, Yoshikawa T, Ozaki T, et al. Effect of oral acyclovir against primary and secondary viraemia in incubation period of varicella. Arch Dis Child 1993;69:639–42.
[98] Wallace MR, Bowler WA, Murray NB, et al. Treatment of adult varicella with oral acyclovir. Ann Intern Med 1992;117:358–63.
[99] Ogilvie MM. Antiviral prophylaxis and treatment in chickenpox. A review prepared for the UK Advisory Group on Chickenpox on behalf of the British Society for the Study of Infection. J Infect 1998;36(Suppl 1):31–8.

[100] Kesson AM, Grimwood K, Burgess MA, et al. Acyclovir for the prevention and treatment of varicella zoster in children, adolescents and pregnancy. J Paediatr Child Health 1996;32: 211–7.
[101] Clark GP, Dobson PM, Thickett A, et al. Chicken pox pneumonia, its complications and management: a report of three cases, including the use of extracorporeal membrane oxygenation. Anaesthesia 1991;46(5):376–80.
[102] Cox SM, Cunningham FG, Luby J. Management of varicella pneumonia complicating pregnancy. Am J Perinatol 1990;7(4):300–1.
[103] Hankins GDV, Gilstrap LC, Patterson A. Acyclovir treatment of varicella pneumonia in pregnancy. Crit Care Med 1987;15:336–7.
[104] Moomaw MD, Cornea P, Rathbun RC, et al. Review of antiviral therapy for herpes labialis, genital herpes and herpes zoster. Expert Rev Anti Infect Ther 2003;1(2):283–95.
[105] Harris RE, Rhoades ER. Varicella pneumonia complicating pregnancy: report of a case and review of the literature. Obstet Gynecol 1965;25:734–40.
[106] Harger JH, Ernest JM, Thurnau GR, et al. Risk factors and outcome of varicella-zoster virus pneumonia in pregnant women. J Infect Dis 2002;185:422–7.
[107] Lee WA, Kolla S, Schreiner Jr RJ, et al. Prolonged extracorporeal life support (ECLS) for varicella pneumonia. Crit Care Med 1997;25(6):977–82.
[108] Steyn DW, Odendaal HJ. Fetal resuscitation in a patient with varicella pneumonia and preterm labor. Int J Gynaecol Obstet 1989;30(2):171–5.
[109] Laforet EG, Lynch CL. Multiple congenital defects following maternal varicella. N Engl J Med 1947;236:534–7.
[110] Higa K, Dan K, Manabe H. Varicella-zoster virus infections during pregnancy: hypothesis concerning the mechanisms of congenital malformations. Obstet Gynecol 1987;69(2): 214–22.
[111] Siegel M, Fuerst HT, Peress NS. Comparative fetal mortality in maternal virus disease. N Engl J Med 1966;274:768.
[112] Preblud SR, Cochi SL, Orenstein WA. Varicella-zoster infection in pregnancy. N Engl J Med 1986;315:1416.
[113] Enders G, Miller E, Cradock-Watson J, et al. Consequences of varicella and herpes zoster in pregnancy: prospective study of 1739 cases. Lancet 1994;343:1548–50.
[114] Cuthbertson G, Weiner CP, Giller RH, et al. Prenatal diagnosis of second-trimester congenital varicella syndrome by virus-specific immunoglobulin M. J Pediatr 1987;111(4):592–5.
[115] Puchhammer-Stöckl E, Kunz C, Wagner C, et al. Detection of varicella virus (VZV) DNA in fetal tissue by polymerase chain reaction. J Perinat Med 1994;22(1):65–9.
[116] Lécuru F, Taurelle R, Bernard JP, et al. Varicella zoster virus infection during pregnancy: the limits of prenatal diagnosis. Eur J Obstet Gynecol Reprod Biol 1994;56:67–8.
[117] Isada NB, Paar DP, Johanson MP, et al. In utero diagnosis of congenital varicella zoster virus infection by chorionic villus sampling and polymerase chain reaction. Am J Obstet Gynecol 1991;165:1727–30.
[118] Verstraelen H, Vanzieleghem B, Defoort P, et al. Prenatal ultrasound and magnetic resonance imaging in fetal varicella syndrome: correlation with pathology findings. Prenat Diagn 2003; 23(9):705–9.
[119] Pretorius DH, Hayward I, Jones KL, et al. Sonographic evaluation of pregnancies with maternal varicella infection. J Ultrasound Med 1992;11:45–63.
[120] Miller E, Cradock-Watson JE, Ridehalgh MK. Outcome of newborn babies given anti-varicella-zoster immunogobulin after perinatal infection with varicella-zoster virus. Lancet 1989; ii(8659):371–3.
[121] American Academy of Pediatrics. Varicella zoster infections. In: Pickering LK, editor. Red book: 2003 report of the Committee on Infectious Diseases. 26th edition. Elk Grove Village (IL): American Academy of Pediatrics; 2003. p. 672–86.
[122] Hanngren K, Grandien M, Granstrom G. Effect of zoster immunoglobulin for varicella prophylaxis in the newborn. Scand J Infect Dis 1985;17(4):343–7.
[123] Centers for Disease Control and Prevention. Prevention of varicella: recommendations of

the Advisory Committee on Immunization Practices. MMWR Morb Mortal Wkly Rep 1996; 45(RR-11):1–25.
[124] Hammerschlag MR, Gershon AA, Steinberg SP, et al. Herpes zoster in an adult recipient of live attenuated varicella vaccine. J Infect Dis 1989;160:535–7.
[125] National Immunization Program. Varicella vaccine—FAQs related to pregnancy. Available at: http://www.cdc.gov/nip/vaccine/varicella/faqs-clinic-vac-preg.htm. Accessed March 21, 2005.

ELSEVIER
SAUNDERS

CLINICS IN
PERINATOLOGY

Clin Perinatol 32 (2005) 697–704

Diagnosis and Management of Human Parvovirus B19 Infection

Mildred M. Ramirez, MD*, Joan M. Mastrobattista, MD

Division of Maternal-Fetal Medicine, Department of Obstetrics, Gynecology, and Reproductive Sciences, University of Texas Health Science Center at Houston, 6431 Fannin, Suite 3.604, Houston, TX 77030, USA

Thirty years have passed since the initial identification of human parvovirus B19 in 1975 by Cossart and colleagues [1]. B19 is a small, nonenveloped, single-stranded DNA virus that causes erythema infectiosum (fifth disease) in children [2,3]. Lacking a lipid envelope makes B19 resistant to antiviral procedures such as detergent and heat treatments [4]. Infection with B19 is limited to humans. Transmission is mainly by respiratory secretions and in some instances by blood products [4]. Winter and spring months are the endemic period for B19. Seroconversion of B19 depends on seasonality and the locale.

The annual incidence of acute B19 infection in pregnancy has been estimated to be 1 in 400 pregnancies [5]. The risk of acute infection is highest in susceptible pregnant women with children ages 6 to 7 years, followed by number of children in household, and school teachers [6]. Because the risk of acquiring B19 infection is highest in women who have school-aged children at home, strategies of decreasing occupational exposure in susceptible pregnant women are ineffective; however, case reports of fetal hydrops and death have occurred after maternal infection with B19 [7]. The obstetrician is often faced with a phone call from a frantic pregnant woman who has been exposed to B19. In this article, the authors review the natural history of B19, pathophysiology, diagnosis, management schemes, and both noninvasive and invasive methods to monitor for fetal anemia.

* Corresponding author.
E-mail address: mildred.m.ramirez@uth.tmc.edu (M.M. Ramirez).

doi:10.1016/j.clp.2005.04.003 ***perinatology.theclinics.com***

Natural history and pathogenesis

B19 can be found worldwide. Once exposed, host viremia peaks during the first 2 days and can last for up to 7 to 12 days. During the first phase of infection, viral replication occurs in human erythroid-progenitor linage cells and induces cell cycle arrests at both G1 and G2 phases [4]. Viral entry into target cells is mediated by a range of cellular receptors, including P antigen and β integrins [8]. P antigen distribution is most commonly found on cells of the erythroid lineage, but is also found on platelets and tissues from the heart, liver, and lungs [9]. Pathogenesis of B19 infection includes lysis of red blood precursors [10], which may lead to severe anemia. During the phase of viral replication and shedding, the patient is generally asymptomatic. When the characteristic rash develops or arthralgias are present, the patient is in the second phase of the disease process. During this phase, the patient is not infectious to others. The pregnant woman may present with a variety of symptoms, such as a flulike syndrome with low-grade fever, sore throat, generalized malaise, and headache. In the study by Hager and colleagues [11], of 618 pregnant women who were exposed to B19, 52 (8.4%) contracted the infection. Of these, 46% presented with arthralgias of the knees, fingers, and wrists. Immunocompromised patients, including those who have AIDS, hemoglobinopathies, cancer, and transplant recipients, may develop a chronic B19 infection resulting in anemia and aplastic crisis [12].

Parvovirus B19 inhibits erythroid cell differentiation by cytotoxic apoptosis. With marked fetal anemia, fetal hydrops may be identified with abnormal fluid collections such as subcutaneous or scalp edema, pericardial or pleural effusions, fetal abdominal ascites, or hydramnios. Additionally, marked hepatosplenomegaly, cardiomegaly, and thickened placenta may be demonstrated [5]. The mechanisms of hydrops include infection of progenitor cells, inducing fetal anemia and tissue hypoxia. This in turn increases cardiac output, and the fetus develops high-output cardiac failure. Approximately 3% of fetuses infected with B19 will develop hydrops [5].

Diagnosis

Physicians must have a high index of suspicion to diagnose a B19 infection during pregnancy. Most frequently, an evaluation is performed after the pregnant woman has been exposed to a child diagnosed with erythema infectiosum (fifth disease). Similarly, a high index of suspicion for B19 should always be considered in the evaluation of a fetus that has nonimmune hydrops. In contrast to children, only about one third of women present with a rashlike illness [11]. In approximately 25% of cases, the patient is asymptomatic. Diagnosis of infection is made by serologic testing, and several immunoassays have been developed over the years. The nature of the antigen incorporated into the serology affects its performance [13]. Currently there is only one US Food and Drug Administration-approved mμ-capture enzyme immunoassay (EIA) that detects specific IgM antibodies (Biotrim Parvovirus B19, Biotrim International LTD, Dublin, Ireland). This assay has a reported sensitivity of 89.1% and a specificity of 99.4%. It uses an EIA-based format incorporating baculovirus-expressed, self-assembled VP2 empty capsid [14]. The benefit of using conformational intact capsid protein VP2 is the reduction of false negative results. Because *Escherichia coli*–expressed B19 antigens that undergo denaturation are used as part of the manufacturing process, false-negative results may occur [13].

IgM antibodies can be detected late in the viremic stage of disease, day 10 to 14 postinfection. These antibodies persist for up to 5 months, but can last longer [15]. With the decline of IgM antibodies, there is a rise in IgG antibodies. These antibodies provide lifelong protection from reinfection in immunocompetent patients. IgG antibodies may remain high for several months and may persist for years. Three possible diagnostic scenarios should be considered (Fig. 1). The first occurs with women who have negative IgG and IgM titers. If exposed, these women may be nonimmune or in a window. Paired sera samples should be repeated in 3 to 4 weeks to rule out seroconversion. If repeat testing is negative, the woman has not been infected with B19 and fetal infection is not a concern. If repeat titers are positive, then there is risk for fetal infection. In a series of 618 patients who had documented exposure to parvovirus B19 [11], there was a 16.7% conversion rate in susceptible patients. This conversion rate is similar to that in other published series [16,17]. Furthermore, the risk of transmission depends whether or not the infection occurs during an endemic versus epidemic time period (1.5% versus 13%, respectively) [6].

The second diagnostic scenario is when the IgG is positive and IgM is negative. This pattern is consistent with prior infection and confers maternal immunity. In this scenario, there is no risk to the fetus for infection. Approximately 50% of women of childbearing age have immunity to parvovirus [18]. The third scenario is positive IgG and IgM antibodies, which represents an acute infection with the risk for fetal hydrops [5].

An additional scenario to consider is new-onset fetal hydrops diagnosed by ultrasound. In many instances, maternal B19 titers may take several days to return if sent to a reference laboratory. Therefore, after targeted ultrasound is performed, amniocentesis can be used to obtain amniocytes to evaluate for various viruses, including B19 by polymerase chain reaction (PCR). Ultimately, fetal blood sampling to assess for fetal anemia and possibly fetal transfusion may be considered, depending on gestational age and results of viral PCR.

Management schemes

The risk of vertical transmission to the fetus is estimated to be approximately 33% [19]. Infection is associated with various fetal outcomes, depending on the gestational age when the infection occurs. Fetal infection has been demonstrated as early as 3 weeks gestation [20]. Infection in the first trimester may result in fetal loss or miscarriage [19]. Transplacental infection in the second and third

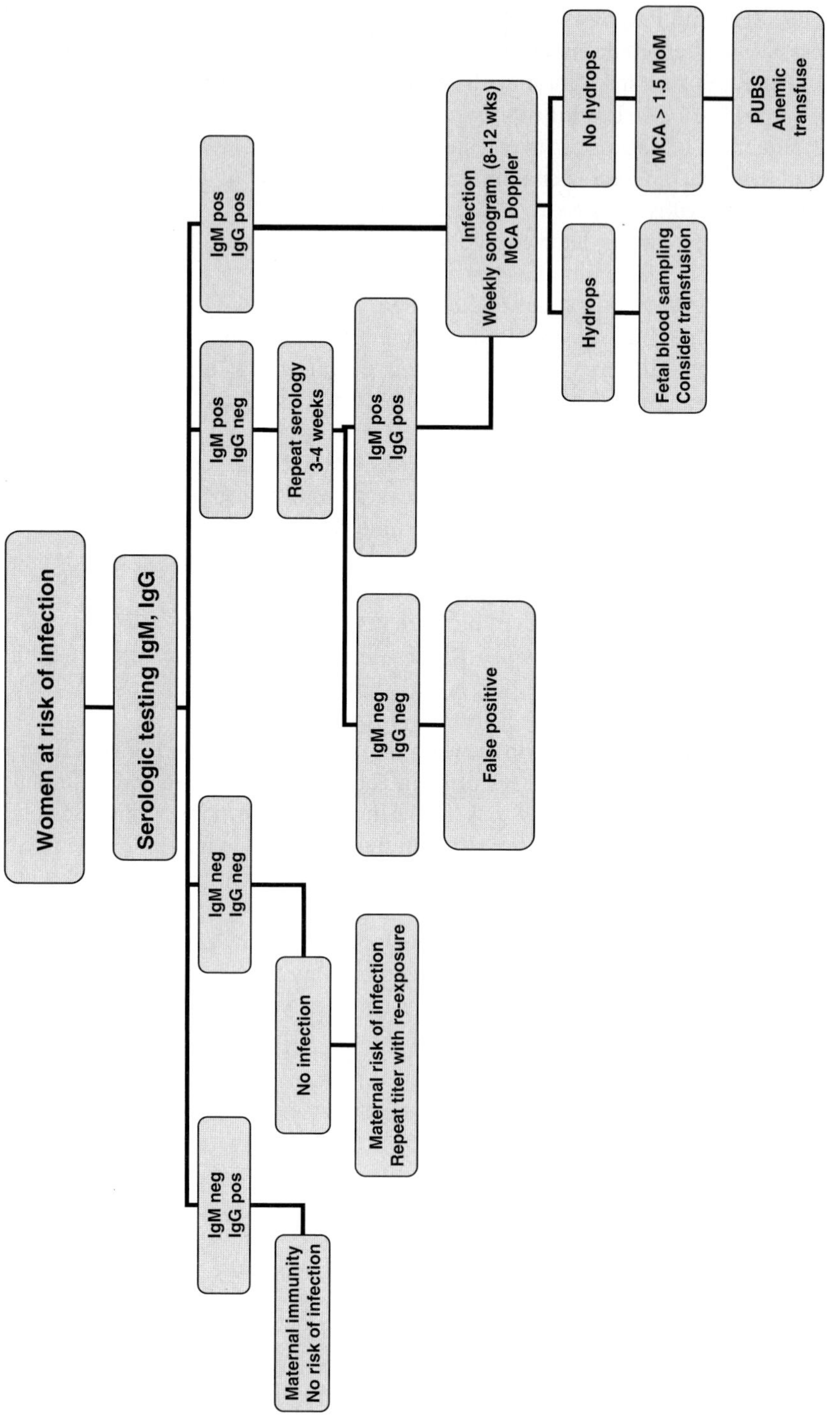

Fig. 1. Diagnostic algorithm for parvovirus B19 infection.

trimester may result in fetal anemia, myocarditis, high-output cardiac failure, fetal hydrops, and stillbirth [5,10,19]. Fetal death may occur in up to 10% of infected fetuses [10,21]. Factors that determine the perinatal course of infection need further elucidation. These factors may involve the viral dose, viral virulence, route of transmission, and the maternal or fetal immune response [20]. The timing of infection may determine whether fetal hydrops develops. Fetal hydrops is rarely seen in cases of intrauterine fetal demise occurring in the third trimester of an infected fetus who has B19. Importantly, we may be overlooking parvovirus as an etiology in these cases. Consideration should be given to evaluating for B19 in cases of second and third trimester fetal demises [22].

Sonographic findings may be lacking in the second and third trimester. In up to one third of fetuses who develop hydrops, spontaneous resolution of hydrops occurs [23]. The associated mortality of fetal hydrops without transfusion was 30% as reported in a survey of maternal-fetal medicine specialists [23]. Viral myocarditis may also occur with further breakdown of red blood cells. The second trimester is a particularly vulnerable time, with its maximal rate of erythropoiesis coupled with the short life span of fetal red blood cells as compared with the adult.

Fetal surveillance schemes vary depending on the trimester of diagnosis. Although fetal death may occur 4 to 6 weeks postinfection, death has been reported up to 12 weeks after B19 infection [24]. Therefore, duration of surveillance varies between 8 and 12 weeks. In the late second and third trimesters, daily fetal movement counting is suggested. Additionally, weekly sonographic evaluations to assess for the development of fetal ascites or hydrops are suggested. At that time, amniotic fluid volume may also be assessed. Complete resolution of fetal hydrops may take weeks.

Noninvasive and invasive prenatal diagnosis

A major concern with a fetal parvovirus B19 infection is the development of fetal anemia. Marked untreated anemia may result in fetal death. Cosmi and colleagues [19] have reported that fetal anemia caused by parvovirus infection could be detected noninvasively. Doppler velocimetry has been used to evaluate for an increase in the peak systolic velocity of blood flow in the middle cerebral artery (MCA) of the fetal brain (Fig. 2); however, fetal hydrops may not always occur with marked fetal anemia, and an intrauterine demise may occur unexpectedly [19]. For these reasons, in addition to weekly fetal testing and assessment for the development of fetal hydrops, a weekly measurement of the peak systolic velocity of the MCA should be assessed. Flow velocity measures the MCA blood viscosity and vascular impedance. From work in Rh isoimmunized women, MCA peak velocity values of greater than 1.50 multiples of the median (MoM) for gestational age have been associated with fetal anemia, and often undergo fetal blood sampling and intravascular transfusion (Fig. 3) [25]. In fetuses undergoing surveillance, if values that are either greater than 1.50 MoM

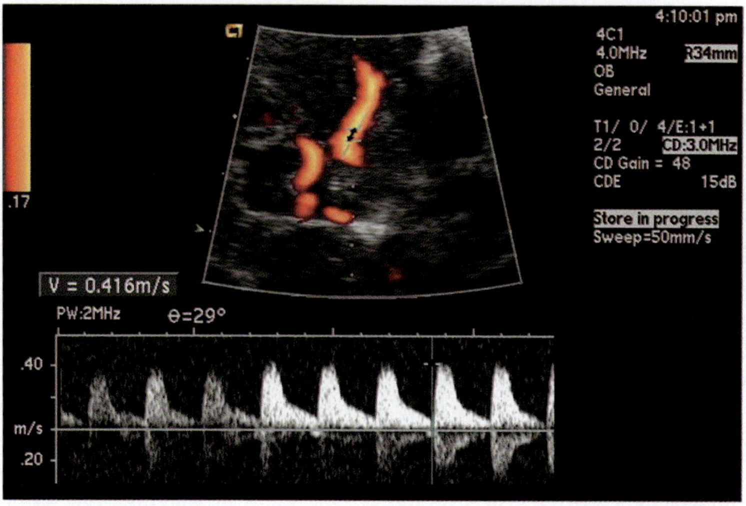

Fig. 2. Doppler velocimetry of fetal middle cerebral artery. Peak systolic velocity (*m/s*) of a fetus undergoing evaluation for fetal anemia. Arrow depicts proper placement of cursor.

are found, or if serial measurements reveal a sharp upward trend or slope, fetal anemia is suspected. Similar results were reported by Cosmi and coworkers [19] using MCA velocity in 32 fetuses at risk for anemia in pregnancies that were complicated by B19 infection. Of the 32 fetuses described, 17 had MCA velocities greater than 1.5 MoM. Sixteen of the 17 fetuses underwent fetal blood sampling, and all were anemic. Peak-velocity MCA measurements are noninvasive, with a reported sensitivity of 94.1% [19]. Because fetuses who have

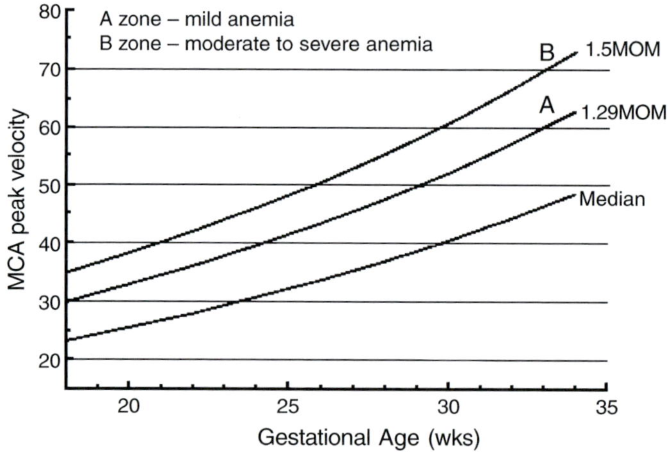

Fig. 3. Middle cerebral artery Doppler peak velocities based on gestational age. MoM, multiples of the median. (*From* Moise KJ. Management of rhesus alloimmunization in pregnancy. Obstet Gynecol 2002;100:605; with permission).

mild anemia may go undetected, weekly assessments for fetuses at risk are a reasonable management plan. With increasing values, however, a more frequent testing schedule may be employed.

With increasing MCA velocities or increasing slope of the curve of MCA values, a fetal blood sampling to assess for fetal anemia may be scheduled. If fetal anemia is confirmed, a fetal blood transfusion can be performed. When preparing for fetal transfusion, both packed red blood cells and platelets must be available to the physician. With a fetal parvovirus infection, thrombocytopenia may be present in addition to anemia. A maternal type and cross-match and mean corpuscular volume (MCV) are sent to the laboratory. Once the cord root is entered and a sample of blood is obtained, fetal origin can be confirmed by comparing the fetal MCV to maternal MCV. Fetal blood is also sent for hemoglobin, hematocrit, and platelet count. If fetal anemia is established with a fetal hematocrit of less than 30%, a fetal transfusion is performed. Platelet backup is made available for cases of significant streaming from the cord because of thrombocytopenia. Complications of fetal blood sampling and fetal transfusion range from 2% to 5%. Such complications include streaming from the cord, umbilical cord hematoma, laceration of the umbilical cord, infection, vaginal bleeding, rupture of membranes, increase in uterine activity, and fetal loss. In hydropic fetuses, the rate of loss may be higher, owing to the severity of the disease as compared with less severe cases. The reported survival after intravascular fetal transfusion may be as high as 60% to 80% [3,26,27].

Summary

The single-stranded DNA virus causing parvovirus B19 is a continuing problem in pregnancy, especially in winter and spring months. Adverse fetal sequelae may include fetal anemia, red blood cell aplasia due to bone marrow suppression, fetal myocarditis, fetal nonimmune hydrops, and fetal death. Contemporary obstetric care consists of the sonographic evaluation of an affected pregnancy for a period of 8 to 12 weeks. New, noninvasive schemes include weekly assessment for the development of fetal hydrops, and a newer modality is the MCA peak-velocity measurements. The MCA velocity measurements should be performed by an operator familiar with the technique. Invasive testing includes fetal blood sampling and fetal transfusion when deemed necessary. Future trends include a vaccination against B19. Until that time, the obstetrician will be routinely confronted with the woman exposed to B19, and needs to be familiar with the diagnosis and management of this condition.

References

[1] Cossart YE, Field AM, Cant B, et al. Parvovirus-like particles in human sera. Lancet 1975;1: 72–3.

[2] Isada NB, Berry SM. In utero diagnosis of congenital infection. In: Gonik B, editor. Viral diseases in pregnancy. New York: Springer-Verlag; 1994. p. 34–49.
[3] Practice Bulletin ACOG. Perinatal viral and parasitic infections. Number 2000;20:2–13.
[4] Chisaka H, Morita E, Yaegashi N, et al. Parvovirus B19 and the pathogenesis of anaemia. Rev Med Virol 2003;13:347–59.
[5] Murphy J, Jones DC. Managing the gravida with parvovirus. OBG Management 2000;Nov:1–7.
[6] Valeur-Jensen AK, Pedersen CB, Westergaard T, et al. Risk factors for parvovirus B19 infection in pregnancy. JAMA 1999;281(12):1099–105.
[7] Brown T, Anand A, Ritchie LD. Intrauterine parvovirus infection associated with hydrops fetalis. Lancet 1984;2:1033–4.
[8] Corcoran A, Doyle S. Advances in the biology, diagnosis and host-pathogen interactions of parvovirus B19. J Med Microbiol 2004;53:459–75.
[9] Cooling LL, Koerner TA, Naides SJ. Multiple glycosphingolipids determine the tissue tropism of parvovirus B19. J Infect Dis 1995;172:1198–205.
[10] Torok TJ, Qi-Yun W, Gary Jr W, et al. Prenatal diagnosis of intrauterine infection with parvovirus B19 by the polymerase chain reaction. Clin Infect Dis 1992;14:149–55.
[11] Hager JH, Alder SP, Koch WC, et al. Prospective evaluation of 618 pregnant women exposed to parvovirus B19: risk and symptoms. Obstet Gynecol 1998;91:412–20.
[12] Young NS. Parvoviruses. In: Fields BN, Knipe BN, Howley PM, editors. Field's virology. 3rd edition. Philadelphia: Lippincott-Raven; 1996. p. 2199–220.
[13] Jordan JA. Appreciating the differences between immunoassays used to diagnose maternal parvovirus B19 infection: understanding the antigen before interpreting the results. Prim Care Update Ob Gyns 2002;9(5):154–9.
[14] Doyle S, Kerr S, O'Keefe G, et al. Detection of parvovirus B19 IgM by antibody capture enzyme immunoassay: receiver operating characteristic analysis. J Virol Methods 2000;90:143–52.
[15] Musiani M, Zerbini M, Gentilomi G, et al. Parvovirus B19 clearance from peripheral blood after acute infection. J Infect Dis 1995;172:1360–3.
[16] Gillespie SM, Cartter ML, Asch S, et al. Occupational risk of human parvovirus B19 infection for school and day-care personnel during an outbreak of erythema infectiousum. JAMA 1990; 263:2061–5.
[17] Kock WC, Adler SP. Human parvovirus B19 infections in women of childbearing age and within families. Pediatr Infect Dis J 1989;8:83–7.
[18] Cohen BJ, Buckley MM. The prevalence of antibody to human parvovirus B19 in England and Wales. J Med Microbiol 1988;25:151–3.
[19] Cosmi E, Mari G, Chiaie LD, et al. Noninvasive diagnosis by Doppler ultrasonography of fetal anemia resulting from parvovirus infection. Am J Obstet Gynecol 2002;187:1290–3.
[20] Nunoue T, Kusuhara K, Hara T. Human fetal infection with parvovirus B19: maternal infection time in gestation, viral persistence, and fetal prognosis. Pediatr Infect Dis J 2002;21(12):1133–6.
[21] Miller E, Fairly CK, Cohen BJ, et al. Immediate and long term outcome of human parvovirus B19 infection in pregnancy. Br J Obstet Gynaecol 1998;106:174–8.
[22] Norbeck O, Papadogiannakis N, Petersson K, et al. Revised clinical presentation of parvovirus B19-associated intrauterine fetal death. Clin Infect Dis 2002;35:1032–8.
[23] Rodis JF, Borgida AF, Wilson M, et al. Management of parvovirus infection in pregnancy and outcome of hydrops: a survey of members of the Society of Perinatal Obstetricians. Am J Obstet Gynecol 1998;179:985–8.
[24] Hedrick J. The effects of human parvovirus B19 and cytomegalovirus during pregnancy. J Perinat Neonatal Nurs 1996;10:30–9.
[25] Moise KJ. Management of rhesus alloimmunization in pregnancy. Obstet Gynecol 2002;100: 600–11.
[26] Humphrey W, Maggon M, O'Shaughnessy R. Severe nonimmune hydrops secondary to parvovirus B-19 infection: Spontaneous reversal in utero and survival of a term infant. Obstet Gynecol 1991;78:900–2.
[27] Fairly CK, Smolenic JS, Caul OE, et al. Observational study of effect of intrauterine transfusions on outcome of fetal hydrops after parvo B19 infection. Lancet 1995;346:1335–7.

ELSEVIER
SAUNDERS

CLINICS IN
PERINATOLOGY

Clin Perinatol 32 (2005) 705–726

Diagnosis and Management of Toxoplasmosis

Jose G. Montoya, MD[a,b,*], Fernando Rosso, MD[a,b,c]

[a]*Department of Medicine, Division of Infectious Diseases and Geographic Medicine, Stanford University School of Medicine, 300 Pasteur Drive, Grant S-169, Stanford, CA 94305-5107, USA*
[b]*Department of Immunology and Infectious Diseases, Research Institute, Palo Alto Medical Foundation, Palo Alto, CA 94301, USA*
[c]*Fundación Clínica Valle del Lili, Cali, Colombia*

Vertical transmission of the parasite *Toxoplasma gondii* can produce significant morbidity and mortality to the fetus and newborn and long-term sequelae to children and adults [1]. Congenital toxoplasmosis primarily occurs in the offspring of women who acquired their primary *T gondii* infection during gestation. Congenital disease is almost never seen in women who acquired their infection in the distant past and before conception. The two major exceptions to the latter dictum include chronically infected women who reactivate their latent *T gondii* infection during gestation because of immunosuppression (eg, AIDS) and women who acquired their primary infection shortly (within 3 months) before conception.

Greater than 90% of pregnant women who acquire their primary *T gondii* infection during gestation are asymptomatic, and approximately 85% of children born having congenital toxoplasmosis do not initially exhibit any signs of disease; however, the parasite has the potential to cause significant long-term damage to infected progeny, and may bring major emotional and economic burdens to parents, relatives, and society. Laboratory diagnosis performed during

* Corresponding author. Department of Medicine, Division of Infectious Diseases and Geographic Medicine, Stanford University School of Medicine, 300 Pasteur Drive, Grant S-169, Stanford, CA 94305-5107.

E-mail address: gilberto@standord.edu (J.G. Montoya).

doi:10.1016/j.clp.2005.04.011

pregnancy and at birth can reveal those mother-baby pairs at risk for congenital toxoplasmosis and those who have infected offspring.

Congenital toxoplasmosis is a preventable and treatable disease [1]. From the time a pregnant woman is at risk of ingesting *T gondii* to the moment her progeny is infected with the parasite, there are many opportunities for health care workers to intervene and stop this potentially tragic cascade of events. Primary prevention (aimed at preventing primary *T gondii* maternal infection during gestation) can be achieved through education targeted at women who have never been exposed to *T gondii* (*T gondii* IgG negative). These women need to be reminded throughout gestation of the behavioral risks that could expose them to acquiring the parasite during gestation. Secondary prevention (aimed at preventing fetal infection during gestation) can be attained by putting in place programs for universal serological screening, as practiced in France and Austria, aimed at detecting women who acquire their primary infection during gestation and who do not experience any symptoms. For these women, an attempt can be made to decrease fetal infection with spiramycin, a prenatal diagnosis of congenital disease can be performed by polymerase chain reaction (PCR) examination of amniotic fluid, and in-utero treatment can be initiated for the fetus suspect or proven to be infected.

This article is intended to serve as a summary of the authors' current approach to diagnosis and management of toxoplasmosis during pregnancy. The roles of commercial nonreference laboratories and reference laboratories are differentiated and emphasized.

The organism and its life cycle

T gondii is an obligate intracellular protozoan that exists in nature in three forms: (1) the oocyst (which releases sporozoites), (2) the tissue cyst (which contains and may release bradyzoites), and (3) the tachyzoite. Oocysts are formed in the small bowel of members of the cat family only, and are excreted in their feces for periods varying from 7 to 20 days. As many as 10 million oocysts may be shed in their feces in a single day, and these become infectious (by sporulation) in 1 to 21 days, depending on temperature and availability of oxygen. Tachyzoites are crescent- or oval-shaped and require an intracellular habitat to survive and multiply. Tachyzoites reside and multiply within vacuoles in their host's cells, and can infect most phagocytic and nonphagocytic cell types, including placental cells. The presence of tachyzoites in human fluids or tissues is the hallmark of acute infection or reactivation of a latent infection.

Following cell entry and replication of the tachyzoite form, encystation and formation of tissue cysts may occur. The conditions that result in cyst formation are not known. The tissue cyst is formed within a host cell and may vary in size from those that contain only a few organisms (bradyzoites) to those 200 μm or greater in size that contain several thousand bradyzoites. The central nervous system, eyes, skeletal system, and smooth and heart muscles appear to be the most common sites of latent infection. Because of this persistence in tissues, demonstration of cysts in histologic sections does not necessarily mean that the infection was recently acquired or that it is clinically relevant.

The parasite undergoes two cycles: an enteroepithelial sexual cycle in the small bowel of members of the cat family; and an extraintestinal asexual cycle in infected animals, including humans. Cats shed oocysts after they ingest any of the three forms of the parasite. Humans get usually infected by ingestion of tissue cysts (in meat) or oocysts (in cat's feces or in contaminated soil or vegetables); the outer walls of cysts or oocysts are disrupted by enzymatic degradation and the parasites are liberated into the intestinal lumen. Bradyzoites released from tissue cysts and sporozoites released from oocysts become tachyzoites and spread to invade virtually all cells and tissues of the human body.

Pathogenesis of toxoplasma infection during pregnancy

Following ingestion of the tissue cyst or oocyst forms by the pregnant woman, her gastric digestive juices disrupt their outer wall, releasing the infective forms, bradyzoites in the case of tissue cysts, and sporozoites in the case of oocysts. respectively. Bradyzoites and sporozoites rapidly invade intestinal lumen enteroepithelial cells, where they become tachyzoites. Further spread of the parasite follows its release from disrupted cells, with invasion of contiguous cells and the lymphatic and blood compartments.

Because *T gondii* can infect essentially all cells and tissues, its dissemination is widespread. It is during the parasitemic phase that the placenta may be infected. Optimal conditions for transmission to the placenta include the onset of parasitemia before the development of adequate humoral or cellular immunity in the mother, and a well-developed placenta blood flow, as exists in the latter part of pregnancy. Transmission is rare early in gestation, but gradually increases in frequency toward the end of pregnancy. Transmission of the parasite when the infection was acquired shortly before conception has been documented, but is an extremely rare event (in these few cases, the infection was acquired within 3 months of the approximate date of conception). Data accumulated from prospective studies indicate that the incidence and severity of congenital toxoplasmosis vary with the trimester during which the infection was acquired by the mother [1]. Moreover, there is an inverse relationship between the frequency of transmission and the severity of disease. Infants born of mothers who acquire their infection in the first trimester more frequently show severe congenital toxoplasmosis [2]. In contrast, the majority of children born of women who acquire their infection during the third trimester are born having the subclinical form of the infection. If left untreated, however, as many as 85% of these latter children develop signs and symptoms of the disease, in most cases chorioretinitis or delays in development [3,4].

Transmission and epidemiology

Toxoplasmosis is a zoonosis of worldwide distribution. The two most common routes of infection in humans are by oral ingestion of the parasite or transplacentally (congenital transmission to the fetus). Primary ingestion of undercooked or raw meat that contains tissue cysts or of water or food contaminated with oocysts results in the acute infection. Less common are transmission by transplantation of an infected organ or transfusion of contaminated blood cells. Transmission has also occurred by accidental sticks with contaminated needles, or through exposing open lesions or mucosal surfaces to the parasite. Coprophagous invertebrates, including cockroaches, filth flies, earthworms, snails, and slugs, may serve as transport hosts for oocysts to reach the gastrointestinal tract of animals or humans.

In humans, the prevalence of the infection increases with age, and there are considerable geographic differences in prevalence rates (eg, 10% in Palo Alto, California; 15% in Boston, Massachusetts; 30% in Birmingham, Alabama; 36% in Strasbourg, France; 81% in the Central African Republic [1]). Differences in the epidemiology of *T gondii* infection in various geographic locales and between population groups within the same locale may be explained by differences in exposure to sources of the infection. Recent epidemiological studies have identified water as a potential source for *T gondii* infection, both in humans and animals [5–7]. Population mapping studies of acutely infected individuals as well as case-control studies linked drinking unfiltered water (presumably contaminated with oocysts) to an outbreak of toxoplasmosis in a municipality in the Western Canadian province of British Columbia [5], and to highly endemic rates of toxoplasmosis in Rio de Janeiro state, Brazil [8]. Coastal freshwater runoff was observed to be a risk factor for *T gondii* infection among southern sea otters along the California coast [9].

The recent overall age-adjusted seroprevalence of *T gondii* infection in the United States (1999–2000, sera collected in the National Health and Examination Survey [NHANES]) [10], based on a survey of 4234 persons aged 12 to 49, was reported at 15.8% (age-adjusted, 95% confidence limits [CL] 13.5, 18.1). Thus, 84.2% of women of childbearing age in the United States are seronegative, and thereby are at risk to acquire *T gondii* infection during gestation. *T gondii* antibody prevalence was higher among nonHispanic black persons than among nonHispanic white persons (age-adjusted prevalence 19.2% versus 12.1%, P=.003), and increased with age. No statistically significant differences were found between *T gondii* antibody prevalence in NHANES (1999–2000), and NHANES III (1988–1994). *T gondii* antibody prevalence has remained stable over the past 10 years in the United States.

Rates of congenital toxoplasmosis have been estimated between 1 per 10,000 and 10 per 10,000 live births [11]. If these rates were extrapolated to the approximately 4 million live births in the United States each year, an estimated 400 to 4000 infants would be born each year having congenital toxoplasmosis [11]. An estimated 400 to 4000 cases of congenital toxoplasmosis do occur each year in the United States. Of the 750 deaths attributed to toxoplasmosis each year, 375 (50%) are believed to be caused by eating contaminated meat, making toxoplasmosis the third leading cause of food-related deaths in this country.

Occasionally outbreaks occur within families or certain populations. The possibility of an outbreak should always be suspected with every patient who presents with a recently acute acquired infection.

The incidence of congenital toxoplasmosis in newborns directly correlates with three factors: (1) the incidence of primary infection among women during pregnancy; (2) the gestational age at which a pregnant woman acquires the infection; and (3) the public health programs instituted for prevention, detection, and treatment of the infection during pregnancy. Although screening for *Toxoplasma* infection is compulsory during pregnancy in some countries, such as Austria and France, in the United States routine serological screening is not performed. The frequency of transmission is approximately 15% for acquisition during the first trimester, 30% for the second trimester, and 60% for the third trimester. It has been reported that spiramycin decreases the incidence of fetal infection by approximately 60%. If the infection is acquired during the first 2 weeks of gestation and spiramycin is administered for the entire pregnancy, the incidence of fetal infection is essentially zero. Recently, a group of European investigators have questioned the utility of spiramycin in preventing vertical transmission of *T gondii* [12,13]. Their studies contain serious methodological limitations and their conclusions are not supported by their published data. Most authorities continue recommending spiramycin for pregnant women who acquire *T gondii* primary infection during gestation, in an attempt to prevent congenital toxoplasmosis.

Clinical manifestations

The possibility of toxoplasmosis during pregnancy should be entertained in the setting of the following clinical scenarios: (1) serological screening of an asymptomatic pregnant woman suggests the possibility of an acute *T gondii* infection acquired recently and during (or shortly before) gestation, (2) painless lymphadenopathy, (3) chorioretinitis, or (4) abnormalities detected on the fetus or the newborn.

The vast majority of pregnant women infected with *T gondii* do not experience any symptoms or signs. The risk to the fetus does not correlate with whether the infection in the mother was symptomatic or asymptomatic during gestation. Significant fetal damage can occur in the offspring of women whose pregnancy was completely uneventful and did not experience any symptoms, which emphasizes the need for universal prenatal serological screening. In approximately 10% of expectant women, few nonspecific symptoms can occur; these include general malaise, low-grade fever, and lymphadenopathy. A single and enlarged cervical lymph node is the most common clinical presentation among women who exhibit symptoms [1]. Diffuse lymphadenopathy might develop, but is rare.

Rarely, pregnant women present with ocular symptoms due to toxoplasmic chorioretinitis [14]. If the ocular involvement by the parasite is due to an acute infection [15] acquired during gestation, the offspring will be at risk for congenital disease, and the patient should be treated to both address her eye disease and to prevent vertical transmission of the parasite. In contrast, if the eye disease is due to reactivation of a chronic infection acquired in the distant past, the fetus is essentially at no risk for congenital disease, and the eye disease should be treated accordingly. In the latter scenario, the risk for vertical transmission is essentially zero (unless the mother is immunosuppressed).

In some cases, the diagnosis of toxoplasmosis during pregnancy is only entertained when ultrasonographic findings reveal the presence of fetal abnormalities, including hydrocephalus, brain or hepatic calcifications, splenomegaly, and ascites [1]. It should be emphasized, however, that a normal fetal ultrasound does not necessarily rule out congenital toxoplasmosis.

In some cases, physicians are asked to establish whether a woman acquired *T gondii* infection during gestation once a child is born having symptoms or signs suggesting congenital infection by one of the infectious agents included in TORCH (toxoplasmosis, others, rubella, cytomegalovirus, herpes) syndrome [1]. It is important to emphasize once more that congenital toxoplasmosis may occur in one of four forms: (1) overt neonatal disease; (2) disease (mild or severe) occurring in the first months of life; (3) sequelae or relapse of a previously undiagnosed infection during infancy, childhood, or adolescence; or (4) subclinical infection. The forms of disease (3) and (4) are by far the most common clinical presentations of congenital toxoplasmosis.

Diagnosis

General approach

The maternal diagnosis of toxoplasmosis during pregnancy is primarily made by the use of serological tests. Presence or absence of symptoms or a detailed epidemiological history suggesting exposure to *T gondii* are not useful tools to decide whether laboratory testing should be performed. Significant fetal damage has been documented in offspring of women who were entirely asymptomatic or who had no apparent exposure to the parasite during gestation. Pregnant women should be systematically screened for *Toxoplasma* IgG and IgM antibodies during their first medical visit (ideally during their first trimester) for obstetrical care. A systematic approach for such program does not exist in the United States, but it is mandated by law in countries such France and Austria. In these countries, serial specimens facilitate the unequivocal diagnosis of a recently acquired infection by demonstration of seroconversion or a significant rise in IgG *Toxoplasma* antibodies accompanied by the presence of detectable IgM test titers. In the United States, physicians most often submit only a single serum sample, from which a diagnosis is expected, but usually is not possible in most situations and laboratories [1].

The problem with serologic diagnosis is further complicated by the fact that antibodies to *T gondii* may persist for years in healthy people. Thus, positive IgG and IgM test results are not necessarily diagnostic of a recently acquired infection. IgG antibodies are detectable for the life of the individual, and IgM antibodies can be detectable for many years in certain patients.

To address the challenge posed by the serological diagnosis of *T gondii* infection and toxoplasmosis, a large number of tests have been described, some of which are available only in highly specialized laboratories [16,17]. Different serologic tests often measure different antibodies that possess unique patterns of rise and fall with the time after infection. Unfortunately, false-positive (up to 60%) results have been a problem with certain commercial kits and laboratories in the United States and Europe [18,19]. In 1996, the US Food and Drug Administration (FDA) and the Centers for Disease Control (CDC) conducted extensive evaluations of the six most commonly used commercial IgM kits in the United States to determine the extent of the problem with the specificity of these kits [19]. Sensitivity rates ranged from 93.3% to 100.0%, and specificity rates ranged from 77.5% to 99.1% for the six kits evaluated.

As a result of these findings, in 1997 the FDA distributed an advisory to physicians in the United States highlighting these test limitations. The agency provided a guide for interpreting test results, and issued a recommendation to laboratory personnel and physicians advising them to be aware of the problems associated with the test kits before making decisions about the clinical management of their patients. In addition, IgM-positive results should be confirmed by a *Toxoplasma* reference laboratory [20].

Toxoplasma serological testing that can be performed at commercial nonreference laboratories

The primary goal of laboratory testing for the possibility of toxoplasmosis during pregnancy is to establish whether an acute infection has been acquired during or shortly before conception.

At present, the most practical approach is to request an initial serological screening comprised of IgG and IgM antibody testing. These tests can be performed at a commercial nonreference laboratory.

Negative results in IgG and IgM tests essentially indicate that the patient has not been exposed to *T gondii*, and therefore is at risk for congenital toxoplasmosis only if the mother acquires a primary infection during gestation.

Education to the mother and household members on infection prevention measures should be provided and emphasized. These are listed in Box 1.

A positive IgG and negative IgM result during the first two trimesters of gestation is in essence consistent with an infection acquired in the distant past and before pregnancy. The incidence of congenital toxoplasmosis in offspring of women infected before gestation has been shown to be extremely rare (approaching zero) unless a woman is immunocompromised (ie, HIV-positive, receiving corticosteroids or immunosuppressive drugs, and so on). A positive IgG and negative IgM result in the third trimester is more difficult to interpret. Although this result is most likely consistent with an infection acquired before pregnancy, in some patients this result can reflect an acute infection acquired early in gestation, with a quick brief rise of IgM titers and their fall to non-detectable levels within a relatively short period of time. A reference laboratory should be consulted in this latter situation.

A positive result in any IgM test (regardless of the IgG test result) should be followed by confirmatory testing at a *Toxoplasma* reference laboratory (eg, the Toxoplasma Serology Laboratory at the Palo Alto Medical Foundation [PAMF-TSL], Palo Alto, California, http://www.pamf.org/serology/), because detectable IgM titers are not necessarily indicative of a recently acquired infection.

Box 1. Measures to prevent primary *Toxoplasma gondii* infection in pregnant women

- Avoid contact with food or water potentially contaminated with cat feces.
- Cook meat to 66°C/150°F or ''well done,'' or that is not pink in the middle (meat that is smoked or cured in brine may be infectious).
- Avoid exposure to soil potentially contaminated with cat feces (eg, in gardening or handling cat liter).
- Disinfect cat litter box with near-boiling water for 5 minutes prior to handling.
- Wear gloves when gardening or handling cat litter.
- Wash hands thoroughly after contact with raw meat.
- Kitchen surfaces and utensils that have come in contact with raw meat should be washed.
- Avoid mucous membrane contact when handling raw meat.
- Avoid ingestion of dried meat.
- Wash fruits and vegetables prior to consumption.
- Refrain from skinning animals.

Toxoplasma serological testing that should be performed at a reference laboratory

Positive IgM test titers can indeed be found in individuals who have been recently infected, but can also be found in others who were infected in the distant past. Persisting IgM antibodies beyond 1 year are not uncommon, and have been described in individuals who have been infected with the parasite for many years [1]. Confirmatory testing of detectable IgM test titers usually requires the use of combination of tests, including alternative methods to detect IgG (ie, dye test, differential agglutination, avidity) and IgM (ie, double-sandwich ELISA) and detection of IgA and IgE antibodies. This combinatorial approach to address the challenge of positive IgM test results has been validated by reference laboratories in Europe and the United States. An example of how a battery of tests can be used for the diagnosis of *T gondii* infection and toxoplasmosis is the *Toxoplasma* serological profile (TSP), which consists of the dye test (DT), IgM ELISA, IgA ELISA, IgE ELISA, and AC/HS (differential agglutination) test (Table 1). The TSP has been reported to be useful in the setting of pregnancy [21] and other clinical scenarios as well, including lymphadenopathy [16], myocarditis and polymyositis [22], and chorioretinitis [22].

TSP has been successfully used at the PAMF-TSL to establish whether a pregnant woman has been infected with the parasite during gestation. Communication of the TSP results and their correct interpretation by an expert to the patient's physician has been reported to decrease the rate of unnecessary abortions by approximately 50% among women for whom positive immunoglobulin M *Toxoplasma* test results had been reported by outside laboratories [21]. The current interpretations of results with the TSP at the PAMF-TSL are described below.

Sera that are obtained within the first two trimesters and are positive with the DT; negative with the IgM, IgA, and IgE ELISAs; and reveal a chronic pattern with the acetone treated/formalin treated (AC/HS) test typically found in patients infected before gestation (chronic TSP pattern). Pregnant women having these results are told that the incidence of congenital toxoplasmosis in the offspring of chronically infected women has been shown to be extremely rare (approaching zero), unless a woman is immunocompromised.

The combination of high titers with the DT; positive IgM, IgA, and IgE ELISAs; and an acute pattern with the AC/HS test is suggestive of a recent infection (acute TSP pattern). Pregnant women who have these serological test results are informed that acute infection during gestation cannot be excluded, and that their offspring may be at risk for congenital toxoplasmosis.

A positive DT and IgM ELISA but a negative, low-positive, or equivocal result with the tests for IgA and IgE antibodies, and an equivocal pattern with the AC/HS test is more difficult to interpret, because it suggests infection acquired before gestation but does not entirely rule out recent infection (equivocal TSP pattern). In the latter setting, a follow-up serum sample has usually been requested and the two sera are run in parallel. If the follow-up sample does not

Table 1
Serological tests used for confirmatory testing of IgM positive titers at the RAMFRI-TSL

Test	Antibody measured	Kinetics during acute infection	Test result excluding acute infection/time window[a]	A typical TSP[b] consistent with a recently acquired infection	A typical TSP[b] consistent with an infection acquired in the distant past
Dye test (DT)	IgG	DT is the "gold standard" for detection of IgG antibodies. It becomes detectable 1–2 weeks after acquisition of infection and peaks between 3 and 6 months. A gradual decline occurs over months to years and lower titers persist for life.	NA	Low (very early in the acute infection) to high titers	Low titers
IgM ELISA	IgM	It appears within the first week or 2 of infection. In some patients IgM antibodies may persist for >1 year after primary infection.	Negative/6 months	High titers	Low or negative titers
IgA ELISA	IgA	It appears within the first week or 2 of infection. In some patients IgA antibodies may persist for or reappear months after primary infection.	ND	High or negative titers	Negative titers

IgE ELISA	IgE	It appears within the first week or two of infection. Duration of detectable IgE antibodies in adults with acute infection is briefer than that of IgM and IgA antibodies. Among patients with detectable titers, IgE antibodies usually disappear 2 to 3 months after primary infection.	ND	High or negative titers	Negative titers
AC/HS	IgG	It compares the titers obtained with formalin-fixed tachyzoites (HS antigen) with those obtained with acetone-fixed tachyzoites (AC antigen). The AC preparation contains stage-specific antigents that are recognized by IgG antibodies early in infection.	Non-acute Pattern/>12 months	Acute pattern	Non-acute pattern
Agglutination	IgG	Most sensitive test to detect rising IgG antibodies	ND	Rising titers in serial samples	Stable titers in serial samples
Avidity	IgG		High/>3 to 5 months[c]	Low or equivocal	High

Abbreviations: NA, not applicable; ND, not determined.

[a] Time window: period of time in months that this serological test result has been shown to exclude acute infection.

[b] TSP = toxoplasma serological profile and is comprised of Dye test, IgM, IgA, IgE, and AC/HS.

[c] Time window depends of the specific kit used.

reveal significant changes with any of the TSP test titers, and if the results from any of the tests of the TSP were lower than one would expect in an acute infection, the diagnosis is most likely infection acquired in the distant past. In some patients, however, despite the testing of serial serum samples in parallel, the interpretation of results from the TSP might remain equivocal. For these patients, the authors have recommend a conservative approach—we suggest that the patient be managed similarly to those patients for whom serology results suggest an infection acquired during gestation. More recently, however, testing for *T gondii*–specific IgG avidity for certain parasite antigens [17,23–29] has been reported to be useful for confirmatory testing in patients who have positive IgG and IgM titers or equivocal TSP results [17].

High-avidity IgG antibodies develop at least 12 to 16 weeks (depending on the test kit used) after acquisition of infection. Thus, the presence of high avidity antibodies indicates that infection was acquired more than 12 to 16 weeks earlier [17,29,30]. The avidity assay should be used in conjunction with other serologic tests (ie, those in the TSP panel) [17,29,31]. The method is most useful (and should be performed) in women in the first 16 weeks of gestation in whom IgM antibodies are found. It is also useful late in gestation to determine whether infection was acquired 4 or more months earlier, thereby allowing for an estimate of the rate of infection of the fetuses at a given time during gestation.

A number of tests for avidity of toxoplasma IgG antibodies have been introduced to help differentiate between recently acquired and distant infection [17,23–29]. This method is based on the observation that during acute *T gondii* infection, IgG antibodies bind antigen weakly (ie, have low avidity), whereas chronically infected patients have more strongly binding (high avidity) antibodies [23]. Protein-denaturing reagents, including urea, are used to dissociate the antibody-antigen complex. Low or equivocal avidity test results can persist for months to years after the primary infection [23,30], and for this reason a low or equivocal avidity test result must not be used to determine whether the infection was acquired recently.

An equivocal IgM test result in the presence or absence of detectable IgG antibodies should also have confirmatory testing performed at a reference laboratory, and most likely requires parallel testing on a follow-up or earlier sample. In this setting, IgG seroconversion (or a significant rise in its titers) is diagnostic of recently acquired and acute *T gondi*i infection.

In summary, serological test results performed at a reference laboratory may have one of three final interpretations: (1) consistent with a recently acquired infection and the possibility of the patient having acquired the infection during pregnancy cannot be excluded. Her offspring is at risk for congenital disease; (2) consistent with an infection acquired before pregnancy. The patient and her physician are told that the incidence of congenital toxoplasmosis in offspring of women infected before gestation has been shown to be extremely rare (approaching zero) unless a woman is immunocompromised (ie, HIV-positive, receiving corticosteroids or immunosuppressive drugs, and so on); (3) serological test results on the available samples are equivocal. To help clarify this interpretation, serum obtained 3 weeks after or before the date of the above specimen should be submitted for further testing to the authors' laboratory (PAMF-TSL). This usually assists in evaluating whether the patient's infection was acquired recently or in the more distant past.

Management of the patient who has suspected or diagnosed acute *Toxoplasma gondii* infection acquired during gestation

Prenatal diagnosis of fetal infection

Prenatal diagnosis of fetal *Toxoplasma* infection should be attempted when a diagnosis of acute maternal infection acquired during pregnancy or just before conception is established, or is highly suspected on the basis of serological test results or abnormal fetal ultrasound examination.

The most reliable method to detect or exclude fetal infection during gestation is amniotic fluid sampling for PCR examination. This test determines whether *T gondii* DNA is present in amniotic fluid. Amniocentesis should be performed, if feasible and safe, at 18 weeks or more of gestation. Amniotic fluid testing for *T gondii* PCR should be avoided at less than 18 weeks gestation, because of the lower sensitivity [32] and higher risk for fetal injury observed earlier in gestation. Romand and colleagues in France [32] evaluated the sensitivity, specificity, and predictive values of prenatal amniotic fluid. They prospectively studied 270 women who had proven primary infection during pregnancy. Definitive infection status of live-born infants was assessed by serologic follow-up until 1 year of age. As expected, the maternal-fetal transmission rate increased according to duration of gestation at maternal infection. Overall sensitivity of PCR on amniotic fluid was estimated at 64% (95% confidence interval [CI] 53.1%, 74.9%), negative predictive value at 87.8% (95% CI 83.5%, 92.1%), whereas specificity and positive predictive value were both 100% (95% CIs 98%, 100% and 92.3%, 100%, respectively). The sensitivity and specificity of the test was significantly influenced by gestational age. Prudence should be exercised when using PCR results for making clinical decisions. PCR results from any laboratory must be reviewed with caution, and if possible, information or data on the reliability and validation data of the PCR tests from that laboratory should be requested [1]. PCR results obtained in different laboratories may differ such that a result reported as positive or negative from one laboratory may be reported as the opposite from another laboratory [1].

Monthly fetal ultrasounds are also recommended for women suspected or diagnosed as having acquired acute toxoplasmosis during pregnancy. Ultrasonographic findings suggestive but not diagnostic of congenital toxoplasmosis include unilateral or bilateral ventricular dilations demonstrated by an increase in the ventricle:hemisphere ratio, ascites, intracranial or intrahepatic calcifications, hepatomegaly, and splenomegaly [1].

Funipuncture, cordocentesis, or periumbilical fetal blood sampling (PUBS) have been largely abandoned because of their inherently higher risk for fetal injury and their lower yield for the diagnosis of congenital infection when compared with amniocentesis for PCR examination [33].

Treatment with spiramycin

The use of the macrolide antibiotic spiramycin (Table 2) during pregnancy in women who acquire acute *T gondii* infection during gestation has been reported to decrease the frequency of vertical transmission. This protection appears to be more distinct in women infected during their first trimester. Its efficacy appears to correlate with the fact that higher concentrations of the drug are achieved in the placenta of mammals [34]. It also appears that its ability to curtail vertical transmission significantly wanes in the late second trimester and in the third trimester. Spiramycin does not cross the placenta reliably, and should be avoided as monotherapy in cases of suspected or established fetal

Table 2
Treatment of *T gondii* in pregnant women

	Medication	Dosage	Duration of therapy
In pregnant women with the diagnosis or suspicion of having acquired acute toxoplasmosis during the first 21 weeks of gestation	Spiramycin	1 g every 8 hours without food	If fetal infection documented or highly suspected, switch to pyrimethamine, sulfadiazine, and folinic acid until term; however, pyrimethamine should not be administered before week 18) If fetal infection excluded by PCR examination of amniotic fluid, continue spiramycin until term
In pregnant women with the diagnosis of having acquired acute toxoplasmosis during the late second trimester or in the third trimester or if fetal infection confirmed or highly suspected	Pyrimethamine +	Loading dose: 100 mg per day in two divided doses for 2 days then 50 mg/d	If fetal infection is highly suspected or confirmed, continue pyrimethamine, sulfadiazine, and folinic acid until term
	Sulfadiazine +	Loading dose: 75 mg/kg per day in two divided doses (maximum 4 g/d) for 2 days , then 100 mg/d in two divided doses (maximum 4 g/d)	If fetal infection is excluded by PCR examination of amniotic fluid and negative follow up ultrasounds, consider switching to spiramycin
	Folinic acid	10–20 mg qd	During and for 1 week after pyrimethamine therapy

infection; there is no evidence that it is teratogenic. Spiramycin is indicated for pregnant women suspected to have or diagnosed with acute *T gondii* infection acquired during the first trimester or early second trimester of gestation. Spiramycin should be administered until delivery, unless a diagnosis of fetal infection is highly suspected or established. Spiramycin needs to be continued throughout pregnancy, even in those patients with negative amniotic fluid PCR results, because of the theoretical possibility that fetal infection can occur later in pregnancy from a placenta that was infected earlier in gestation [1]. For pregnant women in whom the possibility of fetal infection is high or it has been established, spiramycin should be switched to pyrimethamine/sulfadiazine/folinic acid (see Table 2) after the 18th week of gestation.

Spiramycin should not be administered to patients who have known hypersensitivity to the drug or macrolide antibiotics. A small percentage of pregnant women may develop gastrointestinal symptoms or allergic reactions (ie, mild to severe skin rash); however, allergic reactions are rather rare. Spiramcyin is not commercially available in the United States, but it can be obtained at no cost and after consultation with a *Toxoplasma* reference laboratory (PAMF-TSL, 650-853-4828) through the FDA at (301) 827-2127. It should be administered orally at a dose of 1.0 g three times a day (total 3.0 g/d).

Spiramycin's overall efficacy to prevent congenital toxoplasmosis has been recently questioned by a group of European investigators [12,13]. Gilbert and coworkers [12,13,35] concluded in their studies that a significant effect of prenatal treatment (in regard to type—spiramycin versus pyrimethamine/sulfadiazine) and timing (delay in initiation of the drugs) on the risk of mother-to-child transmission of toxoplasmosis was not detected. They have in fact called for placebo-controlled trials to examine the efficacy of such interventions.

These results are not surprising, because the studies have several methodological shortcomings, including very few untreated women in their analysis and the fact that most of these untreated women had been infected during the third trimester [36] and came from centers where only neonatal screening programs were performed. The design of the studies performed to date by Gilbert and colleagues [12,13,35] have not permitted a definitive conclusion. Until appropriately designed studies are performed, most authorities continue to recommend spiramycin for women who have suspected or confirmed acute *T gondii* infection acquired during the first trimester or early in the second trimester of gestation.

Treatment with pyrimethamine/sulfadiazine/folinic acid

The combination of pyrimethamine, sulfadiazine, and folinic acid (see Table 2) is indicated for pregnant women suspected to have or diagnosed with acute *T gondii* infection acquired late in the second trimester (>18 weeks) or during the third trimester of gestation [1]. This combination is also indicated for pregnant women in whom fetal infection by the parasite has been confirmed (ie, positive amniotic fluid PCR result) or in whom abnormal fetal abnormalities consistent with congenital toxoplasmosis have been detected by ultrasound examination. Pyrimethamine is teratogenic, and its use in the first trimester is contraindicated. Pyrimethamine produces reversible, usually gradual, dose-related depression of the bone marrow. All patients who receive pyrimethamine should have their complete blood cell counts monitored. Folinic acid is used for reduction and prevention of the hematological toxicities [1].

Management of the patient who has chronic *Toxoplasma gondii* infection most likely acquired in the distant past and before gestation

Prenatal diagnosis of fetal *Toxoplasma* infection is not indicated when a diagnosis of chronic maternal infection acquired in the distant past and before pregnancy is established, or is highly suspected on the basis of serological test results. The incidence of congenital toxoplasmosis in offspring of women infected before gestation has been shown to be extremely rare (approaching zero) unless a woman is immunocompromised (ie, those who are significantly immunosuppressed due to infection with HIV, ingestion of corticosteroids or immunosuppressive drugs, and so on) [1].

Women who are dually infected with HIV and *T gondii* and have developed AIDS are at risk of reactivating their latent *T gondii* infection and developing maternal toxoplasmosis, as well as of transmitting the parasite to their offspring. The latter has been surprisingly found to be a relatively rare event, however [1,37]. At present, the data are insufficient to define the effectiveness of treatment intended to prevent transmission of *T gondii* to the fetus of an HIV-infected woman. Until, more data become available, the authors consider that *Toxoplasma*-seropositive pregnant women whose CD4 count is less than 200 cells/mm^3 should receive trimethoprim/sulfamethoxazole (ie, TMP/SMX single strength, one tablet per day) to both prevent reactivation of their *Toxoplasma* infection and transmission of the parasite to their offspring.

Management of the pregnant woman who has toxoplasmic chorioretinitis

Pregnant women who have toxoplasmic chorioretinitis as a result of reactivation of chronic disease do not have a higher risk of transmitting the parasite to their offspring than do pregnant women who have been infected before pregnancy and do not have ocular disease. Maternal eye disease should be referred to an ophthalmologist who has experience with the disease [14]. Pregnant women who have toxoplasmic chorioretinitis thought to be a manifestation of recently acquired infection should be treated, because of both the eye disease and the risk of transmission of the infection to their fetus [14]. In the latter scenario, the approach is similar to that outlined in the section "Manage-

and folinic acid, compared with historical controls receiving no or short-course therapy [39–42].

Prevention

Primary prevention (education)

Avoidance of the primary infection using educational tools targeting pregnant women has resulted in reducing rates of seroconversion among pregnant women by 60% [43,44]. It is recommended that educational measures be inserted into existing prenatal programs, visits, and classes. Ultimately, it is the responsibility of health policy makers and physicians to educate both the pregnant woman and the woman who is attempting to conceive in regard to preventive measures. The need for these measures must be continually reinforced throughout pregnancy [43,44]. Box 1 lists the measures that can be taken in an attempt to prevent *T gondii* infection. Physicians are urged to make similar lists available to their pregnant patients.

Secondary prevention (serological screening)

In addition to taking primary prevention measures, it is necessary to identify and treat women who acquire *T gondii* infection during gestation and—if fetal infection is detected by prenatal diagnosis testing—to discuss therapeutic options, including therapeutic abortion and antibiotic treatment of the fetus in utero. Acute toxoplasma infection in pregnant women almost always goes unrecognized, and will continue to be missed unless a universal screening system for the identification of these women is put in place.

Despite the facts that congenital toxoplasmosis continues to occur in the United States and the vast majority of pregnant women who acquire *T gondii* infection during gestation do not exhibit any symptoms, universal screening programs for the detection of toxoplasmosis during pregnancy have never been put in place in the United States. It is interesting to note that for other congenital infections that have been estimated to occur at similar or much lower rates than toxoplasmosis (eg, rubella at 1/100,000 or syphilis at 1/7,000), prenatal routine care does include universal screening for those infections.

In the state of Massachusetts in the United States, as well as in countries such as Denmark, secondary prevention programs that tests cord blood of all newborns for IgM antibodies to *T gondii* have been underway for several years [45,46]. Some of these neonatal screening programs have added screening for neonatal IgA, because presence of IgM in neonates is only present in 50% of congenitally infected babies. Although this method certainly does identify some subclinically infected infants, it misses infants who were infected late in the third trimester but who have yet to form antibodies, and infants infected early in gestation, because the window for detection of fetal/neonatal IgM has elapsed for some of these babies.

Summary

Congenital toxoplasmosis continues to be a tragic outcome of a preventable and treatable infection. Education of patients, physicians, and health policy makers on the primary and secondary preventive measures of the disease, and their execution, will undoubtedly result in lower incidence, morbidity, and mortality rates for congenital disease due to *T gondii*.

References

[1] Remington JS, McLeod R, Desmonts G. Toxoplasmosis. In: Remington JS, Klein JO, editors. Infectious diseases of the fetus and newborn infant. 5th edition. Philadelphia: W. B. Saunders Company; 2001. p. 205–346.
[2] Desmonts G, Couvreur J. Congenital toxoplasmosis. A prospective study of the offspring of 542 women who acquired toxoplasmosis during pregnancy. Pathophysiology of congenital disease [with letter]. In: Thalhammer O, Pollak A, Baumgarten K, editors. Perinatal medicine, 6th European Congress, Vienna. Stuttgart (Germany): Georg Thieme Publishers; 1979. p. 51–60.
[3] Koppe JG, Loewer-Sieger DH, De Roever-Bonnet H. Results of 20-year follow-up of congenital toxoplasmosis. Am J Ophthalmol 1986;101:248–9.
[4] Wilson CB, Remington JS, Stagno S, et al. Development of adverse sequelae in children born with subclinical congenital Toxoplasma infection. Pediatrics 1980;66:767–74.
[5] Bowie WR, King AS, Werker DH, et al. Outbreak of toxoplasmosis associated with municipal drinking water. Lancet 1997;350:173–7.
[6] Miller MA, Grigg ME, Kreuder C, et al. An unusual genotype of *Toxoplasma gondii* is common in California sea otters (*Enhydra lutris nereis*) and is a cause of mortality. Int J Parasitol 2004;34:275–84.
[7] Dubey JP, Graham DH, da Silva DS, et al. *Toxoplasma gondii* isolates of free-ranging chickens from Rio de Janeiro, Brazil: mouse mortality, genotype, and oocyst shedding by cats. J Parasitol 2003;89:851–3.
[8] Bahia-Oliveira LM, Jones JL, Azevedo-Silva J, et al. Highly endemic, waterborne toxoplasmosis in north Rio de Janeiro state, Brazil. Emerg Infect Dis 2003;9:55–62.
[9] Miller MA, Gardner IA, Kreuder C, et al. Coastal freshwater runoff is a risk factor for *Toxoplasma gondii* infection of southern sea otters (*Enhydra lutris nereis*). Int J Parasitol 2002;32:997–1006.
[10] Jones JL, Kruszon-Moran D, Wilson M. *Toxoplasma gondii* infection in the United States, 1999–2000. Emerg Infect Dis 2003;9:1371–4.
[11] Lopez A, Dietz VJ, Wilson M, et al. Preventing congenital toxoplasmosis. MMWR Recomm Rep 2000;49:59–68.
[12] Gilbert RE, Gras L, Wallon M, et al. Effect of prenatal treatment on mother to child transmission of *Toxoplasma gondii*: retrospective cohort study of 554 mother-child pairs in Lyon, France. Int J Epidemiol 2001;30:1303–8.
[13] Gilbert R, Gras L. European Multicentre Study on Congenital Toxoplasmosis. Effect of timing and type of treatment on the risk of mother to child transmission of *Toxoplasma gondii*. BJOG 2003;110:112–20.

[14] Montoya JG, Kovacs JA, Remington JS. *Toxoplasma gondii*. In: Mandell GL, Bennett JE, Dolin R, editors. Principles and practice of infectious diseases, vol. 2. Philadelphia: Elsevier Churchill Livingstone; 2005. p. 3170–98.
[15] Montoya JG, Remington JS. Toxoplasmic chorioretinitis in the setting of acute acquired toxoplasmosis. Clin Infect Dis 1996;23:277–82.
[16] Montoya JG, Remington JS. Studies on the serodiagnosis of toxoplasmic lymphadenitis. Clin Infect Dis 1995;20:781–90.
[17] Montoya JG, Liesenfeld O, Kinney S, et al. VIDAS test for avidity of toxoplasma-specific immunoglobulin G for confirmatory testing of pregnant women. J Clin Microbiol 2002;40: 2504–8.
[18] Liesenfeld O, Press C, Montoya JG, et al. False-positive results in immunoglobulin M (IgM) toxoplasma antibody tests and importance of confirmatory testing: the Platelia Toxo IgM test. J Clin Microbiol 1997;35:174–8.
[19] Wilson M, Remington JS, Clavet C, et al. Evaluation of six commercial kits for detection of human immunoglobulin M antibiodies to *Toxoplasma gondii*. J Clin Microbiol 1997;35:3112–5.
[20] US Public Health Service, Department of Health and Human Services and Food and Drug Administration. FDA public health advisory: limitations of toxoplasma IgM commerical test kits. Rockville (MD): Department of Health and Human Services, Food and Drug Administration; 1997.
[21] Liesenfeld O, Montoya JG, Tathineni NJ, et al. Confirmatory serologic testing for acute toxoplasmosis and rate of induced abortions among women reported to have positive toxoplasma immunoglobulin M antibody titers. Am J Obstet Gynecol 2001;184:140–5.
[22] Montoya JG, Jordan R, Lingamneni S, et al. Toxoplasmic myocarditis and polymyositis in patients with acute acquired toxoplasmosis diagnosed during life. Clin Infect Dis 1997;24:676–83.
[23] Hedman K, Lappalainen M, Seppala I, et al. Recent primary toxoplasma infection indicated by a low avidity of specific IgG. J Infect Dis 1989;159:736–9.
[24] Lappalainen M, Koskela P, Koskiniemi M, et al. Toxoplasmosis acquired during pregnancy: improved serodiagnosis based on avidity of IgG. J Infect Dis 1993;167:691–7.
[25] Cozon GJ, Ferrandiz J, Nebhi H, et al. Estimation of the avidity of immunoglobulin G for routine diagnosis of chronic *Toxoplasma gondii* infection in pregnant women. Eur J Clin Microbiol Infect Dis 1998;17:32–6.
[26] Jenum PA, Stray-Pedersen B, Gundersen A-G. Improved diagnosis of primary *Toxoplasma gondii* infection in early pregnancy by determination of antitoxoplasma immunoglobulin G activity. J Clin Microbiol 1997;35:1972–7.
[27] Gutiérrez J, Rodríguez M, Piédrola G, et al. Detection of IgA and low-avidity IgG antibodies for the diagnosis of recent active toxoplasmosis. Clin Microbiol Infect 1997;3:658–62.
[28] Holliman R, Raymond R, Renton N, et al. The diagnosis of toxoplasmosis using IgG avidity. Epidemiol Infect 1994;112:399–408.
[29] Liesenfeld O, Montoya JG, Kinney S, et al. Effect of testing for IgG avidity in the diagnosis of *Toxoplasma gondii* infection in pregnant women: experience in a US reference laboratory. J Infect Dis 2001;183:1248–53.
[30] Montoya JG, Huffman HB, Remington JS. Evaluation of the immunoglobulin g avidity test for diagnosis of toxoplasmic lymphadenopathy. J Clin Microbiol 2004;42:4627–31.
[31] Remington JS, Thulliez P, Montoya JG. Recent developments for diagnosis of toxoplasmosis. J Clin Microbiol 2004;42:941–5.
[32] Romand S, Wallon M, Franck J, et al. Prenatal diagnosis using polymerase chain reaction on amniotic fluid for congenital toxoplasmosis. Obstet Gynecol 2001;97:296–300.
[33] Daffos F, Forestier F, Capella-Pavlovsky M, et al. Prenatal management of 746 pregnancies at risk for congenital toxoplasmosis. N Engl J Med 1988;318:271–5.
[34] Schoondermark-Van de Ven E, Galama J, Camps W, et al. Pharmacokinetics of spiramycin in the rhesus monkey: transplacental passage and distribution in tissue in the fetus. Antimicrob Agents Chemother 1994;38:1922–9.
[35] Gilbert R, Dunn D, Wallon M, et al. Ecological comparison of the risks of mother-to-child

transmission and clinical manifestations of congenital toxoplasmosis according to prenatal treatment protocol. Epidemiol Infect 2001;127:113–20.

[36] Thulliez P. Commentary: efficacy of prenatal treatment for toxoplasmosis: a possibility that cannot be ruled out. Int J Epidemiol 2001;30:1315–6.

[37] Mitchell CD, Erlich SS, Mastrucci MT, et al. Congenital toxoplasmosis occurring in infants perinatally infected with human immunodeficiency virus 1. Pediatr Infect Dis J 1990;9:512–8.

[38] Stepick-Biek P, Thulliez P, Araujo FG, et al. IgA antibodies for diagnosis of acute congenital and acquired toxoplasmosis. J Infect Dis 1990;162:270–3.

[39] McAuley J, Boyer KM, Patel D, et al. Early and longitudinal evaluations of treated infants and children and untreated historical patients with congenital toxoplasmosis: the Chicago Collaborative Treatment Trial. Clin Inf Dis 1994;18:38–72.

[40] McGee T, Wolters C, Stein L, et al. Absence of sensorineural hearing loss in treated infants and children with congenital toxoplasmosis. Otolarygol Head Neck Surg 1992;106:75–80.

[41] Mets MB, Holfels E, Boyer KM, et al. Eye manifestations of congenital toxoplasmosis. Am J Opthalmol 1996;122:309–24.

[42] Roizen N, Swisher CN, Stein MA, et al. Neurologic and developmental outcome in treated congental toxoplasmosis. Pediatrics 1995;95:11–20.

[43] Wong S, Remington JS. Toxoplasmosis in pregnancy. Clin Infect Dis 1994;18:853–62.

[44] Foulon W, Naessens A, Lauwers S, et al. Impact of primary prevention on the incidence of toxoplasmosis during pregnancy. Obstet Gynecol 1988;72(Part 1):363–6.

[45] Eaton RB, Petersen E, Seppanen H, et al. Multicenter evaluation of a flurometric enzyme immunocapture assay to detect toxoplasma-specific immunoglobulin M in dried blood filter paper specimens from newborns. J Clin Microbiol 1996;34:3147–50.

[46] Petersen E, Eaton RB. Control of congenital infection with *Toxoplasma gondii* by neonatal screening based on detection of specific immunoglobulin M antibodies eluted from phenylketonuria filter-paper blood-spot samples. Acta Paediatr 1999;88(Suppl):36–9.

ELSEVIER
SAUNDERS

Clin Perinatol 32 (2005) 727–738

CLINICS IN
PERINATOLOGY

Influenza and Pneumonia in Pregnancy

Vanessa R. Laibl, MD*, Jeanne S. Sheffield, MD

Division of Maternal-Fetal Medicine, Department of Obstetrics and Gynecology, University of Texas Southwestern Medical Center at Dallas, 5323 Harry Hines Boulevard, Dallas, TX 75390-9032, USA

Influenza is a significant cause of morbidity and mortality from febrile respiratory illness worldwide. Influenza in pregnant women has historically been associated with a higher rate of morbidity and mortality. Pneumonia is the sixth leading cause of death in the United States, and it is the number one cause of death from an infectious disease. Although pregnant women do not get pneumonia more often than nonpregnant women, it can result in greater morbidity and mortality because of the physiologic adaptations of pregnancy. Pregnant patients who have either of these conditions require a higher level of surveillance and intervention.

Influenza

Influenza is caused by two RNA viruses in the family Orthomyxoviridae, influenza A and influenza B. First identified in 1933, they remain a significant cause of morbidity and mortality from febrile respiratory illness worldwide [1]. Influenza A is subtyped using two surface antigens: hemagglutinin (H) and neuraminidase (N). Both viruses are further grouped based on antigenic characteristics. Antigenic drift, the yearly variation in the surface antigens caused by point mutations, results in the need for annual revaccination. Because immunity to surface antigens reduces the chance of becoming infected as well as the severity of symptoms if infected [2], vaccines are developed with subtle alterations each year in anticipation of viral variation. Antigenic shift, seen only in influenza A, occurs when mutations accumulate in the N or H antigens, replacing

* Corresponding author.
E-mail address: vlaibl@parknet.pmh.org (V.R. Laibl).

0095-5108/05/$ – see front matter
doi:10.1016/j.clp.2005.04.009 *perinatology.theclinics.com*

the current antigen with a new subtype. The years associated with antigenic shift report much higher morbidity and mortality rates. Between 1990 and 1999, influenza caused an average of 36,000 deaths per year [3]. The H3N2 strain of influenza A has caused the most hospitalizations during epidemic years since 1968, at approximately 142,000 per year [4]. A patient's response to influenza is multifactorial and cannot be predicted based on viral properties alone [5]. It is this uncertainty that has continued to make influenza a formidable opponent.

Historical perspective

Influenza in pregnant women has historically been associated with a higher rate of morbidity and mortality. The course of influenza in pregnancy was first reported during the epidemic of 1918, when 1350 cases in pregnant women who had an influenza-like illness were evaluated. Pneumonia complicated 585 (43%) of the cases. In 52% of these patients, the pregnancy was interrupted. There were 308 (23%) maternal deaths. Mortality was highest in the last 3 months of pregnancy, and increased if complicated by pneumonia [6]. During the influenza epidemic of 1957, 22 pregnant women in New York City died from complications of the flu. Pregnant women accounted for nearly half the deaths of women of childbearing age [7]. During the same epidemic, 11 pregnant women died in Minnesota. All deaths were attributed to respiratory insufficiency secondary to pulmonary edema and pneumonia [8]. Mullooly and colleagues [9] reviewed influenza complicating pregnancy from 1975 to 1979. There were four epidemics in that 5-year time period. Pregnant women sought outpatient medical attention for acute respiratory disease during the influenza season significantly more often than nonpregnant women; however, unlike the previously reported epidemics, there were no maternal deaths attributable to influenza, and the hospitalization rate was low at 2 per 1000.

Risk factors

It is recommended that high-risk groups be vaccinated annually, because the severity of the season will only be known in retrospect. High-risk groups include children aged 6 to 23 months; people aged 65 or older; residents of long-term care facilities; adults and children who have chronic illnesses, including asthma, diabetes, and immunosuppression; and pregnant women. In 2000, 73 million people in the United States were considered high-risk [4]. Unfortunately, up to 50% of these high-risk patients do not receive annual vaccination.

Pregnant women are felt to be at increased risk for influenza. This risk is higher if they have an underlying medical condition, are of advanced age, or are exposed in the third trimester [10]. In a study by Neuzil and coworkers [10], women in the third trimester were three to four times more likely than postpartum women to be hospitalized for an acute cardiopulmonary illness during influenza season. Asthma in pregnant women increased the rate of hospitalizations for a respiratory illness during influenza season 10-fold [11].

Clinical presentation

The virus is spread from person to person via respiratory droplets. Particles are created when a person coughs, sneezes, or speaks. These particles are filtered by the recipient's nose and pharynx and then reach the alveoli [12].

The clinical presentation of influenza does not appear to be altered by pregnancy. The incubation period for influenza is 1 to 4 days, with an average of 2 days [13]. Patients are generally infectious the day before the onset of symptoms and for 5 days thereafter; however, young children and immunocompromised adults can shed virus for much longer periods of time [4]. Infants infected while in the hospital can shed virus for up to 21 days [12].

Symptoms of influenza include cough, fever, malaise, rhinitis, myalgias, headache, chills, and sore throat. Less common symptoms include nausea and vomiting, otitis, and conjunctival burning. Signs of influenza include fever, tachycardia, facial flushing, clear nasal discharge, and cervical adenopathy. Fever in adults generally lasts for 3 days, with resolution of symptoms normally within 1 week; however, the cough and malaise may persist for greater than 2 weeks [5].

Diagnosis

Influenza is usually diagnosed using clinical features during the influenza season. Rapid testing by either immunofluorescence or immunoassay has the advantage of providing same-day diagnosis; however, it does not have the same sensitivity as culture. There are various rapid tests on the market. Some detect influenza but cannot distinguish influenza A from B. Others detect both and can distinguish them. Nasal samples provide a higher level of sensitivity than do throat samples when performing rapid testing. The positive and negative predictive value of the rapid tests depends on the level of influenza activity in the population being tested. Patients who have a clinical picture highly suggestive of influenza but with a negative rapid test should still be cultured, because false negatives do occur [4,12]. Viral culture is necessary to subtype influenza as well as to perform drug sensitivities.

Complications

Pneumonia, either viral or superimposed bacterial, is a well-recognized complication of influenza. Patients initially present with respiratory distress in the case of viral pneumonia. On chest radiograph, diffuse bilateral infiltrates are seen. Signs of pneumonia include course rales and rhonchi, wheezing, dyspnea, and tachypnea. Superimposed bacterial pneumonia typically occurs 2 to 14 days after symptoms of influenza have resolved. Local consolidation is seen on chest radiograph with superimposed bacterial pneumonia. Myopathy is another complication that has been associated with influenza. Patients may develop rhabdomyolysis and myoglobinuria. In adults, myopathy is more commonly found with influenza A. It has been suggested that a genetic predisposition exists for this complication. Pathology slides of muscle biopsies taken from patients who had suspected influenza-associated myopathy showed lysis of muscle fibers. Carditis has also been reported. The influenza virus has been isolated from the myocardium of patients who died of influenza complications. With carditis there are often EKG changes, including ST changes, inverted T waves, and rate disturbances. Carditis can occur at the same time as the initial respiratory manifestations. Finally, encephalopathy is a rare complication of influenza. The virus has been isolated from cerebrospinal fluid (CSF) and brain tissue at autopsy. Encephalopathy is also thought to be genetically linked [5].

Fetal effects

There is a paucity of prospective data on the effects of intrapartum, laboratory-confirmed influenza on fetal outcome. Irving and colleagues [14] found no significant difference between women who had serum-confirmed influenza and controls in the incidence of congenital malformations. Widelock and coworkers [15] studied the influenza epidemics of 1957 to 1960. They too found no increased incidence of fetal death or malformations in pregnant women who had influenza. Influenza has been associated with limb reduction and neural tube defects, including anencephaly [16–18]. Other investigators have not found an association between influenza and anencephaly [19]. Several studies have noted an increased incidence of schizophrenia in people who were born 2 to 3 months after an influenza epidemic, implying that maternal exposure to influenza in the second trimester, when fetal neurons are migrating, is a risk factor [20,21]. There have also been reports of an increased incidence of cleft lip [22,23]. Unfortunately, many studies are limited by recall and selection bias, making it unclear if there truly is an association.

Treatment

There are four antiviral agents approved for the treatment and prevention of influenza. These medications are no substitute for vaccination, especially in high-risk groups. The adamantanes, M2 ion-channel inhibitors, include amantadine and rimantadine. These drugs have activity only against influenza A [24]. Given as chemoprophylaxis, they are 70% to 90% effective at preventing influenza. They also can be given within the first 48 hours of symptoms to reduce symptom duration. To minimize drug resistance, therapy should be discontinued within 24 to 48 hours after symptoms resolve, or 3 to 5 days. Most notable side effects are of the central nervous system and include confusion, insomnia, and difficulty concentrating [25]. The neuraminidase inhibitors are effective in the treatment of influenza A and B. Oseltamivir, given orally, is approved for both treatment and chemoprophylaxis. It is reported to be 70% to 90% effective at preventing influenza [26]. The most commonly reported side effects are nausea and vomiting [27]. Zanamivir is an inhaled medication approved for treatment only. It should be noted that there have been several reports of bronchospasm in patients who have asthma and who take this drug. Both shorten the duration of symptoms by, on average, 1 day. There are limited data on safety in pregnancy. All four drugs are US Food and Drug Administration category C, and therefore should be used only when the benefits outweigh the risks [28].

Prevention/vaccination

The primary method of influenza prevention is vaccination. Vaccination is most effective when performed in October or November, although unvaccinated patients should not be denied vaccination later in the season. The recommendation of the Advisory Committee on Immunization Practices (ACIP) is that all women who will be pregnant during the influenza season should receive the vaccine. Vaccination can be performed safely in any trimester of pregnancy [29,30]. Breast feeding is not a contraindication to vaccination [4]. There are two different vaccines available. One is a live-attenuated vaccine (LAIV), whereas the other is inactivated. The inactivated vaccine is used for pregnant women as well as all other high risk groups. The LAIV is recommended only for healthy persons ages 5 to 49. The inactivated vaccine is less expensive. Both vaccines are contraindicated in people who have an anaphylactic hypersensitivity to eggs or other components of the vaccine, people who have an acute febrile illness, and people who have a history of Guillain-Barré syndrome within 6 weeks of a previous influenza vaccination. Peak antibody protection develops 2 weeks after vaccination [31,32]. Inactivated vaccine in the United States that is distributed in single-dose syringes is preservative-free and contains only trace amounts of thimerosal, a mercury-containing compound. Thus, there is little concern for mercury exposure because it is limited to less than 0.5 mcg mercury/0.25-mL dose [33]. Vaccine efficacy in healthy adults less than 65 years of age is 70% to 90% if circulating and vaccine viruses are antigenically similar [4].

Secondary prevention strategies should also be implemented. These include hand washing, respiratory and contact isolation, and contact prophylaxis.

Pneumonia

Overall, pneumonia is the sixth leading cause of death in the United States, and it is the number one cause of death from an infectious disease. Over 5 million cases occur annually, with more than 1 million persons requiring hospitalization [34,35]. Although associated with far less mortality, women of reproductive age are susceptible to pneumonia from a bacterial, viral, or fungal source. Although pregnant women do not get pneumonia more often than nonpregnant women, it can result in greater morbidity and mortality because of the physiologic adaptations of pregnancy. These include a decrease in pulmonary functional residual capacity as well as alterations in cell-mediated immunity. Thus, pregnant patients require a higher level of surveillance and intervention. In a study by Jin and colleagues [36] the hospitalization rate for community-acquired pneumonia in pregnant women was 1.51 per 1000 pregnancies. Several recent articles have reported an incidence of 1 per 660 deliveries [36,37].

Bacterial pneumonia

Some of the organisms found to cause bacterial pneumonia include *Streptococcus pneumoniae*, *Hemophilus influenzae*, *Chlamydia pneumoniae*, *Mycoplasma pneumoniae*, and *Legionella pneumophila*. *S pneumoniae* is the most commonly identified bacterial cause, though Richey and coworkers [38] found that in only 27% of cases could the causative organism be identified. The American Thoracic Society notes that even with extensive diagnostic testing, in 50% or more of cases the etiology cannot be identified. A Gram's stain and culture of sputum can be helpful in focusing therapy, but its use is controversial. Bacterial cultures of sputum have poor sensitivity and specificity [39].

Risk factors for pneumonia include asthma and other chronic respiratory diseases, HIV/AIDS, smoking, and drug use [40]. Signs and symptoms of bacterial pneumonia in pregnancy are the same as in nonpregnant individuals. Symptoms include cough (>90%), sputum production (66%), dyspnea (66%), and pleuritic chest pain (50%) [41]. Signs include fever, crackles, and abnormal breath sounds. In patients who have the above findings and in whom pneumonia is suspected, a chest radiograph should be performed. The chest radiograph will confirm pneumonia, rule out other diagnoses, suggest a possible etiology, and aid in determining the severity of illness. Multilobar pneumonia is considered a more severe process than single lobar involvement [39]. Generally, all pregnant women who have pneumonia are hospitalized for observation and initial therapy. Work-up should include a complete blood count, electrolytes, assessment of oxygenation, and blood cultures; however, blood cultures have been found to be positive only 7% to 15% of the time [37,40].

Maternal mortality was greatly reduced with the advent of antibiotics [42,43]. Intravenous antibiotic therapy should be started empirically. Erythromycin is an acceptable initial choice for treatment, because it is considered safe in pregnancy [28]. Treatment success rates up to 99% have been reported [37]. If aspiration, gram-negative organisms, or drug-resistant *S pneumoniae* is suspected, a beta-lactam such as ceftriaxone or ampicillin should be added. Most patients will have a clinical response within 3 days. Therapy should not be changed in the first 72 hours unless there is a marked clinical deterioration [39].

Many different complications of bacterial pneumonia have been reported. Infections at other sites can occur. Meningitis, arthritis, endocarditis, empyema, and pericarditis have all been reported. Severe cases of pneumonia can be complicated by sepsis, heart failure, renal failure, and acute respiratory distress syndrome (ARDS), requiring intensive care admission. Obstetric complications include fetal distress secondary to poor oxygenation and preterm birth. Munn and coworkers [44] found that women who had pneumonia were significantly more likely to deliver before 34 weeks. Preterm birth has been reported to be more common when the woman who has pneumonia also has some underlying comorbid condition [45]. Anemia has also been reported in several studies of pneumonia during pregnancy [37,40,44,46]. Birthweights of infants born to women who have antepartum pneumonia have been found to be significantly less than controls [37,40].

With the increasing number of pregnant women infected with human immunodeficiency virus, *Pneumocystis carinii* pneumonia (PCP) deserves specific mention. Among pregnant women, this is the leading cause of AIDS-related death in the United States [47]. Symptoms include dry cough, dyspnea, and tachypnea. A diffuse infiltrate is seen on chest radiograph. Ahmad and coworkers [48] reported 22 cases of PCP in pregnancy. The mortality rate was extremely high at 50%. Fifty-nine percent required mechanical ventilation. These numbers may be inflated because none of the patients were on antiretroviral therapy, because all were diagnosed with HIV when diagnosed with PCP. Treatment is with trimethoprim-sulfamethoxazole or pentamidine. HIV-infected patients who have a CD4+ T-lymphocyte count less than 200/μL, a history of oropharyngeal candidiasis, or an AIDS-defining illness should receive prophylaxis [49]. The preferred regimen is trimethoprim-sulfamethoxazole, one double-strength tablet per day. Prophylaxis is 90% to 95% effective [50].

Viral pneumonia

Viral pneumonia is most commonly caused by influenza and varicella-zoster virus (VZV). Influenza in pregnancy has been described in great detail earlier in this article. VZV is a DNA virus that affects 0.7 per 1000 pregnancies [51]. Pneumonia is the most common complication in adults, occurring in 10% of cases [52]. Before the availability of antiviral therapy, mortality rates in pregnant women who had VZV pneumonia were quoted as high as 35% to 40% [53,54]. The mortality rate in the era of antiviral therapy is approximately 14% [54,55]. Risk factors for varicella pneumonia include smoking and the presence of 100 or more skin lesions [52]. Pulmonary symptoms begin 2 to 5 days after the onset of rash and fever. Symptoms include cough, hemoptysis, dyspnea, tachypnea, and pleuritic chest pain. Chest radiograph shows diffuse miliary or nodular infiltrates. Treatment is with intravenous acyclovir, although the value of this has not been proven in rigorous scientific studies.

Congenital varicella syndrome occurs in 1% to 2% of cases of maternal varicella, depending on gestational age [56–58]. In a study conducted by the Maternal Fetal Medicine Unit Network of 347 pregnant women who had varicella [59], the rate of congenital varicella was 0.4%. Congenital varicella is characterized by limb hypoplasia, chorioretinitis, cutaneous scars, and cortical atrophy [60,61].

Varicella pneumonia has been associated with preterm labor [60], although this was not substantiated in a later study of 18 women who had varicella pneumonia [52]. Varicella-zoster immunoglobulin given within 96 hours of exposure to varicella can attenuate or prevent infection in susceptible individuals. It is not contraindicated in pregnancy. The varicella vaccine, however, is contraindicated in pregnancy because it is a live-attenuated vaccine [62].

Severe acute respiratory syndrome (SARS) is caused by a novel coronavirus. Since 2002, this atypical pneumonia has affected over 8000 people and resulted in more than 800 deaths worldwide [63]. Transmission is by respiratory droplets or close personal contact. The virus can live in urine and stool for 1 to 2 days. Symptoms are the same in pregnant women as in nonpregnant women, and include fever, chills, rigors, malaise, and myalgias [64]. Patients are most infectious during the second week of illness. Chest radiograph findings are most often generalized, patchy, interstitial infiltrates [63]. Patients have been noted to have lymphopenia [64] as well as thrombocytopenia [63].

Diagnosis can be made by culture, polymerase chain reaction (PCR), enzyme-linked immunosorbent assay (ELISA), and indirect fluorescent antibody (IFA). Guidelines and protocols for diagnostic tests are available on the World Health Organization Web site at http://www.who.int/csr/sars/en/.

Complications of SARS pneumonia include respiratory failure, superimposed bacterial infections, and disseminated intravascular coagulation (DIC). The largest case series of pregnant women who had SARS comes from Wong and coworkers in China [65]. Twelve pregnant women were infected with SARS between February 1, 2003 and July 31, 2003. High rates of morbidity and mortality were noted. The case fatality rate was 25%. A large portion of the cases was complicated by first-trimester spontaneous abortions, preterm births, and intrauterine growth restriction; however, there have been no cases of vertical transmission reported. Treatment includes broad-spectrum antibiotics to cover superimposed bacterial infections, high dose steroids, and possibly ribavirin. Ribavirin has been shown to have teratogenic effects in animals [66,67], and its use in pregnancy has not been established.

Fungal pneumonia

Fungal pneumonia in pregnancy is most often seen in those women who are immunocompromised; however, with the physiologic suppression of cell-mediated immunity in pregnancy, fungal pneumonia can be seen in otherwise healthy women. There have only been a handful of cases of pneumonia secondary to histoplasmosis reported [68]. Although still extremely limited, there are more case reports of blastomycosis. Lemos and colleagues [69] reviewed 19 cases of blastomycosis in pregnancy. Seventy-eight percent had pulmonary involvement, and all recovered or were at least reported as having a "good response." In two cases, the newborn died and was found to have blastomycosis at autopsy. Treatment is with amphotericin B or ketoconazole. Ely and coworkers [70] reported four cases of cryptococcal pneumonia. All were otherwise healthy women. Cryptococcal pneumonia is difficult to diagnosis. In this case series, all women eventually underwent a lung biopsy to make the diagnosis. Symptoms include cough, chest pain, and dyspnea. Chest radiograph findings can vary greatly and include infiltrates, mass lesions, and adenopathy. Treatment is with amphotericin B. Coccidioidomycosis results from the inhalation of *Coccidioides immitis*. One third of infected persons will develop a symptomatic illness.

Complications of coccidioidomycosis include pneumonia and disseminated disease [71]. Symptoms include cough, fever, and erythema nodosum [72]. Erythema nodosum has been reported to be a marker of good outcome in pregnant women [73]. Dissemination of disease in pregnancy is a controversial topic. Historically, dissemination was reported to be 40 to 100 times more frequent in pregnancy [74]. Caldwell and colleagues [72] found the incidence of dissemination in pregnancy to be 9%, three times the rate of the nonpregnant population. In their series, 23/32 recovered without treatment, and there were no deaths. Risk factors include living in an endemic area, smoking, older age, diabetes, and low socioeconomic status [71]. Treatment is with amphotericin B.

Regardless of the type of pneumonia, it is important to be aggressive with monitoring and treatment for the sake of the mother and fetus. Oxygen supplementation should be provided to prevent fetal acidemia. Broad-spectrum empiric antibiotics should be started before identification of the etiologic agent, and antibiotic therapy should be tailored to specific organisms as laboratory tests return. Given that the majority of pregnant women are young and healthy, intense, early treatment is likely to result in a good outcome.

References

[1] Wright PF, Webster RG. Orthomyxoviruses. In: Fields BN, Knipe DM, Howley PM, et al, editors. Fields virology. 4th edition. Philadelphia: Lippincott; 2001. p. 1533–68.

[2] Clements ML, Betts RF, Tierney EL, et al. Serum and nasal wash antibodies associated with resistance to experimental challenge with influenza A wild-type virus. J Clin Microbiol 1986; 24:157–60.

[3] Thompson WW, Shay DK, Weintraub E, et al. Mortality associated with influenza and respiratory syncytial virus in the US. JAMA 2003;289:179–86.

[4] Harper SA, Fukuda K, Uyeki TM, et al. Prevention and control of influenza. Recommendations of the advisory committee on immunization practices. MMWR Recomm Rep 2004;53:1–40.

[5] Kilbourne ED. Influenza. New York: Plenum Publishing Corporation; 1987.

[6] Harris JW. Influenza occurring in pregnant women. JAMA 1919;72:978–83.

[7] Greenberg M, Jacobziner H, Pakter J, et al. Maternal mortality in the epidemic of Asian influenza, New York City, 1957. Am J Obstet Gynecol 1958;76:897–902.

[8] Freeman DW, Barno A. Deaths from Asian influenza associated with pregnancy. Am J Obstet Gynecol 1959;78:1172–5.

[9] Mullooly JP, Barker WH, Nolan TF. Risk of acute respiratory disease among pregnant women during influenza A epidemics. Public Health Rep 1986;101:205–10.

[10] Neuzil KM, Reed GW, Mitchel EF, et al. Impact of influenza on acute cardiopulmonary hospitalizations in pregnant women. Am J Epidemiol 1998;148:1094–102.

[11] Hartert TV, Neuzil KM, Shintani AK, et al. Maternal morbidity and perinatal outcomes among pregnant women with respiratory hospitalizations during influenza season. Am J Obstet Gynecol 2003;189:1705–12.

[12] Saldago CD, Farr BM, Hall KK, et al. Influenza in the acute hospital setting. Lancet Infect Dis 2002;2:145–55.

[13] Cox NJ, Subbarao K. Influenza. Lancet 1999;354:1277–82.

[14] Irving WL, James DK, Stephenson T, et al. Influenza virus infection in the second and third trimesters of pregnancy: a clinical and seroepidemiological study. Br J Obstet Gynaecol 2000; 107:1282–9.

[15] Widelock D, Csizmas L, Klein S. Influenza, pregnancy, and fetal outcome. Public Health Rep 1963;78:1–11.
[16] Aro T, Haapakoski J, Heinonen OP. A multivariate analysis of the risk indicators of reduction limb defects. Int J Epidemiol 1984;13:459–64.
[17] Lynberg MC, Khoury MJ, Lu X, et al. Maternal flu, fever, and the risk of neural tube defects: a population-based case-control study. Am J Epidemiol 1994;140:244–55.
[18] Coffey VP, Jessop WJE. Maternal influenza and congenital deformities. Lancet 1959;2:935–8.
[19] Saxen L, Holmberg PC, Kurppa K, et al. Influenza epidemics and anencephaly. Am J Public Health 1990;80:473–5.
[20] Mednick SA, Machon RA, Huttunen MO, et al. Adult schizophrenia following prenatal exposure to an influenza epidemic. Arch Gen Psychiatry 1988;45:189–92.
[21] Sham PC, O'Callaghan E, Takei N, et al. Schizophrenia following pre-natal exposure to influenza epidemics between 1939 and 1960. Br J Psychol 1992;160:461–6.
[22] Leck I. Incidence of malformations following influenza epidemics. Br J Prev Soc Med 1963; 17:70–80.
[23] Leck I. Further tests of the hypothesis that influenza in pregnancy causes malformations. HSMHA Health Rep 1969;86:265–9.
[24] Hay AJ. The mechanism of action of amantadine and rimantadine against influenza viruses. In: Notkins AL, Oldstone MBA, editors. Concepts in viral pathogenesis III. Berlin: Springer; 1989. p. 561–7.
[25] Money DM. Antiviral and antiretroviral use in pregnancy. Obstet Gynecol Clin N Amer 2003; 30:731–49.
[26] Cooper NJ, Sutton AJ, Abrams KR, et al. Effectiveness of neuraminidase inhibitors in treatment and prevention of influenza A and B: systematic review and meta-analyses of randomized controlled trials. BMJ 2003;326:1235–41.
[27] Monto AS. The role of antivirals in the control of influenza. Vaccine 2003;21:1796–800.
[28] Briggs GG, Freeman RK, Yaffe SJ. Drugs in pregnancy and lactation. Baltimore (MD): Williams and Wilkins; 1998.
[29] Deinard AS, Ogburn PA. NJ/8/76 Influenza vaccination program: effects on maternal health and pregnancy outcome. Am J Obstet Gynecol 1981;140:240–5.
[30] Heinonen OP, Shapiro S, Monson RR, et al. Immunization during pregnancy against poliomyelitis and influenza in relation to childhood malignancy. Int J Epidemiol 1973;2:229–35.
[31] Brokstad KA, Cox RJ, Olofsson J, et al. Parenteral influenza vaccination induces a rapid systemic and local immune response. J Infect Dis 1995;171:198–203.
[32] Gross PA, Russo C, Dran S, et al. Time to earliest peak serum antibody response to influenza vaccine in the elderly. Clin Diagn Lab Immunol 1997;4:491–2.
[33] Centers for Disease Control and Prevention. Recommendations regarding the use of vaccines that contain thimerosal as a preservative. MMWR Morb Mortal Wkly Rep 1999;48: 996–8.
[34] Garibaldi RA. Epidemiology of community-acquired respiratory tract infections in adults: incidence, etiology, and impact. Am J Med 1985;78:32S–7S.
[35] Niederman MS, McCombs JI, Unger AN, et al. The cost of treating community-acquired pneumonia. Clin Ther 1998;20:820–37.
[36] Jin Y, Carriere KC, Marrie TJ, et al. The effects of community-acquired pneumonia during pregnancy ending with a live birth. Am J Obstet Gynecol 2003;188:800–6.
[37] Yost NP, Bloom SL, Richey SD, et al. An appraisal of treatment guidelines for antepartum community-acquired pneumonia. Am J Obstet Gynecol 2000;183:131–5.
[38] Richey SD, Roberts SW, Ramin KD, et al. Pneumonia complicating pregnancy. Obstet Gynecol 1994;84:525–8.
[39] American Thoracic Society. Guidelines for the management of adults with community-acquired pneumonia. Am J Respir Crit Care Med 2001;163:1730–54.
[40] Berkowitz K, LaSala A. Risk factors associated with the increasing prevalence of pneumonia during pregnancy. Am J Obstet Gynecol 1990;163:981–5.

[41] Halm EA, Teirstein AS. Management of community-acquired pneumonia. N Engl J Med 2002; 347:2039–45.
[42] Hopwood HG. Pneumonia in pregnancy. Obstet Gynecol 1965;25:875–9.
[43] Oxorn H. The changing aspects of pneumonia complicating pregnancy. Am J Obstet Gynecol 1955;70:1057–63.
[44] Munn MB, Groome LJ, Atterbury JL, et al. Pneumonia as a complication of pregnancy. J Matern Fetal Med 1999;8:151–4.
[45] Madinger NE, Greenspoon JS, Ellrodt AG. Pneumonia during pregnancy: has modern technology improved maternal and fetal outcome? Am J Obstet Gynecol 1989;161:657–62.
[46] Benedetti TJ, Valle R, Ledger WJ. Antepartum pneumonia in pregnancy. Am J Obstet Gynecol 1982;144:413–7.
[47] Koonin LM, Ellerbrock TV, Atrash HK, et al. Pregnancy-associated deaths due to AIDS in the United States. JAMA 1989;261:1306–9.
[48] Ahmad H, Mehta NJ, Manikol VM, et al. *Pneumocystis carinii* pneumonia in pregnancy. Chest 2001;120:666–71.
[49] Centers for Disease Control. Guidelines for prophylaxis against *Pneumocystis carinii* pneumonia for persons infected with human immunodeficiency virus. MMWR Morb Mortal Wkly Rep 1989;8(S-5):1–9.
[50] Palella Jr FJ, Delaney KM, Moorman AC, et al. Declining morbidity and mortality among patients with advanced human immunodeficiency virus infection. N Engl J Med 1998;338: 853–60.
[51] Esmonde TF, Herdman G, Anderson G. Chickenpox pneumonia: an association with pregnancy. Thorax 1989;44:812–5.
[52] Harger JH, Ernest JM, Thurnau GR, et al. Risk factors and outcome of varicella-zoster virus pneumonia in pregnant women. J Infect Dis 2002;185:422–7.
[53] Haake DA, Zakowski PC, Haake DL, et al. Early treatment with acyclovir for varicella pneumonia in otherwise healthy adults: retrospective controlled study and review. Rev Infect Dis 1990;12:788–98.
[54] Smego RA, Asperilla MO. Use of acyclovir for varicella pneumonia during pregnancy. Obstet Gynecol 1991;78:1112–6.
[55] Brousard RC, Payne DK, George RB. Treatment with acyclovir of varicella pneumonia in pregnancy. Chest 1991;99:1045–7.
[56] Pastusazak A, Levy M, Schick B, et al. Outcome after maternal varicella infection in the first 20 weeks of pregnancy. N Engl J Med 1994;330:901–5.
[57] Enders G, Miller E, Craddock-Watson J, et al. Consequences of varicella and herpes zoster in pregnancy: prospective study of 1739 cases. Lancet 1994;343:1547–51.
[58] Jones KL, Johnson KA, Chambers CD. Offspring of women infected with varicella during pregnancy: a prospective study. Teratology 1994;49:29–32.
[59] Harger JH, Ernest JM, Thurnau GR, et al. Frequency of congenital varicella syndrome in a prospective cohort of 347 pregnant women. Obstet Gynecol 2002;100:260–5.
[60] Paryani SG, Arvin AM. Intrauterine infection with varicella-zoster virus after maternal varicella. N Engl J Med 1986;314:1542–6.
[61] Siegel M. Congenital malformations following chickenpox, measles, mumps, and hepatitis: results of a cohort study. JAMA 1973;226:1521–4.
[62] Atkinson WL, Pickering LK, Schwartz B, et al. General recommendations on immunization. MMWR Recomm Rep 2002;51:1–35.
[63] World Health Organization, SARS Epidemiology Working Group. Consensus document on the epidemiology of severe acute respiratory syndrome (SARS). Geneva, Switzerland: World Health Organization; 2003.
[64] Lam CM, Wong SF, Leung TN, et al. A case-controlled study comparing clinical course and outcomes of pregnant and non-pregnant women with severe acute respiratory syndrome. BJOG 2004;111:771–4.
[65] Wong SF, Chow KM, Leung TN, et al. Pregnancy and perinatal outcomes of women with severe acute respiratory syndrome. Am J Obstet Gynecol 2004;191:292–7.

[66] Kochhar DM, Penner JD, Knudsen TB. Embryotoxic, teratogenic, and metabolic effects of ribavirin in mice. Toxicol Appl Pharmacol 1980;52:99–112.
[67] Ferm VH, Willhite C, Kilham L. Teratogenic effects of ribavirin on hamster and rat embryos. Teratology 1978;17:93–101.
[68] Whitt ST, Koch GA, Fender B, et al. Histoplasmosis in pregnancy. Arch Intern Med 2004; 164:454–8.
[69] Lemos LB, Soofi M, Amir E. Blastomycosis and pregnancy. Ann Diagn Pathol 2002;6:211–5.
[70] Ely EW, Peacock JE, Haponik EF, et al. Cryptococcal pneumonia complicating pregnancy. Medicine 1998;77:153–67.
[71] Rosenstein NE, Emery KW, Werner SB, et al. Risk factors for severe pulmonary and disseminated coccidioidomycosis: Kern County, California, 1995–1996. Clin Infect Dis 2001; 32:708–14.
[72] Caldwell JW, Arsura EL, Kilgore WB, et al. Coccidioidomycosis in pregnancy during an epidemic in California. Obstet Gynecol 2000;95:236–9.
[73] Arsura EL, Kilgore WB, Ratnayake SN. Erythema nodosum in pregnant patients with coccidioidomycosis. Clin Infect Dis 1998;27:1201–3.
[74] Peterson CM, Schuppert K, Kelly PC, et al. Coccidioidomycosis and pregnancy. Obstet Gynecol Surv 1993;48:149–56.

ELSEVIER
SAUNDERS

Clin Perinatol 32 (2005) 739–747

CLINICS IN
PERINATOLOGY

Tuberculosis in Pregnancy

Vanessa R. Laibl, MD*, Jeanne S. Sheffield, MD

Division of Maternal-Fetal Medicine, Department of Obstetrics and Gynecology, University of Texas Southwestern Medical Center at Dallas, 5323 Harry Hines Boulevard, Dallas, TX 75390-9032, USA

Mycobacteria belong to the family *Mycobacteriaceae*. The species most often encountered in humans is *M tuberculosis*. *M tuberculosis* is a rod-shaped, non-spore forming, aerobic bacterium. *M bovis*, *M africanum*, and *M microti*, although less common, can cause human disease as well. It is estimated that 8 to 9 million new cases of tuberculosis occurred worldwide in 2000, with more than half of the cases occurring in Asia [1]. There were approximately 2 million deaths from tuberculosis in 1997, 98% of them in developing countries.

A number of factors were implicated in the resurgence of tuberculosis in the United States in the late 80s and early 90s, including increased immigration from countries with a high prevalence of tuberculosis, HIV infection, emergence of resistant strains, poverty, homelessness, drug abuse, and a decline in tuberculosis-related health services [2]. With better programs directed at the control of tuberculosis, cases began to decrease in 1993. In 1998, 18,361 cases of tuberculosis (6.8 per 100,000 population) were reported to the US Centers for Disease Control and Prevention (CDC). This was a 31% decrease from 1992. Pregnancy is not thought to change the course of tuberculosis [3,4]; however, tuberculosis does pose a risk to the pregnant woman and her fetus.

Transmission and infection

Transmission and infection during pregnancy are felt to be the same as in nonpregnant individuals [5]. *M tuberculosis* is most commonly transmitted from person to person by respiratory droplets that are aerosolized during coughing,

* Corresponding author.
E-mail address: vlaibl@parknet.pmh.org (V.R. Laibl).

0095-5108/05/$ – see front matter
doi:10.1016/j.clp.2005.04.010 *perinatology.theclinics.com*

sneezing, singing, or speaking. The droplets dry rapidly and may remain suspended in the air for several hours. Factors associated with the likelihood of transmission include the intimacy and duration of contact, the degree of infectiousness of the case, and the shared environment of the contact. Patients who have sputum smear-negative/culture-positive tuberculosis are less infectious, and those who have culture-negative pulmonary disease and extrapulmonary tuberculosis are noninfectious.

Droplets gain direct access to the terminal air passages when inhaled, and approximately 10% reach the alveoli. There, activated alveolar macrophages ingest the bacilli. If the bacilli multiply, their growth quickly kills the macrophages, which lyse. These initial stages of infection are usually asymptomatic. Two to 4 weeks after infection, two additional host responses develop: a tissue-damaging response and a macrophage-activating response. Large numbers of activated macrophages accumulate at the site of the primary lesion, and granulomatous lesions are formed [6,7]. These lesions consist of lymphocytes and activated macrophages. Macrophages containing bacilli first travel to the lymph nodes and then the rest of the body.

Many patients are infected with *M tuberculosis* but do not have the active form of disease. In patients that will go on to have active disease, the macrophage-activating response is weak, and therefore mycobacterial growth can be inhibited only by an intensified tissue-damaging response. As the surrounding tissue is

Box 1. Groups at high risk for tuberculosis

Increased risk of exposure

- Immigrants from endemic areas
- Residents of long-term care facilities and nursing homes
- Health care workers
- Incarcerated persons
- Homeless persons
- Intravenous drug users
- People living in crowded conditions

Increased risk of active disease

- Immunocompromised patients, including those with HIV infection
- Elderly, infants
- Patients with diabetes mellitus
- Patients with hemophilia
- Patients with chronic renal failure
- Patients with malignancy
- Patients with silicosis

progressively damaged, the lesion enlarges. The majority of infected individuals who will develop active disease do so within the first 1 or 2 years after infection. Clinical illness shortly after infection is termed primary tuberculosis. Dormant bacilli, however, may persist for years and then become reactivated. This is referred to as secondary or postprimary tuberculosis [8].

It is estimated that about 10% of infected persons will eventually develop active tuberculosis. Groups at risk for infection and at risk for progression to active disease are listed in Box 1. Factors that place patients at high risk for developing active disease include age, HIV coinfection (suppressed cellular immunity), silicosis, malignant neoplasms, hemophilia, chronic renal failure, and insulin-dependent diabetes mellitus [9–13]. Among infected persons, the incidence of tuberculosis is highest during late adolescence and early adulthood. The incidence among women peaks at 25 to 34 years of age [8].

Clinical presentation

Symptoms and signs of tuberculosis include fever, night sweats, cough, weight loss, anorexia, general malaise, and weakness. Massive hemoptysis can occur as a result of erosion into a vessel in the wall of a cavity. Although patients may be asymptomatic, physical findings that have been reported include fever, wasting, rales, and rhonchi. Rarely, patients may have clubbing of their fingers due to hypoxia. On chest radiograph, the classic finding is that of an upper lobe infiltrate or cavity; however, the film may be normal, or may have other findings such as nodules or diffuse infiltrates.

Although any organ system can be affected, the extrapulmonary sites most commonly involved in tuberculosis include lymph nodes, pleura, genitourinary tract, bones and joints, meninges, and peritoneum. Extrapulmonary tuberculosis is being seen more often because of HIV coinfection. Five to ten percent of pregnant women who have tuberculosis have extrapulmonary disease. This is similar to what is found in nonpregnant women [14].

Miliary tuberculosis

Miliary tuberculosis is due to hematogenous spread of tubercle bacilli. It may occur with either recent infection or reactivation of old disseminated foci. Common symptoms include weakness, fever, and weight loss [15]. Miliary tuberculosis can be a difficult diagnosis to make, because there may be no radiographic findings [16]. If present, radiologic findings reported include large infiltrates, interstitial infiltrates, and pleural effusions. A sputum smear is negative in 80% of cases. Hematologic abnormalities seen with miliary tuberculosis include anemia, leukopenia, neutrophilic leukocytosis, and polycythemia [17]. Disseminated intravascular coagulation may be present. In patients who have severe hepatic involvement, abnormal liver enzymes can be seen. A purified protein derivative (PPD) test is negative in up to half of cases. Bronchoalveolar lavage, transbronchial biopsy, or tissue biopsy are often necessary to confirm the diagnosis [8].

Congenital tuberculosis

Congenital tuberculosis is rare. Far more common is for a newborn to become infected after exposure to the infected mother or other family members (neonatal tuberculosis). Congenital tuberculosis is most often seen in a woman who has either tuberculous endometritis or miliary tuberculosis [18]. Tuberculosis can be transmitted to the fetus through the placenta and umbilical vein. Bacilli have been retrieved from the decidua, amnion, and chorionic villi [19]. A fetus may also become infected with *M tuberculosis* by ingesting amniotic fluid [20,21]. Hematogenous acquisition commonly results in granulomatous complexes within the liver. Acquisition via aspiration more often results in complexes in the lungs or gastrointestinal tract [22].

Beitzke [19] has detailed criteria for congenital tuberculosis: (1) firm diagnosis of tuberculosis in the newborn, (2) primary complex in the newborn's liver, (3) if there is no primary complex in the liver identified, tuberculous lesions must be documented in the first few days of life, thus excluding extrauterine infection. In many cases, the newborn is diagnosed before the mother. Hageman and colleagues [23] reviewed cases of congenital tuberculosis. The most common signs and symptoms, in descending order, were respiratory distress, fever, liver/spleen enlargement, poor feeding, lethargy, and lymphadenopathy. In their review, neonatal mortality was 46%; however, in three quarters of the deaths, there was no treatment because the diagnosis was made postmortem. It is important to note that tuberculin testing may initially be negative and remain so for several months.

Diagnosis

The PPD tuberculin skin test is the only test that can reliably detect *M tuberculosis* infection in asymptomatic persons. The test becomes positive 2 to 12 weeks after infection [24]. Sensitized CD4+ lymphocytes travel to the site, proliferate, and produce cytokines. As a result, a raised, erythematous area forms. The size of the reactive area determines whether the test is positive. The size of the reactive area used to define a positive test varies with risk factors.

Table 1 lists the size of induration used for various groups. Induration of 5 mm or greater is used for patients who have HIV infection, recent contact with a person who has active tuberculosis, organ transplant, or fibrotic changes on chest radiograph consistent with old tuberculosis. An induration of 10 mm or greater is used in patients who are recent (within 5 years) immigrants from high-prevalence countries; intravenous drug users; residents or employees of high-risk settings

Table 1
Criteria for a positive tuberculin test

Induration $\geq$5 mm	Induration $\geq$10 mm	Induration $\geq$15 mm
HIV-infected person	Recent immigrant (within 5 years)	Low-risk person
Recent contact with person with TB	Patients at increased risk of active disease (see Box 1)	
Findings on chest radiograph consistent with TB	Health care workers, IV drug users	

such as jails, nursing homes, shelters, and hospitals; or those who have conditions associated with a high risk of disease after infection (see above). An induration of 15 mm or greater is used for low-risk people [25]. Unfortunately, the test has low sensitivity and specificity in the case of active tuberculosis. Also, there are commonly false negatives in immunocompromised patients. Patients who have received the Bacille Calmette-Guérin (BCG) vaccine can have a false-positive test, although rarely will the skin induration exceed 20 mm in cases of false positives [26].

All patients who have a positive test should undergo a chest radiograph with abdominal shield to assess for evidence of disease. Hematologic findings include anemia, leukocytosis, and occasionally hyponatremia. In patients who have suspected active pulmonary tuberculosis, three sputum specimens, collected early in the morning, should be taken for acid-fast bacilli (AFB) smear and mycobacteriology culture. If tissue is obtained for culture, it is very important that it not be put in formaldehyde, because this compromises test accuracy [8]. Definitive diagnosis depends on the isolation and identification of *M tuberculosis* from a diagnostic specimen such as sputum or tissue. Culture is a time-consuming process, because *M tuberculosis* can take up to 4 to 8 weeks to grow; however, it is important, because drug susceptibilities can be determined and treatment optimized for the individual patient [27].

Treatment

The treatment of tuberculosis in pregnancy varies, depending on disease status (ie, PPD-positive alone versus active disease) and drug resistance testing in endemic areas. If a pregnant woman has a positive PPD indicating infection, but no evidence of active disease, some feel that treatment with isoniazid (INH) should be withheld until after delivery because of the increased risk of hepatotoxicity [28,29]. Others feel that it should be given regardless of gestational age. All agree that pregnant women who are HIV-infected should start therapy immediately, and most agree that pregnant women who have other risk factors for progression should not have a delay in initiation of therapy [25].

Management of active pulmonary tuberculosis during pregnancy is similar to that in nonpregnant women. INH, rifampin, and ethambutol (EMB) should be used in initial treatment regimens. If local prevalence of isolates resistant to INH is high, pyrazinamide (PZA) should be added to this regimen until results of susceptibility testing are available. These medications do cross the placenta, but have not been shown to have teratogenic effects [30]. Postpartum women being treated can breast-feed. Though these medications are found in breast milk, the amount of drug does not reach therapeutic levels, and is not sufficient for treatment of the newborn. Pregnant and postpartum women should receive pyridoxine [31]. If the patient misses doses, these must be made up at the end of the treatment period. If the patient misses a significant number of doses, she must be reassessed to determine whether treatment should be extended or restarted from the beginning [32].

Table 2 lists the medications used in the treatment of tuberculosis and their side effects. INH dosing can be daily or two to three times per week. Side effects include aminotransferase elevations, hepatitis, peripheral neurotoxicity, and a lupus-like syndrome. Hepatitis appears to be more common in pregnant patients taking INH, and therefore liver enzymes should be frequently evaluated and pyridoxine should be administered. The dose of pyridoxine found in prenatal vitamins can vary, and generally the dose is inadequate for this purpose [28,33,34]. Rifampin is also a first-line agent with dosing once daily, twice a week, or three times per week. Side effects include rash, nausea/vomiting, and hepatitis. Patients must be warned that rifampin will turn urine, sweat, sputum, and tears orange in color [35,36]. PZA is a first-line agent that is highly active against dormant and semidormant bacterial populations [37]. Hepatotoxicity attributable to PZA used in standard doses occurs in about 1% of cases [38]. Mild anorexia and nausea are common. Transient morbilliform rash can also occur, but is usually self-limited. There is little information about the safety of PZA in pregnancy; however, the benefits of PZA may outweigh the possible risks. The World Health Organization (WHO) and the International Union Against Tuberculosis and Lung Disease (IUATLD) recommend this drug for use in pregnant women who have tuberculosis [39,40]. The US data are very limited; however, there has been a report of PZA use in pregnancy with no bad outcomes [41]. EMB is a first-line drug for treating all forms of tuberculosis. It is included in initial treatment regimens, primarily to prevent emergence of rifampin resistance when primary resistance to INH may be present. Adverse effects

Table 2
Medications for the treatment of tuberculosis in pregnant women and their side effects

Drug	Interval and duration	Side effects and warnings
Isoniazid	Daily or 2–3×/week, 6 or 9 months	Hepatitis, GI distress, seizures, peripheral neuropathy
Rifampin	Daily or 2–3×/week, 2–4 months	Hepatitis, GI distress, purpura febrile reactions, orange secretions
Ethambutol	Daily or 2–3×/week, 2 months	Retrobulbar neuritis, peripheral neuritis, skin reactions
Pyrazinamide	Daily or 3×/week, 2 months	GI distress, rash, arthralgias

Abbreviation: GI, gastrointestinal.

include retrobulbar neuritis, peripheral neuritis (rare), and skin reactions requiring discontinuation of the drug. EMB is considered safe for use in pregnancy [42–46].

There are several drugs, mostly second-line, which are not to be used in pregnancy. They include: ethionamide, which crosses the placenta and is teratogenic in laboratory animals; streptomycin, because of the risk of fetal hearing loss [47–49]; amikacin and kanamycin, because of the risk of fetal nephrotoxicity and congenital hearing loss [47]; capreomycin, because of the risk of fetal nephrotoxicity and congenital hearing loss [47]; and fluoroquinolones, because of teratogenic effects [50,51].

Treatment failure and relapses are a problem that must be addressed as soon as possible. INH is responsible for killing the rapidly dividing cells, which are located mainly in the cavities. This occurs early in treatment, and therefore infectiousness rapidly decreases [52–55]. The rapidly dividing population of bacilli is eliminated early in therapy, as evidenced by the early clinical responses and clearing of live bacilli from sputum within 2 months in about 80% of patients. This same subpopulation is the one most likely to harbor organisms that have random mutations which confer drug resistance [32]. There are also two slower-growing subpopulations of *M tuberculosis* that cause treatment failures and relapses. For this reason, regimens less than 6 months in duration have been shown to have high relapse rates among patients who have smear-positive pulmonary tuberculosis [56,57]. Most relapses occur within 6 to 12 months of completing treatment. In cases of relapse, confirmatory testing must be undertaken quickly, and resistance testing should be performed. In cases of relapse with drug resistance, two to three drugs will need to be added to the regimen. After 3 months of multidrug treatment for a drug susceptible organism, 90% to 95% of patients will have a negative culture and show clinical improvement [32]. A positive sputum culture after 4 months of treatment indicates treatment failure. Reasons for treatment failure include: noncompliance, resistance, drug malabsorption, laboratory error, and biological variation in response. When a treatment failure occurs, resistance testing should be performed so that therapy can be modified.

References

[1] Frieden TR, Sterling TR, Munsiff SS, et al. Tuberculosis. Lancet 2003;362:887–99.
[2] Starke JR. Tuberculosis. Clin Perinatol 1997;24:107–27.
[3] Medchill MT, Gillum M. Diagnosis and management of tuberculosis during pregnancy. Obstet Gynecol Surv 1989;44:81–4.
[4] Miller KS, Miller Jr JM. Tuberculosis in pregnancy: interactions, diagnosis, and management. Clin Obstet Gynecol 1996;39:120–42.
[5] Weinberger SE, Weiss ST, Cohen WR, et al. Pregnancy and the lung. Am Rev Respir Dis 1980;121:559–81.
[6] Schluger NW, Rom WN. The host immune response to tuberculosis. Am J Respir Crit Care Med 1998;157:679–91.

[7] Sodhi A, Gong J, Silva C, et al. Clinical correlates of interferon-gamma production in patients with tuberculosis. Clin Infect Dis 1997;25:617–20.
[8] Braunwald E, Fauci AS, Kasper DL, et al. Harrison's principles of internal medicine. 16th edition. New York: McGraw-Hill; 2005.
[9] Markowitz N, Hansen NI, Hopewell PC, et al. Incidence of tuberculosis in the United States among HIV-infected persons. Ann Intern Med 1997;126:123–32.
[10] Westerholm P, Ahlmark A, Maasing R, et al. Silicosis and risk of lung cancer or lung tuberculosis: a cohort study. Environ Res 1986;41:339–50.
[11] Lundin AP, Adler AJ, Berlyne GM, et al. Tuberculosis in patients undergoing maintenance hemodialysis. Am J Med 1979;67:597–602.
[12] Andrew OT, Schoenfeld PY, Hopewell PC, et al. Tuberculosis in patients with end-stage renal disease. Am J Med 1980;68:59–65.
[13] Boucot KR, Dillon ES, Cooper DA, et al. Tuberculosis among diabetics: the Philadelphia Survey. Am Rev Tuberc 1952;65(Suppl):1–50.
[14] Wilson EA, Thelin TJ, Dilts PV. Tuberculosis complicated by pregnancy. Am J Obstet Gynecol 1972;115:526–9.
[15] Sahn S, Neff T. Miliary tuberculosis. Am J Med 1974;56:495–505.
[16] Grieco MH, Chmel H. Acute disseminated tuberculosis as a diagnostic problem. Am Rev Respir Dis 1974;109:554–60.
[17] Menitove S, Harris HW. Miliary tuberculosis. In: Schlossberg D, editor. Tuberculosis. 2nd edition. New York: Springer-Verlag; 1988. p. 179–89.
[18] Cooper AR, Heneghan W, Matthew JD. Tuberculosis in a mother and her infant. Pediatr Infect Dis 1985;4:181–3.
[19] Beitzke H. Ueber die angeborene tuberkuloese infection [About the congenital tuberculosis infection]. Ergeb Gesamten Tuberkuloseforsch 1935;7:1–30.
[20] Vallejo JG, Starke JR. Tuberculosis in pregnancy. Clin Chest Med 1992;13:693–707.
[21] Hertzog AJ, Chapman S, Herring J. Congenital pulmonary aspiration-tuberculosis. Am J Clin Pathol 1940;19:1139–42.
[22] Cantwell MF, Shehab ZM, Costello AM, et al. Brief report: congenital tuberculosis. N Engl J Med 1994;330:1051–4.
[23] Hageman J, Shulman S, Schreiber M, et al. Congenital tuberculosis: critical reappraisal of clinical findings and diagnostic procedures. Pediatrics 1980;66:980–4.
[24] Huebner RE, Schein W, Bass Jr JB. The tuberculin skin test. Clin Infect Dis 1993;17:968–75.
[25] Centers for Disease Control and Prevention. Targeted tuberculin testing and treatment of latent tuberculosis infection. American Thoracic Society. MMWR Recomm Rep 2000;49(RR-6):1–51.
[26] Sepulveda RL, Ferrer X, Latrach C, et al. The influence of Calmette-Guerin bacillus immunization on the booster effect of tuberculin testing in healthy young adults. Am Rev Respir Dis 1990;142:24–8.
[27] American Thoracic Society. Diagnostic standards and classification of tuberculosis in adults and children. Am J Respir Crit Care Med 2000;161:1376–95.
[28] Franks AL, Binkin NJ, Snider Jr DE, et al. Isoniazid hepatitis among pregnant and postpartum Hispanic patients. Public Health Rep 1989;104:151–5.
[29] Snider Jr DE, Caras GJ. Isoniazid-associated hepatitis deaths: a review of available information. Am Rev Respir Dis 1992;145:494–7.
[30] Briggs GG, Freeman RK, Yaffe SJ. Drugs in pregnancy and lactation. 5th edition. Baltimore (MD): Williams & Wilkins; 1998. p. 400–1, 562–4, 918–9, 945–6.
[31] Snider DE, Powell KE. Should women taking antituberculosis drugs breast-feed? Arch Intern Med 1984;144:589–90.
[32] American Thoracic Society, Centers for Disease Control and Prevention, and Infectious Diseases Society of America. Treatment of tuberculosis. MMWR Morb Mortal Wkly Rep 2003;52(RR11):1–77.
[33] Snider DE. Pyridoxine supplementation during isoniazid therapy. Tubercle 1980;61:191–6.
[34] Ludford J, Doster B, Woolpert SF. Effect of isoniazid on reproduction. Am Rev Respir Dis 1973;108:1170–4.

[35] Dickinson JM, Mitchison DA. Experimental models to explain the high sterilizing activity of rifampin in the chemotherapy of tuberculosis. Am Rev Respir Dis 1981;123:367–71.
[36] Steen JS, Stainton-Ellis DM. Rifampicin in pregnancy. Lancet 1977;ii:604–5.
[37] Girling DJ. The role of pyrazinamide in primary chemotherapy for pulmonary tuberculosis. Tubercle 1984;65:1–4.
[38] Døssing M, Wilcke JTR, Askgaard DS, et al. Liver injury during antituberculosis treatment: an 11-year study. Tuber Lung Dis 1996;77:335–40.
[39] World Health Organization. Treatment of tuberculosis: guidelines for national programmes. 2nd edition. Geneva (Switzerland): World Health Organization; 1997.
[40] Enarson DA, Rieder HL, Arnodottir T, et al. Tuberculosis guide for low income countries. 4th edition. Paris: International Union against Tuberculosis and Lung Diseases; 1996.
[41] Davidson PT. Managing tuberculosis during pregnancy. Lancet 1995;346:199–200.
[42] Bobrowitz ID. Ethambutol in pregnancy. Chest 1974;66:20–4.
[43] Lewit T, Nebel L, Terracina S, et al. Ethambutol in pregnancy: observations on embryogenesis. Chest 1974;66:25–6.
[44] Snider DE, Layde PM, Johnson MW, et al. Treatment of tuberculosis during pregnancy. Am Rev Respir Dis 1980;122:65–79.
[45] Doster B, Murray FJ, Newman R, et al. Ethambutol in the initial treatment of pulmonary tuberculosis. Am Rev Respir Dis 1973;107:177–90.
[46] Tugwell P, James SL. Peripheral neuropathy with ethambutol. Postgrad Med J 1972;48:667–70.
[47] United States Pharmacopeial Dispensing Information. Drug information for the health care professional, vol. I. Englewood (CO): Micromedex; 1999.
[48] Conway N, Birt BD. Streptomycin in pregnancy: effect on the foetal ear. BMJ 1965;2:260–3.
[49] Robinson GC, Cambon KG. Hearing loss in infants of tuberculous mothers treated with streptomycin during pregnancy. N Engl J Med 1964;271:949–51.
[50] Peloquin CA. Antituberculosis drugs: pharmacokinetics. In: Heifets LB, editor. Drug susceptibility in the chemotherapy of mycobacterial infections. Boca Raton (FL): CRC Press; 1991. p. 59–88.
[51] Lipsky BA, Baker CA. Fluoroquinolone toxicity profiles: a review focusing on newer agents. Clin Infect Dis 1999;28:352–64.
[52] Jindani A, Aber VR, Edwards EA, et al. The early bactericidal activity of drugs in patients with pulmonary tuberculosis. Am Rev Respir Dis 1980;121:939–49.
[53] Chan SL, Yew WW, Ma WK, et al. The early bactericidal activity of rifabutin measured by sputum viable counts in Hong Kong patients with pulmonary tuberculosis. Tuber Lung Dis 1992; 73:33–8.
[54] Sirgel FA, Botha FJH, Parkin DP, et al. The early bactericidal activity of rifabutin in patients with pulmonary tuberculosis measured by sputum viable counts: a new method of drug assessment. J Antimicrob Chemother 1993;32:867–75.
[55] Hafner R, Cohn JA, Wright DJ, et al. Early bactericidal activity of isoniazid in pulmonary tuberculosis. Am J Respir Crit Care Med 1997;156:918–23.
[56] East Africa/British Medical Research Council. Controlled clinical trial of five short-course (4 month) chemotherapy regimens in pulmonary tuberculosis: second report of the 4th study. Am Rev Respir Dis 1981;123:165–70.
[57] Singapore Tuberculosis Service/British Medical Research Council. Long-term follow-up of a clinical trial of 6-month and 4-month regimens of chemotherapy in the treatment of pulmonary tuberculosis. Am Rev Respir Dis 1986;133:779–83.

ELSEVIER
SAUNDERS

Clin Perinatol 32 (2005) 749–764

CLINICS IN
PERINATOLOGY

Urinary Tract Infections in Pregnancy

Pooja Mittal, MD[a,*], Deborah A. Wing, MD[b]

[a]*Division of Maternal-Fetal Medicine, Department of Obstetrics-Gynecology, Hutzel Women's Hospital, Wayne State University, 3990 John R Road, 7 Brush North, Detroit, MI 48201, USA*

[b]*Division of Maternal-Fetal Medicine, Department of Obstetrics-Gynecology, University of California, Irvine Medical Center, 101 The City Drive, South, Building 56, Suite 800, Orange, CA 92868, USA*

Urinary tract infections (UTIs) represent the most common bacterial infection in pregnant and nonpregnant women [1,2]. Eight million women visit a physician annually for evaluation of UTIs [3] at a direct cost of $659 million [4] and aggregate cost of $1.6 billion [4,5]. Physiologic changes of pregnancy increase a woman's susceptibility to UTI. Progesterone effects and mechanical compression by the gravid uterus impair emptying of the bladder and lead to increased bladder residual volume and vesicoureteral reflux. Relative stasis of urine in the ureters results in hydronephrosis. Furthermore, pregnancy-related changes in glomerular filtration rate increases the urinary glucose concentration and alkalinity, thereby facilitating bacterial growth [6]. In addition, alterations in maternal immunologic defense mechanisms occur in pregnancy [7]. The signs and symptoms of UTIs vary by the type of infection. UTI in pregnancy is classified by the site of bacterial proliferation as follows: asymptomatic bacteriuria (ASB; urine), cystitis (bladder), pyelonephritis (kidney).

Asymptomatic bacteriuria

ASB is defined as significant bacterial colonization of the lower urinary tract without symptoms. Traditional diagnostic criteria of significant bacteriuria include culture of 10^5 colony forming units (CFUs)/mL of a single uropathogen on two consecutive clean catch urine specimens [6,7]. Recent evidence suggests that

* Corresponding author.
E-mail address: pmittal@med.wayne.edu (P. Mittal).

doi:10.1016/j.clp.2005.05.006 ***perinatology.theclinics.com***

lower colony counts ($\geq 10^2$–10^3 CFUs/mL) may demonstrate active infection and eventually lead to pyelonephritis in pregnant women [8–10]. The incidence of ASB during pregnancy is 2% to 14%—similar to that of nonpregnant women—and translates into 80,000 to 400,000 cases in the United States each year [10,11]. Predisposing factors to ASB include low socioeconomic status, increasing age, multiparity, sexual behavior, and a history of childhood UTIs (with or without scarring). The prevalence of ASB also is increased markedly in certain preexisting medical conditions, such as diabetes mellitus, sickle cell disease, immunocompromised states (eg, AIDS), urinary tract anatomic anomalies, and spinal cord injuries. UTI before pregnancy is a predictor of the diagnosis of ASB at the first prenatal visit [12].

Without treatment, ASB progresses to pyelonephritis in 20% to 40% of pregnant women. In contrast, progression to pyelonephritis in nonpregnant women is only 1% to 2%. Furthermore, the incidence of pyelonephritis in pregnant women without ASB complicating early pregnancy is less than 1%. With appropriate treatment in pregnancy, progression to pyelonephritis can be decreased to 3% [13].

The causative organisms that are isolated in ASB, cystitis, and pyelonephritis are similar in pregnant and nonpregnant women. Enterobacteriae, a group of gram-negative rods, encompass most colonizing organisms, including *Escherichia coli*, the primary pathogen in 80% to 90% of initial UTIs and 70% to 80% of recurrent infections [6,12,14,15]. Other gram-negative pathogens include *Klebsiella pneumoniae* and *Proteus mirabilis*. Further pathogens include *Pseudomonas aeruginosa* and gram-positive organisms, *Streptococcus agalacticae*, and *Staphylococcus saphrophyticus*. The most virulent strains of *E coli* possess toxins and adhesins, pili, or fimbriae to allow adherence to uroephithelium [12]. These protect the bacteria from urinary lavage and allow bacterial multiplication and renal tissue invasion. Specific O-serotypes of *E coli* have been epidemiologically related to the occurrence of acute pyelonephritis, recurrent infection, parenchymal scarring, and renal failure [16]. Fimbriae P, found in uropathogenic strains of *E coli*, aids in adherence to vaginal and renal epithelium and causes upper UTI [17]. Recently, the class of DR adhesins also has been associated with pyelonephritis in pregnancy, and a high rate of preterm delivery in mice [18].

Screening for ASB in pregnancy is recommended by the U.S. Preventative Services Task Force and the American College of Obstetricians and Gynecologists [19,20]. A urine culture should be obtained between 12 and 16 weeks of pregnancy. Appropriate therapy for positive urine culture at this time leads to the highest number of bacteria-free weeks in pregnancy. This recommendation is based on a large epidemiologic study from Sweden [13]. Urine culture detects approximately 80% of cases of ASB. The average cost of urine culture ranges from $16 to $45. In a cost analysis, screening with urine culture is cost-effective if the risk of ASB is greater than 2%, the risk of resultant pyelonephritis is greater than 13%, or if the efficacy of treatment in preventing pyelonephritis is 38% [21]. In populations with a prevalence of ASB of at least 9%, urine culture was the most cost-effective screening method [22]. Globally, disadvantages to urine culture lie in the delay to results (24–48 hours) and low yield with high cost in areas of low prevalence. Other screening modalities have been suggested as expedient, more cost-effective alternatives for detection of urinary tract infection but the usefulness is variable. Alternative modes of testing, such as urinary dipstick testing to screen for pyuria by the presence of nitrites and leukocyte esterase (ChemstripN test, Biodynamics, Indianapolis, Indiana), has a sensitivity that ranges from 50% to 92% and a negative predictive value of 99.2% [22]. Although rapid screening tests are less expensive and faster than urine culture, they are limited by their requirement of high bacterial concentrations ($\geq 10^5$ CFU/mL) for positive results [8]. In light of the current opinion to treat ASB at a much lower bacterial count in pregnancy, these tests would be inadequate as initial screening methods; urine culture remains the screening test of choice [6].

Treatment of asymptomatic bacteriuria in pregnancy

A variety of antibiotics has been used to treat ASB and seem to have similar efficacy [7] as seen in meta-analysis of various regimens in the Cochrane Database [23]. Treatment is empiric because causative bacteria are predictable. Increasing antimicrobial resistance among uropathogens poses a challenge to therapy. Although the susceptibility of these pathogens to antimicrobial therapy has changed, their prevalence has not. The pattern of resistance varies geographically. In the United States, resistance increases from east to west, with the highest prevalence of multi-drug-resistant phenotypes on the Pacific Coast [24]. This should be taken into account when determining appropriate therapy. Other factors to be considered in the selection of appropriate antimicrobial therapy include the spectrum of activity of the agent, potential side effects, duration of therapy, cost, and pharmacokinetics [25]. β-Lactam antibiotics, including ampicillin, are among the oldest antibiotics that are used to treat bacterial infection; however, the pharmacokinetic changes of pregnancy decrease plasma concentrations of β-lactams by up to 50% [7]. Although well-tolerated orally, increasing resistance levels of *E coli* limits its use in the treatment of UTI. For example, *E coli* resistance to ampicillin is greater than 60% in some centers [8]. Cephalosporins also are well-tolerated and safe in pregnancy; cephalexin is the most commonly used cephalosporin in pregnancy. Penicillins and cephalosporins are associated with allergic, and at times, anaphylactic reactions. Nitrofurantoin achieves therapeutic concentration only in urine. Therefore, it only is indicated for the treatment of uncomplicated UTIs [7]. With the low level of resistance to nitrofurantoin among uropathogens, it remains an ideal therapeutic agent and is safe for use in pregnancy. In an evaluation of national practice patterns from 1989 to 1998, nitrofurantoin was the most frequently used antimicrobial agent for UTIs among obstetrician-gynecologists [26]. The limitation of nitrofurantoin is its poor activity against *Proteus* spp. The main side effects are gastrointestinal, and have been mitigated by the current macrocrystalline formulations. Nitrofurantoin also may incite hemolytic anemia in patients who have glucose-

6–phosphate dehydrogenase deficiency. Trimethoprim-sulfamethoxazole, the primary agent used in the general population, is contraindicated in the first trimester of pregnancy because of its inhibitory effect on folate metabolism and resultant association with neural tube defects. Sulfonamides are not recommended in the third trimester because of the risk of kernicterus in the newborn and their effects on folate metabolism. Although fluoroquinolones attain high renal concentration and are used commonly in nonpregnant patients, the risk of arthropathy in the newborn contraindicates their use in pregnancy [7,10].

A longtime traditional preventative and therapeutic agent for UTI is cranberries, either in juice or tablet form. Cranberries contain proanthocyanidins which prevent the adherence of bacterial pathogens to uroepithelium, and thereby prevent UTIs. In a recent Cochrane Review, cranberries, in both forms, significantly reduced the incidence of UTIs in women over a 12-month period (relative risk 0.61; 95% CI: 0.40–0.91) when compared with placebo. Difficulty with compliance was noted in all evaluated trials [27]. No trials exist that describe the preventative effects of cranberry ingestion in pregnancy.

The current standard of practice is to treat pregnant patients who have ASB with at least 7 days of an oral antimicrobial agent [6,7,12,14]. If bacteriuria persists, a second 7- or 14-day course of the same or different antimicrobial agent is used. In nonpregnant women, short-course treatment (single-dose or 3 days) of uncomplicated lower UTI is as effective as a 7- to 14-day course. Committee guidelines of the Infectious Disease Society of America (IDSA), after a meta-analysis of the literature, support the effectiveness of 3-day oral antimicrobial treatment in nonpregnant women [28], which is the current standard of care [15]. Persistent bacteriuria and reinfection rates are similar with short-course treatment when compared with more conventional therapy; however, single-dose regimens seem to be associated with a higher rate of early recurrence by the original strain than the 7- to 14-day regimen [29]. Failure to eradicate uropathogens from the vaginal reservoir results in earlier recurrence. Three-day courses seem to be more effective than single-dose regimens in preventing early reinfection. Although firmly established in nonpregnant women, short-course therapy of ASB in pregnancy has not been evaluated adequately. Short-course regimens are preferable because of fewer side effects, decreased health care costs, and increased patient compliance [30]. Multiple studies suggest that short-course therapy is appropriate in pregnancy; a variety of 3-day and single-dose regimens has been proposed (Table 1). In general, no significant difference in recurrence rates has been seen between short-course and conventional therapies. Because of inadequate power in these studies, there is insufficient evidence to recommend this approach [31].

After ASB has been diagnosed in pregnancy—regardless of the chosen antimicrobial agent or the duration of therapy—repeat urine cultures should be obtained monthly throughout gestation because of the significant risk of recurrent bacteriuria [8,30]. Up to one third of pregnant women experience a recurrence [13,14,16].

Upon diagnosis of recurrence with the same uropathogen or reinfection with a new uropathogen, a second full course of antimicrobial therapy should be given.

Table 1
Suggested three-day regimens for the treatment of asymptomatic bacteriuria in pregnancy

Antimicrobial agent	Regimen	Drug class
Cephalexin	500 mg po qid	Class B
Nitrofurantoin macrocrystals	100 mg po qid	Class B
Nitrofurantoin monohydrate-macrocrystals	100 mg po bid	Class B
Amoxicillin[a]	500 mg po qid	Class B
Ampicillin[a]	500 mg po qid	Class B

Abbreviations: bid, twice a day; po, by mouth; qid, four times a day.

[a] Must check hospital susceptibilities before prescribing β-lactam monotherapy.

Treatment should be based on urine culture and sensitivities. With either situation, consideration should be given to implementing long-term nightly suppressive therapy with low-dose cephalexin (125–250 mg) or nitrofurantoin (50–100 mg) throughout the pregnancy and including the puerperium [32]. Suppression therapy also should be considered in women who have persistent bacteriuria, despite multiple courses of antimicrobial treatment, to prevent progression to symptomatic infection. Care must be used because prolonged use of antimicrobials, such as cephalosporins, may predispose women to chronic vaginal candidiasis [7]. Postpartum radiologic evaluation for urinary tract anomalies or urolithiasis should be considered in patients who have recurrent UTIs.

Health consequences of asymptomatic bacteriuria in pregnancy

The presence of ASB in pregnancy places patients at increased risk for the development of cystitis and pyelonephritis with their respective morbidities. A critical meta-analysis by Romero and colleagues [33] showed the relationship between ASB alone and preterm delivery and low birth weight infants. The risk of preterm delivery in women who had ASB during gestation was twofold greater than those who never were affected. With adequate treatment of ASB, the relative risk of low birth weight infants was 0.56 compared with an untreated group [33]. These findings were confirmed in a recent Cochrane review of available data which demonstrated the decreased incidence of pyelonephritis and low birth weight infants when ASB is treated [23]. Several theories have been suggested to explain the mechanism by which uncomplicated UTI triggers preterm labor and delivery. Bacterial endotoxin release is believed to provoke labor directly or through a prostaglandin-mediated cascade. Alternatively, it is believed that UTI predisposes women to amnionitis, and thus, preterm labor. Although previously suggested, ASB does not seem to be related to preeclampsia or anemia [34].

Cystitis

Acute bacterial cystitis presents with clinical signs and symptoms of urgency, frequency, dysuria, pyuria, and hematuria without evidence of systemic illness

[35]. Cystitis complicates 1% to 4% of all pregnancies [8]. Diagnosis, although mostly clinical, includes a positive urine culture with at least 10^5 CFU/mL of a single uropathogen. Although routine surveillance during prenatal care is designed to minimize bacteriuria, this has had no effect on the incidence of cystitis. This suggests that most infections arise without antecedent bacteriuria [36]. On initial prenatal evaluation, most women who will have cystitis in pregnancy have negative screening cultures [37]. Unlike ASB, the diagnosis of cystitis in pregnancy does not increase the risk for developing pyelonephritis.

Risk factors for developing cystitis in pregnancy include those stated for ASB as well as a history of *Chlamydia trachomatis*, illicit drug use, and less than 12 years of education [38]. The spectrum of uropathogens that have been isolated in cystitis is similar to that seen in ASB. Therefore, the treatment modality of dosing and duration of therapy is the same. Follow-up surveillance, including monthly urine cultures for the duration of the pregnancy, is recommended. As with ASB, cystitis is associated with preterm labor and delivery [35].

Women may present with symptoms that are consistent with cystitis but with a negative urine culture. After confirming the lack of recent antibiotic use, the diagnosis of urethral syndrome should be considered. Urethral cultures for *Chlamydia* should be performed, followed by appropriate treatment [39].

Pyelonephritis

Acute pyelonephritis complicates 1% to 2% of all pregnancies and affects approximately 100,000 women in the United States annually [40]. Associated with marked fetal and maternal morbidity, it is the most severe form of UTI and the most common indication for antepartum hospitalization [2]. Risk factors for the development of pyelonephritis include those of ASB and cystitis as well as a history of pyelonephritis, urinary tract malformations, and calculi [13]. Patients who are at increased risk should be screened with monthly urine cultures. Because of the increasing mechanical compression of the enlarging uterus, pyelonephritis is most common during the second half of pregnancy; only 4% of cases present in the first trimester, 67% present in the second and third trimesters, and 27% present in the postpartum period [8]. Usually unilateral, pyelonephritis affects the right kidney more frequently secondary to dextrorotation of the uterus [6].

Diagnosis of pyelonephritis in pregnancy

Pyelonephritis presents with predominantly systemic signs and symptoms. These include fever; flank pain; costovertebral angle tenderness (CVAT); shaking chills; nausea; vomiting; and less commonly, symptoms of cystitis, such as dysuria and frequency. Most patients who have pyelonephritis also present with dehydration. The most common presenting symptoms are fever and flank pain [13]. Therapy largely is empiric and begun upon clinical diagnosis. Diagnosis is confirmed with urine culture. Per the IDSA consensus, pyelonephritis is defined as the identification of at least 10^4 CFU/mL of a single uropathogen in a midstream sample [28]. Microscopically, the diagnosis can be confirmed with the presence of 1 or 2 bacteria per high-power field on an unspun catheterized urine sample, or 20 bacteria per high-power field on a spun sample. These parameters correlate with more than 10^5 CFU/mL of bacteria on urine culture. Additional diagnostic signs include the presence of pyuria or leukocyte casts [13].

Further laboratory investigation should include a complete blood cell count and serum chemistry evaluation. Hypokalemia, elevated serum creatinine, anemia, thrombocytopenia, and elevated lactate dehydrogenase due to endotoxin-mediated hemolysis may be encountered. Transient renal insufficiency with at least a 50% decrease in creatinine clearance is observed in more than 25% of patients [41]. Electrolyte abnormalities should be corrected. Most abnormalities should normalize spontaneously with treatment of the primary disease. Although self-limited, anemia often requires several weeks to resolve. Renal scarring has been described as a long-term sequela of acute pyelonephritis in pregnancy. The magnitude of renal scarring may be related to the inflammatory process. Interleukin-6, an endogenous pyogen, correlates with the level of urinary tract inflammatory response [42], whereas interleukin-8, a chemoattractant for neutrophils, corresponds to the degree of pyuria and is related to renal scarring [43]. In a recent report, antimicrobial therapy significantly decreased these inflammatory markers within 6 hours. Normalization is almost achieved at 24 hours [44]. These findings emphasize the importance of rapid diagnosis and institution of therapy. Radiographic examination of women 10 to 20 years after diagnosis of pyelonephritis showed that those who were pregnant at the time of diagnosis were four times more likely to develop renal scarring [45]. However, functional renal impairment was not different between the pregnant and non-pregnant groups. One in 3000 women who have pyelonephritis in pregnancy develops renal failure, and pregnancy remains one of the most common conditions in which isolated pyelonephritis leads to renal failure [46]. Long-term follow-up of these patients is essential.

Although blood cultures are obtained frequently on initial evaluation, their usefulness in the assessment of pyelonephritis is limited. Bacterial pathogens that are isolated from blood cultures rarely differ from those that are found in the corresponding urine culture [47]. Furthermore, in a retrospective study of 156 cases of pyelonephritis in pregnancy, 90% of pathogens were sensitive to the initial empiric treatment; only 2% of blood cultures and 3% of urine cultures precipitated an adjustment in therapy [48]. Most changes in therapy were governed by clinical indications, such as persistent fever or CVAT. These findings were supported by a recent retrospective review of 391 cases of pyelonephritis in pregnancy; a change in management because of bacteremia alone occurred in only 1% of cases [49]. Although blood culture may help to guide antimicrobial therapy when faced with inadequate clinical response, limiting the use of cultures in the evaluation of pyelonephritis in pregnancy was estimated to result in an annual savings of $10 to $20 million [48]. Blood cultures have been and are advocated in cases that are complicated by sepsis, temperature of at least 39°C, or respiratory distress syndrome.

Routine renal ultrasound evaluation is of limited clinical benefit and should be reserved for women who are unresponsive to initial treatment [50].

The uropathogens that are found in pyelonephritis are similar to those that cause ASB and cystitis. *E coli* predominates, and is isolated in 70% to 80% of cases [49,51,52]. *Klebsiella pneumoniae* and *Proteus* spp appear less frequently, but play an important role in cases of recurrent pyelonephritis [53]. Gram-positive and anaerobic bacteria usually do not ascend to the upper urinary tract except in cases of instrumentation or obstruction.

Treatment of pyelonephritis in pregnancy

Because most patients who have pyelonephritis are dehydrated, initial management should include adequate intravenous hydration and close monitoring of urine output. Cooling blankets and antipyretics may be used to alleviate pyrexia [13]. The current standard of care includes hospitalization and parenteral antimicrobial therapy.

Initial antimicrobial treatment is empiric. Intravenous antimicrobial therapy, including regimens of ampicillin, plus gentamicin, cefazolin, and ceftriaxone, are equally efficacious (Table 2) [35,55]. First-line therapy often includes a first-generation cephalosporin. A commonly used regimen is cefazolin, 1–2 g intravenously every 6 to 8 hours. Cefazolin possesses the same spectrum of activity against the common causative organisms as do the broader-spectrum cephalosporins and penicillins and is less expensive. Although there have been reports of in vitro resistance to cephalosporins, clinical efficacy seems to be unchanged [16]. Ampicillin monotherapy has fallen into disfavor because of the high incidence of resistant bacteria, and therefore, usually is used in conjunction with gentamicin [53]. To avoid exacerbation of the renal insufficiency that commonly accompanies pyelonephritis, drug serum levels should be followed when using aminoglycosides, such as gentamicin. Other options include broader-spectrum penicillins, such as mezlocillin or piperacillin, and second- or third-generation cephalosporins [13].

Table 2
Suggested antimicrobial regimens for the treatment of pyelonephritis in pregnancy

Antimicrobial agent	Regimen	Drug class
Ampicillin (+) Gentamicin	2 grams IV q6 h	Class B
Gentamicin	2 mg/kg load, then 1.7mg/kg in 3 divided doses	Class C
Ampicillin-sublactam	3 grams IV q6 h	Class B
Ceftriaxone	1 gram IV/IM q24 h	Class B
Cefuroxime	0.75–1.5 grams IV q8 h	Class B
Cefazolin	1–2 grams IV q6–8 h	Class B
Mezlocillin	3 grams IV q6 h	Class B
Piperacillin	4 grams IV q8 h	Class B

Abbreviations: IM, intramuscularly; IV, intravenously; q, every.

With appropriate antimicrobial management, 75% of patients become asymptomatic and afebrile within 48 hours, whereas 95% will defervesce within 72 hours of treatment [13,16]. Failure to respond clinically after 72 hours of therapy most likely indicates a resistant pathogen, urinary tract anomaly, or urolithiasis. In case of poor response, management should include the addition or substitution of an aminoglycoside as well as radiographic evaluation to rule out other etiologies. Renal ultrasonography is used often but is of limited value because of its decreased sensitivity for detection of calculi during pregnancy [56]. Intravenous pyelography (IVP) may be used safely in pregnancy with one shot at 20 to 30 minutes to maximize detection and minimize radiation exposure to the fetus (Fig. 1) [56]. MRI also may garner information regarding urinary tract obstruction safely.

In an inpatient setting, parenteral antimicrobial therapy usually is continued until the patient is afebrile for 48 hours. The patient is switched to oral antimicrobial therapy for 2 weeks. A follow-up urine culture, or test of cure, is performed to ensure eradication of the bacteria [13].

Outpatient management for pyelonephritis in pregnancy has been proposed with the benefits of decreased health care costs and increased patient convenience [51,52,57–59]. Wing and colleagues described a series of randomized controlled trials that compared inpatient with outpatient management of pyelonephritis in pregnancy at less than 24 weeks and more than 24 weeks [51,52]. Patients who were randomized to outpatient management at less than 24 weeks received two

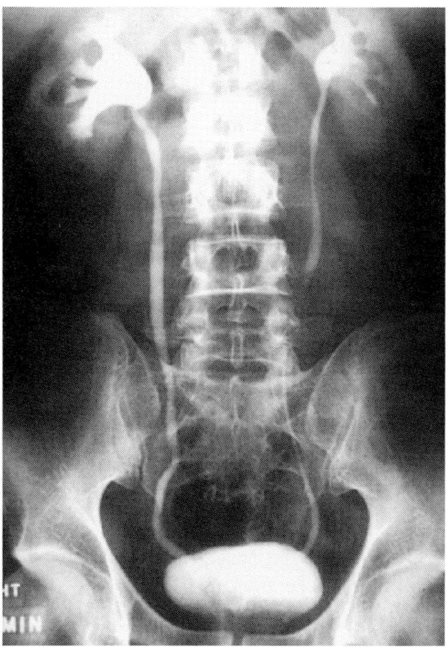

Fig. 1. Intravenous pyelogram (IVP) in pregnancy. IVP "one-shot" after 20 minutes demonstrates mild right hydronephrosis and hydroureter.

doses of ceftriaxone, 1 g intramuscularly, whereas inpatients received cefazolin, 1 g every 8 hours. Ninety-five percent of patients qualified for outpatient treatment and no significant differences in clinical or delivery outcomes was observed. In a separate investigation of women who were more than 24 weeks' gestation, inpatient and outpatient enrollees received two doses of ceftriaxone, 1 g over 24 hours. Ninety percent of women were treated safely with ambulatory care; however at greater than 24 weeks' gestation the number of patients who qualified for outpatient therapy was decreased by 50% because of evidence of complications that were due to pyelonephritis and necessitated inpatient management. Additionally, 51% of those women who were greater than 24 weeks who were randomized to outpatient therapy could not complete the study assignment or had to be readmitted for complications that were related to the primary infection. They concluded that in pregnancies beyond 24 weeks, outpatient management of pyelonephritis had limited usefulness. Although studies demonstrate the usefulness of ambulatory management of pyelonephritis in pregnancy, they also strongly advise that careful consideration must be made in selecting appropriate candidates to maximize efficacy and safety [13,16,51,52]. Selection criteria should include compliant patients with pregnancies at less than 24 weeks' gestation at diagnosis, with no evidence of comorbid disease (eg, diabetes mellitus). In addition they should not exhibit signs or symptoms of sepsis, temperature greater than 38°C, recurrent upper urinary tract disease, inability to tolerate oral intake, or signs of preterm labor. For appropriate candidates, an initial observation period of 24 hours is needed to confirm maternal and fetal well-being. During this time, antimicrobial therapy, hydration, and laboratory evaluation is initiated. Upon discharge, adherence to close outpatient follow-up must be stressed. Instructions should be given to return to the emergency room immediately if signs of sepsis, respiratory insufficiency, or preterm labor develop. Twenty-four hours after discharge, patients should be evaluated for appropriate clinical response. As with inpatient therapy, a urine culture should be obtained after 2 weeks to confirm adequate treatment.

Because of the 20% recurrence rate of pyelonephritis before delivery [13], nightly suppression therapy after documented cure is advocated for all women who have a diagnosis of pyelonephritis in pregnancy. Continuous prophylaxis with low-dose nitrofurantoin, 100 mg daily, reduces recurrence by 95% [60]. In a retrospective review, a recurrence rate of 60% without suppression was reduced to 2.7% with daily suppressive treatment [61]. Suppression therapy should be continued until 4 to 6 weeks post partum. In addition, urine cultures to screen for recurrent bacteriuria should be obtained monthly for the remainder of the pregnancy.

Complications of pyelonephritis in pregnancy

Bacteremia occurs in 15% to 20% of cases of pyelonephritis; the most common pathogen is *E coli* [62]. Gram-negative bacteria possess endotoxin within their cell wall. Endotoxin-mediated damage includes that of capillary endothelium, diminished vascular resistance, and changes in cardiovascular output. When the active component of endotoxin—lipid A—is released into the maternal circulation, it precipitates a cascade response of proinflammatory cytokines, histamine, and bradykinins that may lead to the more serious complications of septic shock, disseminated intravascular coagulation, respiratory insufficiency, and adult respiratory distress syndrome (ARDS).

Pyelonephritis is the most common cause of septic shock in pregnancy [62]. Patients who have septic shock require admission to intensive care, immediate fluid resuscitation, and antimicrobial therapy. In cases of hypotension and oliguria, the use of dopamine support may be necessary. Increased alveolar-capillary membrane permeability—mediated by endotoxemia—results in pulmonary edema and respiratory insufficiency. Although patients generally respond well to oxygen therapy, worsening dyspnea, tachypnea, and hypoxemia may signify progression to the highly morbid condition of ARDS [63]. ARDS, defined as a disease of acute onset with bilateral infiltrates on chest radiograph and hypoxemia without evidence of pulmonary hypertension [63], complicates 1% to 8% of cases of pyelonephritis in pregnancy [13]. Pulmonary injury manifests within 48 hours of beginning antimicrobial therapy. Management includes maternal stabilization and fetal monitoring. Baseline chest radiograph and arterial blood gas should be obtained. Although adequate supplemental oxygen therapy combined with diuresis often is sufficient, mechanical ventilation may be required. Delivery does not decrease maternal or fetal morbidity/mortality globally and should be considered on a case-by-case basis [64]. In one retrospective analysis, pulmonary injury in antepartum pyelonephritis was associated with temperature of greater than 103°F in gestations of more than 20 weeks, and tachycardia of more than 100 beats per minute [65]. ARDS also was diagnosed more frequently in patients who had received β-sympathomimetic tocolytic agents and excessive intravenous hydration. Tocolytics predispose women to pulmonary edema through cardiovascular changes. Although all virulent bacteria pose a threat for pulmonary injury, *Klebsiella pneumoniae*, a common community and nosocomially acquired pulmonary pathogen, more frequently leads to ARDS [65]. The incidence of preterm delivery in pyelonephritis is reported from 6% to 50%, depending on gestational age at presentation and the use of antimicrobial therapy [13]. Although uterine contractions often accompany pyelonephritis, there often is little or no acute cervical change. A controversy exists in the literature regarding the etiology of these contractions, fever versus endotoxin release after antibiotic treatment, and their relationship to preterm delivery. Antibiotic treatment alone of pyelonephritis significantly decreased the frequency of contractions with no resultant association with pyrexia [54]; however, recent murine models of gravid myometrium demonstrated a direct effect of endotoxin release upon uterine contractility. The effect occurs through the release of endogenous prostaglandins; an influx of calcium ions; and to a lesser extent, inhibition of sodium pumps [66]. Yet similar murine models show that although endotoxin-mediated inflammatory response increases the amplitude of uterine contractions, it has no effect on their frequency [67]. Studies continue to examine this topic. Because treatment of the primary disease often mitigates the uterine contractions that are seen with acute pyelonephritis, tocolysis use should be reserved for cases of documented cervical change [54].

Neonatal effects of urinary tract infections in pregnancy

There also has been a suggestion that UTI during pregnancy is associated with developmental delay and mental retardation in the neonate. Long-term infant follow-up per the National Collaborative Perinatal Project revealed that preschool intelligence quotient scores were 2.38 points lower in white male infants of mothers who had a UTI in pregnancy when compared with an unexposed cohort; however, no significant difference was noted among African American males or females [68,69]. Given the multifactorial nature of developmental delay and mental retardation, determining the cause is difficult, and no firm consensus has been reached on this apparent relationship. Recently, McDermott and colleagues [70] revisited this controversy. They found that the relative risk of infant cognitive delay with untreated UTI in pregnancy was 1.31 (95% CI, 1.12–1.54) when compared with unexposed infants. Furthermore, when comparing untreated women with treated women, the relative risk of infants who had mental retardation or developmental delay was 1.22 (95% CI, 1.02–1.46). These results support the association between UTI in pregnancy and cognitive delay and emphasize the importance of rapid diagnosis and treatment.

New directions

Ongoing research strives to improve prevention, detection of risk factors, and efficacy of treatment. In this era of increasing multidrug resistance, novel approaches that are directed at prevention of infection are underway. Methods to combat *E coli* colonization, in particular, are under investigation; as a result, a myriad of vaccines directed against *E coli* has emerged. Roberts and colleagues [17] described the efficacy of vaccination with purified *E coli* PapDG protein. Pap G, an adhesion, is a crucial component of P fimbriae, which allows bacterial binding to vaginal and renal epithelium. Upon intraperitoneal administration of purified PapDG to cynomolgus monkeys, significant levels of specific antibody against PapDG were noted. On histologic comparison of renal tissue with a control group following inoculation of *E coli* containing P fimbriae, vaccinated monkeys showed no evidence of pyelonephritis, whereas the control group had 22% to 33% positive histologic sections. Other vaccines that are under development include a parenteral formulation against *E coli* type I fimbriae (MedImmune, Inc., Gaithersburg, Maryland) [71], which is commonly found in UTI isolates, and Urovac (Solco Basel Ltd., Basel, Switzerland) [72], a vaginally administered preparation which is directed against multiple uropathogens. These vaccines hold promise for the future in mitigating and potentially eradicating the disease burden and societal costs of UTIs.

Summary

UTIs frequently complicate pregnancy with their concomitant morbidities. ASB, if left unrecognized and untreated, frequently progresses to pyelonephritis, and is associated with preterm delivery and low birth weight infants. A possible association exists between ASB and cognitive delay. Pyelonephritis is a serious medical condition in pregnancy and poses a significant medical risk to maternal, and, therefore, fetal well-being. Patients should be treated immediately and failure of response should be evaluated promptly. Close observation is necessary to detect complications, such as septic shock and respiratory insufficiency. When afebrile for 48 hours, patients may be discharged home with increased surveillance for the duration of the pregnancy. The risk of recurrence may be minimized with suppression therapy, or alternatively, monthly urine cultures.

References

[1] Foxman B. Epidemiology of urinary tract infections: incidence, morbidity, and economic costs. Dis Mon 2003;49(2):53–70.
[2] Foxman B, Klemstine K, Brown P. Acute pyelonephritis in US hospitals in 1997: hospitalization and in-hospital mortality. Ann Epidemiol 2003;13(2):144–50.
[3] Schappert S. National Ambulatory Medical Care Survey: 1994 summary. Adv Data 1996; 10(273):1–18.
[4] Rosenberg M. Pharmacoeconomics of treating uncomplicated urinary tract infection. Int J Antimicrob Agents 1999;11(3–4):247–51.
[5] Foxman B, Barlow R, D'Arcy H, et al. Urinary tract infection: self-reported incidence and associated costs. Ann Epidemiol 2000;10(8):509–15.
[6] Connolly A, Thorp JM. Urinary tract infections in pregnancy. Urol Clin North Am 1999;26(4): 779–87.
[7] Christensen F. Which antibiotics are appropriate for treating bacteriuria in pregnancy? J Antimicrob Chemother 2000;46(Suppl 1):29–34.
[8] Le J, Briggs FF, McKeown A, et al. Urinary tract infections during pregnancy. Ann Pharmacother 2004;38(10):1692–701.
[9] Lenke RR, VanDorsten JP, Schifrin BS. Pyelonephritis in pregnancy: a prospective randomized trial to prevent recurrent disease evaluating suppressive therapy with nitrofurantoin and close surveillance. Am J Obstet Gynecol 1983;146(8):953–7.
[10] Krcmery S, Hromec J, Demesova D. Treatment of lower urinary tract infection in pregnancy. Int J Antimicrob Agents 2001;17(4):279–82.
[11] Millar LK, Cox SM. Urinary tract infections complicating pregnancy. Infect Dis Clin North Am 1997;11(1):13–26.
[12] Ovalle A, Levancini M. Urinary tract infections in pregnancy. Curr Opin Urol 2001;11(1):55–9.
[13] Wing DA. Pyelonephritis. Clin Obstet Gynecol 1998;41(3):515–26.
[14] Gilstrap LC, Ramin SM. Urinary tract infections during pregnancy. Obstet Gynecol Clin North Am 2001;28(3):581–91.

[15] Hooton TM. Fluoroquinolones and resistance in the treatment of uncomplicated urinary tract infection. Int J Antimicrob Agents 2003;22(Suppl 2):65–72.

[16] Wing DA. Pyelonephritis in pregnancy: treatment options for optimal outcomes. Drugs 2001; 61:2087–96.

[17] Roberts JA, Kaack MB, Baskin G, et al. Antibody responses and protection from pyelonephritis following vaccination with purified *Escherichia coli* PapDG protein. J Urol 2004;171:1682–5.

[18] Selvarangan F, Goluszko P, Singhal J, et al. Interaction of Dr adhesion with collagen type IV is a critical step in *Escherichia coli* renal persistence. Infect Immun 2004;72(8):4827–35.

[19] American College of Obstetricians and Gynecologists. Antimicrobial therapy for obstetric patients. Washington DC: American College of Obstetricians and Gynecologists; 1998 [ACOG Technical Bulletin No. 117].

[20] United States Preventive Services Task Force. Guide to clinical preventive services. Periodic updates. 3 edition. Rockville: Agency for Healthcare Quality and Research; 2004 [AHRQ Publication #04–IP003].

[21] Wadland WC, Plante DA. Screening for asymptomatic bacteriuria in pregnancy. A decision-cost analysis. J Fam Pract 1989;29(4):233–6.

[22] Rouse DJ, Andrews WW, Goldenberg RL, et al. Screening and treatment of asymptomatic bacteriuria of pregnancy to prevent pyelonephritis: a cost-effectiveness and cost-benefit analysis. Obstet Gynecol 1995;86(1):119–23.

[23] Smaill F. Antibiotics for asymptomatic bacteriuria during pregnancy. Cochrane Database Syst Rev 2001;2:CD000490. p. 1–22.

[24] Sannes MF, Kuskowski MA, Johnson JR. Geographical distribution of antimicrobial resistance among Escherichia coli causing acute uncomplicated pyelonephritis in the United States. FEMS Immunol Med Microbiol 2004;42(2):213–8.

[25] Nicolle LE. Urinary tract infection: traditional pharmacologic therapies. Am J Med 2002; 113(1A):35S–44S.

[26] Huang ES, Stafford RS. National patterns in the treatment of urinary tract infections in women by ambulatory care physicians. Arch Intern Med 2002;162:41–7.

[27] Jepson RG, Mihaljevic L, Craig J. Cranberries for preventing urinary tract infections. Cochrane Database Syst Rev 2004;2:CD001321. p. 1–10.

[28] Warren JW, Abrutyn E, Hebel JR, et al. Guidelines for antimicrobial treatment of uncomplicated acute bacterial cystitis and acute pyelonephritis in women. Infectious Diseases Society of America (IDSA). Clin Infect Dis 1999;29:745–58.

[29] Rubin RH, Shapiro DS, Andriole VT, et al. Evaluation of new anti-infective drugs for the treatment of urinary tract infection. Clin Infect Dis 1992;15:S216–27.

[30] Tan JS, File TM. Treatment of bacteriuria in pregnancy. Drugs 1992;44(6):972–80.

[31] Villar J, Lydon-Rochelle MT, Gulmezoglu AM, et al. Duration of treatment for asymptomatic bacteriuria during pregnancy. Cochrane Database Syst Rev 2000;2:CD000491. p. 1–29.

[32] Pfau A, Sacks TG. Effective prophylaxis for recurrent urinary tract infections during pregnancy. Clin Infect Dis 1992;14(4):810–4.

[33] Romero R, Oyarzun E, Mazor M, et al. Meta-analysis of the relationship between asymptomatic bacteriuria and preterm delivery/low birth weight. Obstet Gynecol 1989;73:576–82.

[34] MacLean AB. Urinary tract infection in pregnancy. Int J Antimicrob Agents 2001;17:273–7.

[35] Vazquez JC, Villar J. Treatments for symptomatic urinary tract infections during pregnancy. Cochrane Database Syst Rev 2003;4:CD002256. p. 1–55.

[36] Harris RE, Gilstrap III LC. Cystitis during pregnancy: a distinct clinical entity. Obstet Gynecol 1981;57:578.

[37] North DH, Speed JE, Weinter WB, et al. Correlation of urinary tract infection with urinary screening at the first antepartum visit. J Miss State Med Assoc 1990;31:331–3.

[38] Pastore LM, Savitz DA, Thorp JM, et al. Predictors of symptomatic urinary tract infection after 20 weeks' gestation. J Perinatol 1999;19(7):488–93.

[39] Renal and urinary tract disorders. In: Cunningham FG, Gant N, Leveno KJ, Gilstrap III LC, Hauth JC, Wenstrom KD, editors. Williams obstetrics. 21st edition. New York: McGraw-Hill; 2001. p. 1251–72.

[40] Gilstrap III LC, Cunningham FG, Whalley PJ. Acute pyelonephritis in pregnancy: an anterospective study. Obstet Gynecol 1981;57:409–13.
[41] Whalley PJ, Cunningham FG, Martin FG. Transient renal dysfunction associated with acute pyelonephritis of pregnancy. Obstet Gynecol 1975;46:174–7.
[42] Otto G, Braconiew J, Andreasson A, et al. Interleukin-6 and disease severity in patients with bacteremic and nonbacteremic febrile urinary tract infection. J Infect Dis 1999;179:172–9.
[43] Haraoka M, Senoh K, Ogata N, et al. Elevated interleukin-8 levels in the urine of children with renal scarring and/or vesicoureteral reflux. J Urol 1996;155:678–80.
[44] Horcajada JP, Velasco M, Filella X, et al. Evaluation of inflammatory and renal-injury markers in women treated with antibiotics for acute pyelonephritis caused by *Escherichia coli*. Clin Diagn Lab Immunol 2004;11(1):142–6.
[45] Raz R, Sakran W, Chazan B, et al. Long-term follow-up of women hospitalized for acute pyelonephritis. Clin Infect Dis 2003;37:1014–20.
[46] Nahar A, Akom M, Hanes D, et al. Pyelonephritis and acute renal failure. Am J Med Sci 2004; 328(2):121–3.
[47] Velasco M, Martinez JA, Moreno-Martinez A, et al. Blood cultures for women with uncomplicated acute pyelonephritis: are they necessary? Clin Infect Dis 2003;37:1127–30.
[48] MacMillan MC, Grimes DA. The limited usefulness of urine and blood cultures in treating pyelonephritis in pregnancy. Obstet Gynecol 1991;78:745–8.
[49] Wing DA, Park AS, DeBuque L, et al. Limited clinical utility of blood and urine cultures in the treatment of acute pyelonephritis during pregnancy. Am J Obstet Gynecol 2000;182:1437–41.
[50] Seidman DS, Soriano D, Dulitzki M, et al. Role of renal ultrasonography in the management of pyelonephritis in pregnant women. J Perinatol 1998;18(2):98–101.
[51] Millar LK, Wing DA, Paul RH, et al. Outpatient treatment of pyelonephritis in pregnancy: a randomized controlled trial. Obstet Gynecol 1995;86:560–4.
[52] Wing DA, Hendershott CM, DeBuque L, et al. Outpatient treatment of acute pyelonephritis in pregnancy after 24 weeks. Obstet Gynecol 1999;94:683–8.
[53] Dunlow S, Duff P. Prevalence of antibiotic-resistant uropathogens in obstetric patients with acute pyelonephritis. Obstet Gynecol 1990;76:241.
[54] Millar LK, DeBuque L, Wing DA. Uterine contraction frequency during treatment of pyelonephritis in pregnancy and subsequent risk of preterm birth. J Perinat Med 2003;31(1): 41–6.
[55] Wing DA, Hendershott CM, DeBuque L, et al. A randomized trial of three antibiotic regimens for the treatment of pyelonephritis in pregnancy. Obstet Gynecol 1998;92:149–53.
[56] Butler EL, Cox SM, Eberts E, et al. Symptomatic nephrolithiasis complicating pregnancy. Obstet Gynecol 2000;96:753.
[57] Angel JL, O'Brien WF, Finan MA, et al. Acute pyelonephritis in pregnancy: a prospective study of oral versus intravenous antibiotic therapy. Obstet Gynecol 1990;76:28–32.
[58] Brooks AM, Garite TG. Clinical trial of the outpatient management of pyelonephritis in pregnancy. Inf Dis Obstet Gynecol 1995;3:50–5.
[59] Sanchez-Ramos L, McAlpine KJ, Adair DC, et al. Pyelonephritis in pregnancy: once-a-day ceftriaxone versus multiple doses of cefazolin: a randomized, double blind trial. Am J Obstet Gynecol 1995;172:129–33.
[60] Sandberg T, Brorson JE. Efficacy of long-term antimicrobial prophylaxis after acute pyelonephritis in pregnancy. Scand J Infect Dis 1991;23(2):221–3.
[61] Harris RE, Gilstrap LC. Prevention of recurrent pyelonephritis during pregnancy. Obstet Gynecol 1974;44:637.
[62] Mabie WC, Barton JR, Sibai B. Septic shock in pregnancy. Obstet Gynecol 1997;90:553–61.
[63] Graves CR. Acute pulmonary complications during pregnancy. Clin Obstet Gynecol 2002;45(2): 369–76.
[64] Tomlinson MW, Caruthers TJ, Whitty JE, et al. Does delivery improve maternal condition in the respiratory-compromised gravida? Obstet Gynecol 1998;91:108–11.
[65] Towers CV, Kaminskas CM, Garite TJ, et al. Pulmonary injury associated with antepartum pyelonephritis: can patients at risk be identified? Am J Obstet Gynecol 1991;164(4):974–8.

[66] Ross RG, Sathishkumar K, Naik AK, et al. Mechanism of lipopolysaccharide induced changes in effects of contractile agonists on pregnant rat myometrium. Am J Obstet Gynecol 2004;190(2): 532–40.

[67] Mackler AM, Ducsay TC, Ducsay CA, et al. Effects of endotoxin and macrophage-related cytokines on the contractile activity of the gravid mouse uterus. Biol Reprod 2003;69(4):1165–9.

[68] Broman SH, Nichols PL, Kennedy WA. Preschool IQ: prenatal and early developmental correlates. New York: John Wiley & Sons; 1975.

[69] Broman SH. Prenatal risk factors for mental retardation in young children. Public Health Rep 1987;102:55–7.

[70] McDermott S, Callaghan W, Szwejbka L, et al. Urinary tract infections during pregnancy and mental retardation and developmental delay. Obstet Gynecol 2000;96(1):113–9.

[71] Langermann S, Mollby R, Burlein JE, et al. Vaccination with FimH adhesin protects cynomolgus monkeys from colonization and infection by uropathogenic *Escherichia coli*. J Infect Dis 2000; 181:774.

[72] Uehling DT, Hopkins WJ, Elkahwaji J, et al. Phase 2 clinical trial of vaginal mucosal immunization for recurrent urinary tract infection. J Urol 2003;170:867.

ELSEVIER
SAUNDERS

Clin Perinatol 32 (2005) 765–776

CLINICS IN
PERINATOLOGY

Emerging Infections and Pregnancy: West Nile Virus, Monkeypox, Severe Acute Respiratory Syndrome, and Bioterrorism

Denise J. Jamieson, MD, MPH[a,*],
Daniel B. Jernigan, MD, MPH[b], Jane E. Ellis, MD, PhD[c],
Tracee A. Treadwell, DVM, MPH[b]

[a]*Division of Reproductive Health, National Center for Chronic Disease Prevention and Health Promotion, Centers for Disease Control and Prevention, 4770 Buford Highway, Atlanta, GA 30341, USA*

[b]*National Center for Infectious Diseases, Centers for Disease Control and Prevention, 1600 Clifton Road, Atlanta, GA 30333, USA*

[c]*Department of Gynecology and Obstetrics, Emory University School of Medicine, 69 Jesse Hill Jr. Drive, S.E., Atlanta, GA 30303, USA*

In 1991, the National Academy of Science's Institute of Medicine convened a 19-member multidisciplinary panel to study the emergence of infectious disease threats. This expert panel issued a landmark report, entitled *Emerging Infections—Microbial Threats to Health in the United States* [1], which described a host of factors that contribute to the introduction and spread of novel infectious diseases. In 2003, a follow-up report was issued, entitled *Microbial Threats To Health: Emergence, Detection, and Response* [2]. These two reports emphasize the urgent threat posed by the introduction and spread of novel infectious disease agents in the United States. Furthermore, they describe the critical role that globalization plays in the rapid and efficient spread of these infectious diseases. As global borders blur, and people, animals, food, and other products are rapidly transported, the infectious diseases that they harbor may also be

* Corresponding author.
E-mail address: djamieson@cdc.gov (D.J. Jamieson).

doi:10.1016/j.clp.2005.04.008

efficiently transported to new locations. In addition to the unintentional spread of disease, we also now face the possibility of intentional disease spread by bioterrorist attacks.

As new infectious diseases, such as West Nile virus, monkeypox, and severe acute respiratory syndrome (SARS) are recognized in the United States, there are critical questions about how these infectious diseases will affect pregnant women and their infants. In addition, the implications of bioterrorist attacks for exposed pregnant women need to be considered. In this article, the authors address the following questions for a number of infectious disease threats: (1) Does pregnancy affect the clinical course of these novel infectious diseases? (2) What are the implications for prophylaxis and treatment of exposed or infected pregnant women? (3) Are these novel infectious diseases transmitted during pregnancy, labor and delivery, or breastfeeding?

West Nile virus

West Nile virus is a mosquito-borne flavivirus that is transmitted to humans primarily through the bite of infected mosquitoes [3]. Infection in humans is varied: it can be asymptomatic; it can result in a mild illness with fever, rash, and headache; or it can be severe, with meningoencephalitis and other neurologic sequelae, because the virus has a predilection for the human nervous system [4]. Information about West Nile virus in pregnancy is fairly limited, with only six cases of West Nile virus in pregnancy having been reported to date [5–10], although the Centers for Disease Control and Prevention (CDC) has been tracking more than 70 pregnant women infected with West Nile virus since 2003 [6].

There has been only one documented case of probable intrauterine infection with West Nile virus [5,7]. A 20-year-old woman at 27 weeks gestation presented with fever, severe headache, blurred vision, abdominal and back pain, and vomiting. She was treated with intravenous antibiotics. On the fourth day of hospitalization, the patient was afebrile, but had pain and symmetric weakness in her legs. After more than 2 weeks of hospitalization, the patient left against medical advice and was readmitted 2 days later after having fallen. Electromyelography (EMG) indicated widespread involvement of the lower motor neurons. Serologic testing revealed West Nile virus-specific (WNV-specific) IgM antibodies in the serum and in cerebrospinal fluid, consistent with the diagnosis of meningoencephalitis. At 38 weeks of gestation, the patient had a spontaneous vaginal delivery of a viable infant. At delivery, WNV-specific IgM was detected in maternal serum, cord blood, infant serum, and infant cerebrospinal fluid. The infant also had WNV-specific IgM antibody in the serum. The placenta was polymerase chain reaction (PCR)-positive for West Nile virus at one of two reference laboratories. In addition, the infant had evidence of bilateral chorioretinitis and cerebral tissue destruction. This is the only reported case of documented intrauterine transmission of West Nile virus. The infant ocular and neurologic abnormalities that were noted at birth likely resulted from the infection with West Nile virus.

In another reported case of West Nile virus infection in pregnancy complicated by meningoencephalitis, there was no evidence of fetal infection, although the work-up of the infant for infection was incomplete [8]. A 28-year-old having a history of chronic hypertension and sickle cell trait presented at 16 weeks gestation with headache, neck pain, fever, nausea, and vomiting. She reported recently being bitten by mosquitoes, and WNV-specific IgM was detected in her cerebrospinal fluid, consistent with the diagnosis of West Nile virus meningoencephalitis. She was treated with antibiotics and antivirals, and required mechanical ventilation. At 32 weeks, she was induced for superimposed preeclampsia and fetal growth restriction. The infant appeared normal and did well, although a serologic evaluation for possible West Nile virus infection in the infant was not undertaken. In this case, it is likely that the maternal hypertensive disease contributed substantively to the fetal growth restriction. What is unclear is whether infection with West Nile virus could have also contributed to the fetal growth restriction.

In four other cases of West Nile virus infection in pregnancy that have been reported in the literature [9,10], there has been no evidence of fetal infection or fetal effects from maternal infection. In each of these cases, infant serologic testing for WNV-specific IGM was negative. In addition to the cases during pregnancy, there has also been one reported case of probable West Nile virus infection to an infant through breastfeeding [11].

Based on the limited information reported to date, it is not clear whether pregnant women are more susceptible to infection to West Nile virus, or if they have a more severe clinical course. With the CDC now actively collecting information on cases in pregnancy, we hope that there will be additional information addressing these issues in the near future. The fetal effects of maternal infection are also unclear, with one probable case of congenital anomalies associated with intrauterine infection and one possible case of fetal growth restriction, although the growth restriction could also easily be attributed to the maternal hypertensive disease. West Nile virus is a flavivirus with antigenic similarities to Japanese encephalitis and St. Louis encephalitis [3]. Other flaviviruses have been associated with spontaneous abortion and neonatal illness, but they have not been known to cause birth defects [6]. In terms of preventing illness, pregnant women should be advised to use protective clothing, avoid outdoor exposure during times of the day when mosquitoes are most active (ie, dawn and dusk), and use insect repellants containing N,N-diethl-m-tolumide (DEET) [6].

Monkeypox

Monkeypox, which belongs to the orthopoxvirus group of viruses [12], was so-called because it was discovered in laboratory monkeys in 1958 [13].

Monkeypox was first identified as the cause of a smallpox-like illness in humans in Africa in 1970 [13], and subsequent outbreaks were reported, including one large series of 88 cases reported from the Democratic Republic of the Congo [14]. Information about monkeypox infection among pregnant women is extremely limited, because most prior descriptions of monkeypox outbreaks in Africa do not include a description of the natural history of outbreaks among pregnant woman. One probable case of perinatal infection has been reported from Zaire. At approximately 24 weeks gestation, a pregnant woman developed a febrile illness with a rash, and monkeypox virus was subsequently isolated from a vesicular lesion. Six weeks later she delivered a 1500 g infant who had a generalized skin rash resembling monkeypox [13].

In June 2003, the first evidence of community-acquired monkeypox infection was reported in the United States [12]. By July 8, 2003, a total of 71 monkeypox cases had been reported from six states [15]. This outbreak resulted from contact with infected pet prairie dogs, who acquired monkeypox after being housed or transported with infected African rodents. Because some of these infected pets were in households with pregnant mothers, there was concern about how to advise pregnant women [16].

Because smallpox (vaccinia) vaccine had been reported to reduce the risk of monkeypox among previously vaccinated persons in Africa, the CDC recommended that persons exposed to a sick prairie dog or an infected person be vaccinated, regardless of their pregnancy status [16].

Severe acute respiratory syndrome

SARS is an acute viral infection with a novel coronavirus [17,18], which in 2003 caused outbreaks of more than 50 cases in 6 countries, but affected 25 countries [19]. The largest case series of pregnant women comes from Hong Kong, where 12 pregnant women who had SARS were hospitalized in 2003 [20–23]. Three of the 12 pregnant patients who had SARS died, for a case-fatality rate of 25%. Among the 7 women who presented in their first trimester of pregnancy, 4 had spontaneous abortions between 2 and 5 weeks after onset of illness, and 2 electively terminated their pregnancies after recovery from SARS. Among the 5 women who presented in the late second or third trimesters, 4 had preterm deliveries, with 3 patients delivered by emergency cesarean section due to inadequate maternal oxygenation and 1 due to fetal distress. Two patients had evidence of intrauterine growth restriction and oligohydramnios. Six patients were admitted to the intensive care unit [22]. Among the five newborn infants, there was no evidence of clinical or serologic evidence of perinatal transmission, as assessed by SARS-associated coronavirus reverse-transcriptase PCR and viral culture on cord blood, placenta tissue, and amniotic fluid [21]. A matched study in Hong Kong [20] comparing the clinical course and outcomes of 10 pregnant SARS patients with 40 nonpregnant controls found that pregnant and nonpregnant patients had similar clinical symptoms and presentation, but that pregnant patients had evidence of more severe illness. Pregnant patients were more likely to require endotracheal intubation and admission to the intensive care unit, and they were more likely to develop renal failure and disseminated intravascular coagulopathy compared with nonpregnant patients. There were three deaths among the pregnant patients compared, with no deaths in the non-pregnant group.

Two of the eight people who had laboratory-confirmed SARS in the United States in 2003 were pregnant women [24–26]. Both had traveled to Hong Kong and stayed in the same hotel as the physician who is thought to be the source of infection for index case-patients in a variety of countries. A 36-year-old woman traveled to Hong Kong at 19 weeks gestation. Upon her return to the United States she was hospitalized for pneumonia, and subsequently required mechanical ventilation. Serum specimens were tested at the CDC and found to be positive for SARS-coronavirus antibody. She recovered and did well until 38 weeks gestation, when she underwent cesarean delivery for a complete placenta previa. The infant was normal-appearing and had no evidence of infection; however, clinical specimens from the infant were not tested for SARS coronavirus [24,25]. The second patient in the United States was a 38-year-old who traveled to Hong Kong at 7 weeks gestation. She and her husband also stayed at the Hong Kong hotel implicated in the spread of SARS to a number of countries. Both the pregnant woman and her husband were diagnosed with SARS upon their return to the United States. The pregnant woman was hospitalized for 9 days and recovered fully from her illness. At 36 weeks gestation, she had preterm premature rupture of membranes and delivered a healthy infant without evidence of infection [26].

Although not confirmed by the two cases in the United States, the cases reported from Hong Kong suggest that pregnant women who have SARS may have a more severe clinical course compared with nonpregnant women. In addition, SARS during pregnancy may be associated with increased rates of spontaneous abortion, preterm delivery, and intrauterine growth restriction. There has been no evidence, however, of perinatal transmission of SARS. In terms of treatment, although ribavirin has been used empirically to treat SARS, it has not been studied systematically to determine whether it is effective treatment [27]. There are concerns about using ribavirin early in pregnancy; embryocidal and teratogenic effects of ribavirin have been noted in animal studies and ribavirin is designated as pregnancy category X, indicating that it should not be used in pregnancy [28]. Although there are few data regarding use early in pregnancy, in the few women given ribavirin later in pregnancy for measles or influenza, no fetal adverse effects have been noted [29,30]. Eleven of the 12 pregnant SARS patients in Hong Kong received ribavirin, including 6 of the 7 patients diagnosed in the first trimester [23]. It is possible that the high rates of spontaneous abortion observed in Hong Kong could be due to treatment with ribavirin rather than the SARS infection.

Bioterrorism

In this new age of heightened concern about terrorist attacks, the possibility of intentional attacks in the United States using biologic weapons has been of increased concern recently, particularly after the anthrax attacks of 2001 [31]. The Working Group on Civilian Biodefense, which is an expert panel composed of representatives from academic, government, military, public health, and emergency management agencies and institutions, has identified a limited number of biologic agents that are of particular concern. These include anthrax, smallpox, botulism, tularemia, plague, and the viral hemorrhagic fevers [32–38]. Physicians and public health officials have been developing strategies for how to respond to potential bioterrorist attacks, including identifying that an attack has occurred, prophylaxing those exposed, diagnosing and treating cases, and implementing containment measures to minimize the number of people exposed. It is critical that these comprehensive response plans include specific guidance for pregnant women, so that pregnant women who are exposed or who are cases can be treated appropriately. For some of these bioterrorist agents, such as smallpox, we have some information about infection in pregnancy; however, for many of these potential bioterrorist agents there is limited information about these infections in pregnancy.

Anthrax

Anthrax infections can be cutaneous, inhalational, or gastrointestinal, and are caused by *Bacillus anthracis*, an aerobic, gram-positive, spore-forming bacillus species [36,38]. Although anthrax has been around since the time of ancient Rome [39], information about anthrax in pregnancy is limited. There were two recent cases of anthrax infection in pregnancy reported from Turkey in 2003 [40]. In one case, a 33-year old woman at 32 weeks gestation presented with a submandibular eschar and extensive edema of the face, neck, and upper thorax. Her report of flaying a dead cow 7 days earlier was consistent with exposure, because herbivores are often infected after ingesting anthrax spores from the soil. She was treated with penicillin and prednisolone, recovered 10 days later, and delivered prematurely at 34 weeks gestation. The second case was a 29-year-old woman at 33 weeks of gestation who had a lesion on her elbow, was treated with penicillin, and delivered at 34 weeks gestation. In both cases, *B anthracis* was isolated from their lesions, they recovered quickly without sequelae, and their neonates did not have any evidence of infection.

There have been several other cases of anthrax infection in pregnancy from Iran and India [41,42]. In two cases, pregnant women presented with gastrointestinal anthrax after ingesting contaminated meat. In both cases the women died from peritonitis. Of over 140 maternal death autopsies performed at a hospital in Iran, four women had anthrax [41]. There are no reported cases of perinatal transmission of anthrax in the literature, and no cases of inhalational anthrax in pregnancy.

During the anthrax attacks of 2001, which resulted in 22 cases and five deaths [38], guidelines were rapidly developed and disseminated to address prophylaxis for exposed persons as well as recommendations for treatment. Both the American College of Obstetricians and Gynecologists (ACOG) and the CDC recommend that pregnant women who have a high-risk environmental exposure should receive prophylaxis [43,44]; however, decisions about whether an exposure is risky enough to merit prophylaxis for a pregnant woman should be made by public health officials, not by the woman's obstetrician-gynecologist or other care provider [44]. The first-line regimen for prophylaxis of pregnant women should be a 60-day course of ciprofloxacin. If the specific strain of *B anthracis* is found to be penicillin-sensitive, then a switch to amoxicillin may be considered. Due to effects on fetal bone and dental enamel, doxycycline, the other first-line agent for anthrax prophylaxis among nonpregnant adults, should be used with caution in asymptomatic pregnant women, and only when contraindications proscribe use of other drugs. If doxycycline is used in pregnant women, periodic liver function testing should be performed because of the small increased risk of maternal hepatic necrosis. Although anthrax vaccine supplies are currently limited, anthrax vaccination has been proposed as an adjunct to microbial prophylaxis for optimal postexposure prophylaxis [38]; however, there are no animal or human safely studies of the anthrax vaccine during pregnancy, and the vaccine is not recommended for use in pregnancy [45]. For initial therapy of inhalational anthrax among nonpregnant adults, intravenous ciprofloxacin or doxycycline, along with one or two additional agents, is recommended [38]. For pregnant women, the recommendations for treatment are similar to those of nonpregnant adults, although ciprofloxacin would be generally preferable to doxycycline.

Smallpox

Due to its high fatality rate and its ease of transmission, as well as the general lack of immunity currently in the US population, smallpox is one of the most feared potential agents of bioterror. Smallpox is caused by variola virus, a DNA virus of the genus *Orthopoxvirus*, the same genus as monkeypox, cowpox, and vaccinia. Variola differs from the other orthopox viruses in that it is readily transmitted from person-to-person [35].

Smallpox is generally more severe in pregnant women than in nonpregnant women or in men [46]. In several reports from India, pregnant women had a higher case-fatality rate and a sevenfold increased risk of a severe hemorrhagic type of smallpox compared with nonpregnant adults [47]. Rates of spontaneous abortion, stillbirth, and preterm delivery are very high among women who have smallpox [46]. In addition, congenital cases of smallpox have been reported [46]. Therefore, the potential impact that an intentional attack with smallpox in the United States would have specifically on pregnant women is particularly concerning.

Vaccinia vaccine, the highly effective vaccine against smallpox, was recommended for all US children until 1972. Currently, only those laboratory workers and health care workers at high risk of exposure are being offered vaccinia vaccination [48]; however, vaccination during pregnancy is generally contraindicated because of documented cases of fetal vaccinia following maternal vaccination. Although pregnancy is a contraindication to routine nonemergency vaccination, in the case of an intentional attack, pregnancy should not be a contraindication to postexposure vaccination [48]. Vaccinia immune globulin (VIG) is recommended for persons who have severe, life-threatening complications from vaccinia vaccination. VIG is not contraindicated in pregnancy if severe adverse vaccine reactions occur [48].

Other agents

Several other agents, such as botulism, tularemia, plague, and hemorrhagic fever viruses, have been highlighted by the Working Group on Civilian Biodefense as potential biologic weapons. Botulism is an extremely potent biological toxin that comes from *Clostridium botulinum*. Once absorbed, botulism toxin binds irreversibly to peripheral cholinergic synapses and blocks acetylcholine release, causing paralysis. Recovery may take weeks to months to complete, and results from reinnervation of paralyzed muscle fibers [32]. There have been several cases of botulism in pregnancy reported in the literature. In the most dramatic case [49], a 37-year-old woman at 23 weeks gestation who had consumed home-produced green beans was hospitalized for progressive weakness and eventual paralysis, requiring assisted ventilation for 2 months. Botulism antitoxin was administered. Although she became increasingly paralyzed, fetal growth was normal and fetal movement was apparent. She recovered fully and delivered a healthy infant at term. In another case, an Alaskan native was hospitalized at 16 weeks gestation with botulism after ingesting contaminated whitefish. After receiving antibotulism toxin, she was discharged home on the tenth hospital day. She delivered a healthy infant at term [50]. There has been no evidence to date of transplacental transport of botulism toxin to the fetus, nor have there been any reports of adverse fetal effects of maternal treatment with botulism antitoxin [49–51]. Based on limited information, pregnant women should receive the same treatment for botulism as nonpregnant adults, which consists of supportive care and passive immunization with equine antitoxin [32].

Tularemia is a plaguelike disease of rodents caused by *Francisella tularensis*. For prophylaxis of tularemia after an intentional attack, ciprofloxacin, one of the two preferred regimens for nonpregnant adults, is recommended for pregnant women,. For treatment of tularemia, gentamicin, also one of the two preferred choices for nonpregnant adults, is recommended [34].

Yersinia pestis, the causative agent of plague, is an enzootic infection of rodents that most commonly causes bubonic plague. In an intentional attack using *Y pestis*, the recommendation for pregnant women is to use gentamicin for prophylaxis [37].

The viral hemorrhagic fevers, which are caused by several families of viruses, are a clinical illness associated with fever and a bleeding diathesis. Several of these such as Ebola, Marburg, Lassa, and yellow fever have been identified by the Working Group on Civilian Biodefense as potential biologic weapons [33]. There is some evidence that the mortality of some viral hemorrhagic fevers appears to be higher in pregnancy. Although there are no antiviral drugs approved by the US Food and Drug Administration for treatment of viral hemorrhagic fevers, ribavirin may reduce mortality of several of them, including Lassa fever. As previously mentioned, ribavirin is designated as pregnancy category X and is contraindicated in pregnancy; however, given the severity of the hemorrhagic fevers, the Working Group on Civilian Biodefense feels that the benefits appear likely to outweigh the risks and recommends ribavirin use for severely ill pregnant women [33].

Summary

As we face emerging and re-emerging health threats, we will need to understand how these novel diseases will affect pregnant women. In some cases, such as SARS, the hemorrhagic fevers, and smallpox, it appears that pregnant women may have more severe clinical courses compared with nonpregnant adults. In some cases, it appears that the rapid diagnosis of the disease may be delayed due to pregnancy. For example, in one of the reported anthrax cases, there was probably a delay in diagnosis of anthrax peritonitis because the pregnancy complicated the presenting clinical picture [41]. In terms of prophylaxis and treatment of emerging diseases, in many cases, such as anthrax, tularemia, and plague, first-line therapies and postexposure prophylaxis is similar in pregnant and nonpregnant adults. Although vaccinations such as those for smallpox and anthrax are not generally recommended for pregnant women, in some cases they may be used for postexposure prophylaxis. For example, for pregnant women exposed to monkeypox or smallpox, use of the vaccinia vaccine is recommended. In some cases, such as with ribavirin, which is generally contraindicated in pregnancy due to its teratogenic and embyrocidal effects, decisions about use in pregnancy need to be carefully weighed. In the case of SARS, where treatment is generally supportive and the effectiveness of ribavirin has not been convincingly demonstrated, use of ribavirin may not be indicated. By contrast, ribavirin has been shown to be effective treatment for some of the viral hemorrhagic fevers, such as Lassa fever, and despite the risks, treatment of pregnant women may be warranted given the severity of illness. In terms of perinatal transmission, there are cases of intrauterine transmission of West Nile virus, monkeypox, and smallpox virus reported in the literature.

There are a growing number of new or newly recognized pathogens in the United States that threaten our health. As new disease threats emerge, it will be critical to evaluate and understand how these diseases affect pregnant women, so that reasonable response plans for diagnosis and treatment of pregnant women can be rapidly developed.

References

[1] Institute of Medicine. Emerging infections: microbial threats to health in the United States. Washington (DC): National Academy Press; 1992.
[2] Institute of Medicine. Microbial threats to health: emergence, detection, and response. Washington (DC): National Academies Press; 2003.
[3] Petersen LR, Marfin AA, Gubler DJ. West Nile virus. JAMA 2003;290(4):524–8.
[4] Granwehr BP, Lillibridge KM, Higgs S, et al. West Nile virus: where are we now? Lancet Infect Dis 2004;4(9):547–56.
[5] Centers for Disease Control and Prevention. Intrauterine West Nile virus infection—New York, 2002. MMWR Morb Mortal Wkly Rep 2002;51(50):1135–6.
[6] Centers for Disease Control and Prevention. Interim guidelines for the evaluation of infants born to mothers infected with West Nile virus during pregnancy. MMWR Morb Mortal Wkly Rep 2004;53(7):154–7.
[7] Alpert SG, Fergerson J, Noel LP. Intrauterine West Nile virus: ocular and systemic findings. Am J Ophthalmol 2003;136(4):733–5.
[8] Chapa JB, Ahn JT, DiGiovanni LM, et al. West Nile virus encephalitis during pregnancy. Obstet Gynecol 2003;102(2):229–31.
[9] Hayes EB, O'Leary DR. West Nile virus infection: a pediatric perspective. Pediatrics 2004; 113(5):1375–81.
[10] Bruno J, Rabito Jr FJ, Dildy III GA. West nile virus meningoencephalitis during pregnancy. J La State Med Soc 2004;156(4):204–5.
[11] Centers for Disease Control and Prevention. Possible West Nile virus transmission to an infant through breast-feeding—Michigan, 2002. MMWR Morb Mortal Wkly Rep 2002;51(39):877–8.
[12] Centers for Disease Control and Prevention. Multistate outbreak of monkeypox—Illinois, Indiana, and Wisconsin, 2003. MMWR Morb Mortal Wkly Rep 2003;52(23):537–40.
[13] Jezek Z, Fenner F. Human monkeypox. New York: Karger; 1988.
[14] Hutin YJ, Williams RJ, Malfait P, et al. Outbreak of human monkeypox, Democratic Republic of Congo, 1996 to 1997. Emerg Infect Dis 2001;7(3):434–8.
[15] Centers for Disease Control and Prevention. Update. Multistate outbreak of monkeypox—Illinois, Indiana, Kansas, Missouri, Ohio, and Wisconsin, 2003. MMWR Morb Mortal Wkly Rep 2003;52(27):642–6.
[16] Jamieson DJ, Cono J, Richards CL, et al. The role of the obstetrician-gynecologist in emerging infectious diseases: monkeypox and pregnancy. Obstet Gynecol 2004;103(4):754–6.
[17] Drosten C, Gunther S, Preiser W, et al. Identification of a novel coronavirus in patients with severe acute respiratory syndrome. N Engl J Med 2003;348(20):1967–76.
[18] Ksiazek TG, Erdman D, Goldsmith CS, et al. A novel coronavirus associated with severe acute respiratory syndrome. N Engl J Med 2003;348(20):1953–66.
[19] Peiris JS, Chu CM, Cheng VC, et al. Clinical progression and viral load in a community outbreak of coronavirus-associated SARS pneumonia: a prospective study. Lancet 2003; 361(9371):1767–72.
[20] Lam CM, Wong SF, Leung TN, et al. A case-controlled study comparing clinical course and outcomes of pregnant and non-pregnant women with severe acute respiratory syndrome. BJOG 2004;111(8):771–4.
[21] Shek CC, Ng PC, Fung GP, et al. Infants born to mothers with severe acute respiratory syndrome. Pediatrics 2003;112(4):e254.
[22] Wong SF, Chow KM, Leung TN, et al. Pregnancy and perinatal outcomes of women with severe acute respiratory syndrome. Am J Obstet Gynecol 2004;191(1):292–7.

[23] Wong SF, Chow KM, de Swiet M. Severe acute respiratory syndrome and pregnancy. BJOG 2003;110(7):641–2.
[24] Centers for Disease Control and Prevention. Severe acute respiratory syndrome (SARS) and coronavirus testing—United States, 2003. MMWR Morb Mortal Wkly Rep 2003;52(14): 297–302.
[25] Robertson CA, Lowther SA, Birch T, et al. SARS and pregnancy: a case report. Emerg Infect Dis 2004;10(2):345–8.
[26] Stockman LJ, Lowther SA, Coy K, et al. SARS during pregnancy, United States. Emerg Infect Dis 2004;10(9):1689–90.
[27] Wenzel RP, Edmond MB. Managing SARS amidst uncertainty. N Engl J Med 2003; 348(20):1947–8.
[28] Watts DH. Antiviral agents. Obstet Gynecol Clin North Am 1992;19(3):563–85.
[29] Atmar RL, Englund JA, Hammill H. Complications of measles during pregnancy. Clin Infect Dis 1992;14(1):217–26.
[30] Kirshon B, Faro S, Zurawin RK, et al. Favorable outcome after treatment with amantadine and ribavirin in a pregnancy complicated by influenza pneumonia. A case report. J Reprod Med 1988;33(4):399–401.
[31] Lane HC, Fauci AS. Bioterrorism on the home front: a new challenge for American medicine. JAMA 2001;286(20):2595–7.
[32] Arnon SS, Schechter R, Inglesby TV, et al. Botulinum toxin as a biological weapon: medical and public health management. JAMA 2001;285(8):1059–70.
[33] Borio L, Inglesby T, Peters CJ, et al. Hemorrhagic fever viruses as biological weapons: medical and public health management. JAMA 2002;287(18):2391–405.
[34] Dennis DT, Inglesby TV, Henderson DA, et al. Tularemia as a biological weapon: medical and public health management. JAMA 2001;285(21):2763–73.
[35] Henderson DA, Inglesby TV, Bartlett JG, et al. Smallpox as a biological weapon: medical and public health management. Working Group on Civilian Biodefense. JAMA 1999;281(22): 2127–37.
[36] Inglesby TV, Henderson DA, Bartlett JG, et al. Anthrax as a biological weapon: medical and public health management. Working Group on Civilian Biodefense. JAMA 1999;281(18): 1735–45.
[37] Inglesby TV, Dennis DT, Henderson DA, et al. Plague as a biological weapon: medical and public health management. Working Group on Civilian Biodefense. JAMA 2000;283(17): 2281–90.
[38] Inglesby TV, O'Toole T, Henderson DA, et al. Anthrax as a biological weapon, 2002: updated recommendations for management. JAMA 2002;287(17):2236–52.
[39] Dirckx JH. Virgil on anthrax. Am J Dermatopathol 1981;3(2):191–5.
[40] Kadanali A, Tasyaran MA, Kadanali S. Anthrax during pregnancy: case reports and review. Clin Infect Dis 2003;36(10):1343–6.
[41] Handjani AM. Case records of the Pahlavi hospitals. Pahlavi Med J 1976;7:147–59.
[42] Sujatha S, Parija SC, Bhattacharya S, et al. Anthrax peritonitis. Trop Doct 2002;32(4):247–8.
[43] Centers for Disease Control and Prevention. Updated recommendations for antimicrobial prophylaxis among asymptomatic pregnant women after exposure to *Bacillus anthracis*. MMWR Morb Mortal Wkly Rep 2001;50(43):960.
[44] Committee ACOG. Opinion number 268, February 2002. Management of asymptomatic pregnant or lactating women exposed to anthrax. American College of Obstetricians and Gynecologists. Obstet Gynecol 2002;99(2):366–8.
[45] The Centers for Disease Control. Status of US Department of Defense preliminary evaluation of the association of anthrax vaccination and congenital anomalies. JAMA 2002;287(9):1107.
[46] Fenner F, Henderson DA, Arita I, et al. Smallpox and its eradication. Geneva (Switzerland): World Health Organization; 1988.
[47] Suarez VR, Hankins GD. Smallpox and pregnancy: from eradicated disease to bioterrorist threat. Obstet Gynecol 2002;100(1):87–93.

[48] Centers for Disease Control and Prevention. Vaccinia (smallpox) vaccine. MMWR Recomm Rep 2001;50:1–10.
[49] Polo JM, Martin J, Berciano J. Botulism and pregnancy. Lancet 1996;348(9021):195.
[50] Robin L, Herman D, Redett R. Botulism in a pregnant women. N Engl J Med 1996; 335(11):823–4.
[51] Centers for Disease Control and Prevention. Wound botulism—California, 1995. MMWR Morb Mortal Wkly Rep 1995;44(48):889–92.

ELSEVIER
SAUNDERS

Clin Perinatol 32 (2005) 777–787

CLINICS IN
PERINATOLOGY

Epidural Analgesia for Labor Pain and Its Relationship to Fever

James M. Alexander, MD

Department of Obstetrics and Gynecology, University of Texas Southwestern Medical Center at Dallas, 5323 Harry Hines Boulevard, Dallas, TX 75390-9032, USA

When epidural analgesia is given for pain relief during labor, it is associated with a rise in maternal temperature. Fusi and colleagues [1] first reported this association in 1989. They showed that women who receive labor epidurals have a slight increase in their temperature related to the amount of time the epidural is in place; women in their study who had longer labors and had an epidural in place for greater than 4 hours had an increase in temperature of approximately 0.5°C. No women in the study who received a labor epidural had an increase in temperature that resulted in overt fever (temperature greater than 38.0°C), leading the study authors to conclude that the temperature effect of labor epidural was not clinically significant. In 1991, a second report appeared showing that epidural analgesia increases maternal temperature, but does not result in clinical fever, findings similar to the Fusi group's [2]. Since the appearance of these two reports, other investigators have studied the effect of labor epidural on maternal temperature, and have not only confirmed the association, but have found that in some cases the increase in temperature is clinically significant and results in overt fever [3–8].

Determining the mechanism for the rise in maternal temperature seen with epidural is made difficult by the characteristics of women in labor who receive them. It is not clear whether a cause-and-effect relationship between epidural and fever exists, or whether epidural is a marker for other factors that place a woman at risk. For example, longer labor is associated with a higher incidence of epidural use, which in turn is associated with fever and chorioamnionitis [9–11]. Determining whether maternal fever is due to the epidural or the circumstances leading to its administration can be difficult.

E-mail address: jamesalexander@utsouthwestern.edu

0095-5108/05/$ – see front matter
doi:10.1016/j.clp.2005.04.004

The association between labor epidural and fever has led to concern about its effect on maternal and fetal well being. This concern received widespread attention after the report published by Lieberman and colleagues in 1997 [3]. In their report, 34% of the neonates born to women receiving epidurals underwent sepsis evaluation, compared with 10% in the nonepidural group, and 15% received antibiotics, compared with 4% in the nonepidural group. Although the overall exposure of neonates to antibiotics was high, the actual incidence of clinically significant sepsis was quite low at 0.2%, and independent of the type of labor analgesia used. In their conclusion, the study authors pointed out that women who receive labor epidurals should be made aware that they are placing their neonate at increased risk for sepsis evaluation and antibiotic therapy that would otherwise be unnecessary, which may lead to unanticipated complications. They suggested that efforts to decrease these unnecessary interventions should include re-examination of which neonates receive sepsis evaluation, modification of the epidural effect on maternal temperature using different epidural techniques, and reconsidering the use of epidural analgesia in labor. Critics of this study point out that the study design was retrospective, that women self-selected their analgesia, that the study participants were already at risk for fever (the epidural group had much longer labors as well as larger babies), and that some of the women may have had fever before epidural administration [12]. Many critics felt that the data reported had too many confounders to make recommendations against labor epidurals due to adverse neonatal effects [13].

Normal temperature regulation

The hypothalamus is responsible for maintaining normal body temperature [14]. It does this by integrating information it receives about core and peripheral temperature with processes that result in heat loss and gain. Peripheral nerves transmit information from the skin and the anatomic nervous system transmits information from the internal organs to the hypothalamus. Typically, the normal metabolic activities of the body result in net heat production. The hypothalamus controls temperature by counterbalancing heat production with processes that promote heat loss. The primary mechanisms triggered by the hypothalamus to accomplish this include peripheral vasodilation and sweating. Heat loss also can occur through an increase in ventilation. Behavior can affect body temperature as well, and is often modified when the hypothalamus sends the message to the cortex, resulting in one feeling hot. This sensation leads to behavior modification, such as the shedding of clothes or moving to a cooler environment. Interference with any of these mechanisms can result in heat retention leading to fever.

Fever also occurs when the hypothalamus changes its set point. Normally the hypothalamus tries to maintain a core body temperature of 37°C. In the setting of infection, this set point is increased, and mechanisms are activated to increase body temperature. The most common process leading to an increase in the set point is infection. Microbes lead to activation of an immune response that involves monocytes, macrophages, the endothelial, and other cells. Pyrogenic cytokines including interleukin 1 and 6, tumor necrosis factor, and interferon are released from these cells, which stimulates the hypothalamus to change its set point.

Heat production and heat loss during labor

Labor was first associated with fever in the absence of infection in 1875 [15]. The activity of the uterus in labor contributes to core temperature and processes that interfere with heat dispersion can lead to fever. Marx and Loew [16] quantified temperature increases associated with uterine contractions in 1975. In that study, they measured the rise in maternal temperature associated with uterine contractions in active labor. During each individual contraction, a rise of 0.03°C to 0.2°C was seen, resulting in a cumulative increase of the core body temperature up to 2°C over 5 hours. This increase correlated well to the changes in oxygen consumption and acid metabolite production with uterine activity that the study authors had learned about from a prior study [7]. In that prior study, uterine contractions were associated with an increase in oxygen consumption as well as lactate and pyruvate, with every contraction, reaching a peak at the time of delivery. The maximum lactate values were seen in nulliparous women who experienced longer labors.

Heat production in the laboring patient is countered by heat loss to the environment. The temperature of the ambient air in which women labor is lower than their core body temperature by approximately 25°F. Women in labor also receive large amounts of intravenous fluid, which infuses at room temperature, further decreasing core body temperature. Another mechanism by which heat loss occurs is through ventilation. The tremendous surface area of the alveoli allows significant dissipation of heat to the environment. Labor pain often leads to hyperventilation, magnifying this effect. These processes all serve to dissipate heat and typically counterbalance the effect of heat production in labor.

Epidural analgesia and noninfectious fever

Epidural anesthesia can effect thermoregulation through multiple mechanisms that, depending on the circumstances, can result in an increase in core temperature. Sympathectomy results in a redistribution of blood flow from the core to the periphery, initially leading to heat loss and a decrease in temperature. This effect is typically counterbalanced by intense shivering, resulting in heat production and negating the effect of redistribution of blood flow to the periphery [17]. In addition, sympathectomy can limit or even eliminate sweating, further contributing to heat retention. Furthermore, effective pain relief in labor can also decrease the hyperventilation often experienced by laboring women, and can interfere with the ability to dissipate heat [18]. These processes in the setting of labor, a thermogenic event, can lead to a rise in temperature.

As noted previously, in 1989 Fusi and colleagues [1] were the first to report that labor epidural analgesia is associated with hyperthermia. These investigators had previously observed that women in labor for longer than 12 hours often become febrile independent of infection. They also found that these women were likely to have received epidural analgesia. They hypothesized that the fever was due to epidural analgesia interfering with the ability to dissipate heat. To test their hypothesis, they designed a prospective study of pyrexia in labor in women using either epidural or pethidine for analgesia, using vaginal temperature probes. Thirty-three patients were studied and included in the final analysis. Fig. 1 shows the mean vaginal temperature in the two groups of patients during labor. Epidural placement occurred at 4.2 hours from the start of labor, and those women who received a labor epidural had an increase in temperature starting within 1 hour of epidural administration. The temperature steadily increased to about 1.0°C over the course of labor, and no women experienced an increase over 38°C. Fusi and his coworkers concluded that epidural analgesia is associated with elevations in maternal temperature, likely due to an interference with the ability to dissipate heat during labor.

The Fusi study measured vaginal temperature, which can be affected by sympathectomy and vasodilation in the vaginal mucosa and may not be an accurate reflection of the overall core temperature. Tympanic temperature, however, provides a measure of core temperature that is independent of these effects, and may provide a more accurate assessment of epidural effect. Camann and colleagues [2] prospectively studied fever during labor in 53 women in active labor who received parenteral opioid (nalbuphine) or epidural using tympanic membrane temperature. They found a temperature increase in women who received an epidural when compared with intravenous opioid. Two epidural techniques were studied, one using bupivacaine only and one with both bupiva-

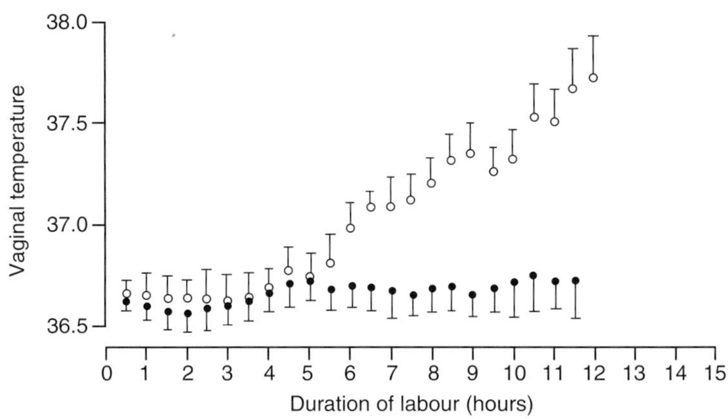

Fig. 1. Mean vaginal temperature (°C) in the two groups of patients during labor. (*From* Fusi L, Steer PJ, Maresh MJ, et al. Maternal pyrexia associated with the use of epidural analgesia in labour. Lancet 1989;Jun 3;1(8649):1250–2; with permission.)

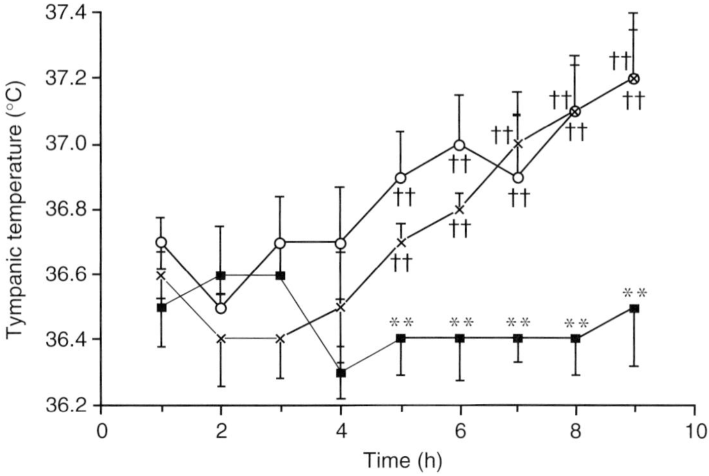

Fig. 2. Mean tympanic temperatures during labor in the extradural-BF (○), extradural-B (×), and opioid (■) groups. (*From* Camann WR, Hortvet LA, Hughes N, et al. Maternal temperature regulation during extradural analgesia for labour. Br J Anaesth 1991;67:565–8; with permission).

caine and fentanyl. As shown in Fig. 2, an increase in maternal temperature occurred in women using epidural analgesia, beginning at 4 hours and progressively rising from there, regardless of the technique used. Similar to the findings reported by Fusi and coworkers [1], the rise did not exceed 1°C or 38°C. This rise in temperature was not associated with evidence of infection. Because of the small increase in temperature seen, Camann and colleagues [2] felt that it was not associated with an adverse intrauterine environment or subsequent fetal compromise.

Ploeckinger and coworkers [4] reported on a much larger group of patients in 1995, and showed similar results to the above. They retrospectively analyzed 7317 women who delivered at the University Hospital in Vienna, Austria. The 1056 women who received an epidural were more likely to have a fever higher than 38°C compared with those who did not (1.6% versus 0.2%). Importantly, the epidural group had several other risk factors for fever, including an increased incidence of labors resulting in operative delivery (suggesting the presence of labor dystocia) and a greater number of nulliparous patients. The question this study and others like it raise is whether the epidural itself or patient characteristics associated with epidural analgesia itself are responsible for the increase in fever—a question raised by much of the literature on the subject.

Epidural and infectious fever

The studies by Fusi [1] and Camaan [2] and their coworkers reported a noninfectious effect of epidural on fever. The small temperature elevations seen in these studies were not thought to be associated with adverse effects on the mother or fetus. Later studies, however, have associated epidural with conditions associated with infection, raising concerns about maternal and especially fetal effects. In an effort to determine the effect of epidural on maternal fever and its potential association with infection, Dashe and colleagues [19] studied the placenta. These researchers reasoned that fever in the presence of placental inflammation supports the clinical diagnosis of infection. Conversely, fever without placental inflammation is less likely to be infection-related and more likely an effect of epidural on thermoregulation. To that end, they examined 149 placentas from term, singleton gestations that had a minimum of 6 hours of membrane rupture. They found that maternal fever was more common with epidural analgesia (46% versus 26%), as was fever with placental inflammation (35% versus 17%). As shown in Table 1, fever was uncommonly seen in women who did not have placental inflammation (11% in women who had epidural, 9% in women who did not have epidural). This finding led the study authors to conclude that epidural is associated with intrapartum fever, but only in the presence of placental inflammation; thus the fever associated with epidural analgesia is due to infection and not analgesia.

It seems unlikely that epidural analgesia is directly responsible for infection; however, epidural may be indirectly related through its association with prolonged labor. The randomized controlled trial of epidural analgesia versus intravenous narcotic analgesia reported by Sharma and coworkers [9] showed that epidural was associated with an approximately 1-hour increase in labor and an increase in the diagnosis of chorioamnionitis. It is reasonable to assume that the increase in the diagnosis of chorioamnionitis in the epidural group is related to the length of labor, an epidural effect. This study and others like it support the concept that the effect of epidural on maternal temperature may be more indirect than initially supposed. Philip and colleagues [5] published a study in 1999 examining the effect of epidural, parity, and length of labor on fever. Their study was a secondary analysis of a previously randomized trial of epidural and meperidine analgesia. The analysis included 715 women, 68 of whom had fever during labor. As shown in Fig. 3, 47 (69%) of the women who had fever were nulliparous. Of these, the majority had labors of 12 hours or more. Women who

Table 1
Markers of potential intrapartum infection

Marker	Epidural (%) (n = 80)	No epidural (%) (n = 69)	*P*
Placental inflammation[a]	49 (61)	25 (36)	.002
Maternal fever[b]	37 (46)	18 (26)	.01
Fever with placental inflammation	28 (35)	12 (17)	.02
Fever without placental inflammation	9 (11)	6 (9)	.61

Data are presented as n (%).

[a] Placental inflammation $\geq$grade 2 inflammation of the chorionic plate.

[b] Maternal fever $\geq$38°C in labor or within 6 hours of delivery.

Data from Dashe JS, Rogers BB, McIntire DD, et al. Epidural analgesia and intrapartum fever: placental findings. Obstet Gynecol 1999;93:341–4.

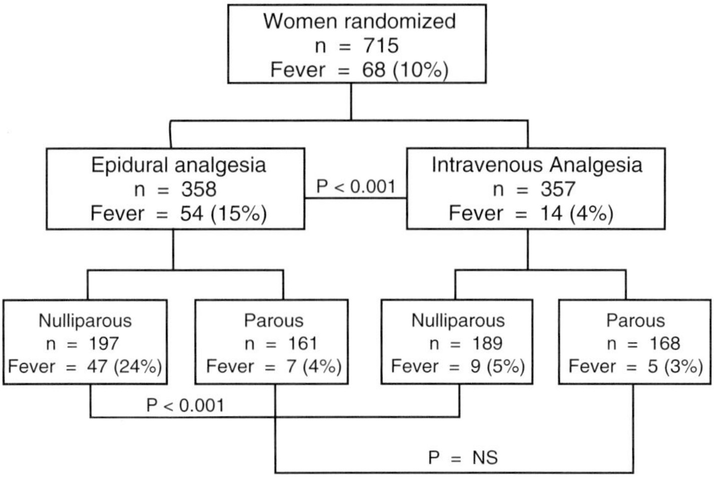

Fig. 3. Maternal fever in relation to type of analgesia and parity. (*From* Philip J, Alexander JM, Sharma SK, et al. Epidural analgesia during labor and maternal fever. Anesthesiology 1999;90:1273; with permission.)

had shorter labors (<6 hours) had a very low incidence of fever (4%) as did multiparous women. Multivariate analysis showed that nulliparity, epidural analgesia, and prolonged labor were all independently associated with fever. Importantly, the study authors found that epidural analgesia-associated fever was only associated with the subset of nulliparous women who had labors that extended beyond 6 hours. This subset of women represented 7% of the cohort; thus the majority of women who were not at risk for fever.

Neonatal effects of epidural-related fever in labor

Shortly after reports of fever in labor appeared associating epidural analgesia with fever, concern about neonatal effects rose. Morishima and coworkers [20] reported that maternal hyperthermia was associated with fetal acidosis and hypoxia. In their study, 23 near-term pregnant baboons were subjected to hyperthermia, with a maternal temperature elevation to between 41°C and 42°C. Serial arterial blood samples were drawn from the fetus with pO_2 and pH determination. A progressive deterioration was seen in both the fetal pH and oxygenation that corresponded well to the increase in maternal temperature. The importance of this experiment is the finding of an adverse effect of fever in and of itself on the fetus that was independent of infection.

Macaulay and colleagues [21] assessed the effect of epidural or fetal temperature in labor using an intrauterine probe that directly assessed fetal skin temperature. The study reported findings on 57 patients who were in active labor with ruptured membranes. Of the 33 women who received an epidural, 10 of their fetuses had a temperature higher than 38°C, compared with none of the 24 fetuses of the women who did not receive an epidural in labor. None of the women had a diagnosis of chorioamnionitis. The increased fetal temperatures were not associated with a low Apgar score or cord pH. Despite the inability to demonstrate a direct effect on the fetus, these findings are cause for concern when one considers the ramifications of elevated fetal temperatures reported by Morishima and colleagues [20].

Two studies in the late 1990s [3,22] suggested that epidural fever may indirectly place the neonate at risk for adverse outcome. Mayer and coworkers [22] studied 300 nulliparous women who had uncomplicated pregnancies and who received three different types of analgesia in labor: epidural, narcotic, or both. They found a 6% incidence of antibiotic use in the opioid group, compared with a 16% TO 22% incidence of use in the epidural group. Only 10 patients had culture or pathology proven chorioamnionitis; all 10 had other signs of infection. These authors suggest that large numbers of women are exposed to antibiotics unnecessarily, based on elevated temperatures alone. Furthermore, they point out that the downstream risk of this practice is to overexpose neonates to antibiotic therapy for presumed sepsis. The authors concluded that limiting antibiotic therapy to those women who have fever and additional risk factors for infection would decrease antibiotic use in mothers and neonates by 50% without under-treatment of chorioamnionitis.

This study [22] points out the difficulty the clinician has in establishing the cause of temperature elevation in labor. Traditional signs of infection are unreliable in the laboring woman. White blood cell (WBC) counts are often elevated well above normal in labor and are unreliable. Cultures of the endometrial cavity are difficult to collect without contamination by vaginal flora. Furthermore, the culture results are not available for several days, long after labor is complete and treatment has been initiated. Uterine tenderness, a physical sign commonly associated with infection, is difficult to interpret in laboring patients [23]. For all these reasons, the diagnosis of chorioamnionitis in labor is problematic, and often fever is the only sign of infection.

In 1997, Lieberman and colleagues [3] documented an increase in neonatal sepsis workups in infants born to mothers who received a labor epidural. Their study was a secondary analysis of a previously published trial of the active management of labor [24], a randomized trial conducted at Brigham and Women's hospital from 1990 to 1994 to examine the effect of an active management of labor program on cesarean rates. In their analysis [3], women who received epidural were compared with those who did not. Although the management of labor technique (traditional versus an active management of labor protocol) was randomized in the primary trial, analgesia was not. As one might expect, characteristics of those women who received epidural were significantly different that those who did not. They had larger babies, were more likely to undergo induction of labor, were less likely to undergo treatment with the active management of labor, and most importantly, had longer labors (12.1 hours versus 6.3 hours). Women receiving epidural more commonly experienced intrapartum fever higher than 100.4°F (14.5% versus 1%, $P < .001$). The incidence of fever in the epidural group was related to the length of labor, with more than 30% of women receiving epidural having fever at more than 18 hours. The incidence of fever in the no epidural group was low (1%) regardless of the length of labor; however, only 8% of this group had a labor that was longer than 12 hours, making direct comparison to the epidural group difficult. This study [3] also reported a significant association between epidural and neonatal sepsis evaluations. Neonates born to mothers who received an epidural were more likely to undergo sepsis evaluation (34% versus 9.8%) and antibiotic therapy (15.4% versus 3.8%). These differences persisted after multiple regression analysis; however, the analysis did not adjust for the length of labor, probably the most significant difference in the two groups. The most intriguing data presented in this study were those supporting the finding that neonatal sepsis workups in those women who received epidural were elevated even in those women who did not have fever (25% versus 9%).

The Lieberman and coworkers study [3] created significant discussion and controversy. Although the association between fever and epidural had been previously reported, and it stood to reason that this could result in neonates being exposed to sepsis workups, the direct association between epidural and neonatal sepsis workups in the absence of fever was a novel observation. The lay press took great interest in this finding, and headlines such as "When labor pain drugs cause fevers, babies face tests" and "Epidurals lead to more infant tests" appeared in publications and on television. Critics pointed to several problems with the study design. It has been established in randomized controlled trials that epidural prolongs labor, which in turn increases the risk for chorioamnionitis [9]. It has also been shown that women who request epidural (as in the Lieberman study) are at risk for labor dystocia [14,25]. Critics suggest that Lieberman's retrospective study design did not account for these confounders, and mistakenly associated epidural with neonatal sepsis when in fact other factors were more important. Critics also point out that although neonatal sepsis workups were increased in the epidural group, confirmed cases of sepsis were rare and not related to labor analgesia. In addition, the criteria for neonatal sepsis workups were not described, and it is not clear how this effected the overall findings, especially in those women whose infants received a workup in the absence of fever. In the end, the study by Lieberman and colleagues [3] has raised serious concerns about the indirect effect of epidural analgesia on neonates, and has led to more questions than answers.

Summary

The association between labor epidural and maternal fever has become well-established. The effects of epidural on maternal temperature are both direct and indirect. The direct effect of epidural on maternal temperature appears due to its interference with heat dissipation and rarely seems to result in overt fever. The data suggest that this effect is unlikely to adversely affect the fetus. More commonly, the effect of labor epidural on temperature is indirect and associated with conditions such as labor dystocia that place a woman at risk for infection. As shown by Lieberman and coworkers [3], this may translate into unnecessary interventions in the neonate, including antibiotic exposure and prolonged hospitalization, but does not appear to place the neonate at risk for overt sepsis.

At this juncture, it seems unreasonable to avoid labor epidurals due to the risk of fever. The majority of women in labor do not appear to be at risk, and the full ramification of the fever is not yet well understood. Furthermore, steps can be taken to modify the effect of epidural on unnecessary interventions such as neonatal sepsis evaluation [13]. It has been suggested that pediatricians and neonatologists develop guidelines that limit neonatal sepsis evaluations to infants who are at increased risk for infection. Likewise, efforts should be made to further refine the diagnosis of chorioamnionitis, and further research along these lines is warranted. Until then, epidural analgesia remains one of the most effective forms of pain relief in labor, and remains a reasonable option for most women.

References

[1] Fusi L, Steer PJ, Maresh MJA, et al. Maternal pyrexia associated with the use of epidural analgesia in labour. Lancet 1989;1:1250–2.

[2] Camann WR, Hortvet LA, Hughes N, et al. Maternal temperature regulation during extradural analgesia for labour. Br J Anaesth 1991;67:565–8.

[3] Lieberman E, Lang JM, Frigoletto F, et al. Epidural analgesia, intrapartum fever, and neonatal sepsis evaluation. Pediatrics 1997;99:415–9.

[4] Ploeckinger B, Ulm MR, Chalubinski K, et al. Epidural anaesthesia in labour: influence on surgical delivery rates, intrapartum fever and blood loss. Gynecol Obstet Invest 1995;39:24–7.

[5] Philip J, Alexander JM, Sharma SK, et al. Epidural analgesia during labor and maternal fever. Anesthesiology 1999;90:1271–5.

[6] Herbst A, Wolner-Hanssen P, Ingemarsson I. Risk factors for fever in labor. Obstet Gynecol 1995;86:790–4.

[7] Yancey MK, Zhang J, Shcwarz J, et al. Labor epidural analgesia and intrapartum maternal hyperthermia. Obstet Gynecol 2001;98:763–70.

[8] Vinson DC, Thomas R, Kiser T. Association between epidural analgesia during labor and fever. J Fam Pract 1993;36:617–22.

[9] Sharma SK, Alexander JM, Messick G, et al. Cesarean delivery. A randomized trial of epidural analgesia versus intravenous meperidine analgesia during labor in nulliparous women. Anesthesiology 2002;96:546–51.

[10] Ramin SM, Gambling DR, Lucas MJ, et al. Randomized trial of epidural versus intravenous analgesia during labor. Obstet Gynecol 1995;86:783–9.

[11] Thorp JA, Eckert LO, Ang MS, et al. Epidural analgesia and cesarean section for dystocia: risk factors in nulliparas. Am J Perinatol 1991;8(6):402–10.

[12] Pleasure JR, Stahl GE. Epidural analgesia and neonatal fever [letter]. Pediatrics 1998;101(3): 490–4.

[13] Chestnut DE. Fever and infection. In: Obstetric anesthesia: principles and practice. 2nd edition. St. Louis (MO): Mosby Inc.; 1999. p. 711–24.

[14] Braunwald E, Fauci AS, Kasper DL, et al. Harrison's principles of internal medicine. 15th edition. New York: McGraw-Hill Companies; 2001.

[15] Goodlin RC, Chapin JW. Determinants of maternal temperature during labor. Am J Obstet Gynecol 1982;143:97–103.

[16] Marx GF, Loew DAY. Tympanic temperature during labour and parturition. Br J Anaesth 1975;47:600–2.

[17] Hynson JM, Sessler DI, Glosten B, et al. Thermal balance and tremor patterns during epidural analgesia. Anesthesiology 1991;74:680–90.

[18] Marx GF, Green NM. Maternal lactate, pyruvate, and excess lactate production during labor and delivery. Am J Obstet Gynecol 1964;90:786–93.

[19] Dashe JS, Rogers BB, McIntire DD, et al. Epidural analgesia and intrapartum fever: placental findings. Obstet Gynecol 1999;93:341–4.

[20] Morishima HO, Glaser B, Niemann WH, et al. Increased uterine activity and fetal deterioration during maternal hyperthermia. Am J Obstet Gynecol 1975;121(4):531–8.

[21] Macaulay JH, Bond K, Steer PJ. Epidural analgesia in labor and fetal hyperthermia. Obstet Gynecol 1992;80:665–9.

[22] Mayer DC, Chescheir NC, Spielman FJ. Increased intrapartum antibiotic administration associated with epidural analgesia in labor. Am J Perinatol 1997;14(2):83–6.

[23] Cunningham FG, Gant NF, Leveno KJ, et al. Williams obstetrics. 21st edition. New York: McGraw-Hill Companies; 2001.

[24] Frigoletto Jr FD, Lieberman E, Lang JM, et al. A clinical trial of active management of labor. N Engl J Med 1995;333:745–50.

[25] Alexander JM, Sharma SK, McIntire DD, et al. Intensity of labor pain and cesarean delivery. Anesth Analg 2001;92:1524–8.

ELSEVIER
SAUNDERS

Clin Perinatol 32 (2005) 789–802

CLINICS IN
PERINATOLOGY

The Use of Radiographic Modalities to Diagnose Infection in Pregnancy

Jason A. Pates, MD[a,*], Diane M. Twickler, MD[a,b]

[a]*Department of Obstetrics & Gynecology, University of Texas Southwestern Medical Center at Dallas, 5323 Harry Hines Boulevard, Dallas, TX 75390-9032, USA*
[b]*Department of Radiology, University of Texas Southwestern Medical Center at Dallas, 5323 Harry Hines Boulevard, Dallas, TX 75390-8896, USA*

Several radiographic modalities are available to the obstetrician to assist in the diagnosis of infection during pregnancy. Typically, these imaging techniques are used when the diagnosis is not evident from history, physical examination, and laboratory data. Radiological studies often are helpful to discriminate between differential diagnoses and guide therapy. Most diagnostic radiological procedures are associated with little, if any, known significant fetal risks [1].

The use of diagnostic imaging provokes anxiety among physicians and patients. To counter these concerns, several centers institute procedures to optimize maternal and fetal well-being while minimizing the number of unnecessary tests that is ordered. One center recently published details of such a system which includes technician education, dose specifications for gravid patients, imaging algorithms for different disease processes, shielding instructions, and detailed consent forms [2]. Our institution requires formal obstetric and general surgical consults before imaging that requires ionizing radiation in pregnancy. System-wide protocols for evaluating pregnant women with imaging resources minimize confusion and streamline care to achieve timely, accurate diagnoses.

* Corresponding author.
E-mail address: jason.pates@utsouthwestern.edu (J.A. Pates).

doi:10.1016/j.clp.2005.05.004 ***perinatology.theclinics.com***

Imaging modalities

Ultrasound, MRI, nuclear imaging, and ionizing radiation may be used effectively for the diagnosis and treatment of infection in pregnancy. Each organ system may be studied optimally with one or multiple imaging techniques but clinicians must be knowledgeable regarding a particular study's risks and the information it provides.

Ionizing radiation

Ionizing radiation can result in the following harmful effects: cell death and teratogenic effects, carcinogenesis, and genetic effects or mutations in germ cells [1]. There is little or no information to estimate the frequency or magnitude of adverse genetic effects on future generations [1]. The conventional unit that is used most often in pregnancy is the Gray (Gy) or centiGray (cGy). The recommended maximum threshold for cumulative dose for an entire gestation is approximately 5 cGy [1]. Radiation exposure occurs most commonly with plain film, CT, fluoroscopy, angiography, and nuclear medicine. Table 1 shows the fetal exposure for common studies that are used in pregnancy [1].

A plain film generally exposes the fetus to small amounts of radiation [1]. Radiation exposure from CT varies, depending on the number and spacing of adjacent image sections [1]. Spiral CT is a recent advance that allows for exposure that is similar or less than previous estimates of conventional CT [3]. Fetal exposure with this method is highly dependent on the pitch—the degree of stretching or tightening of the spiral [3].

Dosimetry calculations for fluoroscopy and angiography prove difficult because of variations in the number of films obtained, fluoroscopy time, and the length of fetal exposure to the radiation field [3]. Commonly performed fluoroscopy studies related to infection in pregnancy include intravenous pyelography (IVP) and endoscopic retrograde cholangiopancreatography. Many

Table 1
Estimated fetal exposure of common studies

Procedure	Fetal exposure
Chest radiograph (2 views)	.00002 cGy
Abdominal film	0.2 cGy
Intravenous pyelography	0.1 cGy or greater
Hip film (single view)	0.2 cGy
Mammography	.0007 to .002 cGy
Barium enema or small bowel series	2–4 cGy
CT scan of head or chest	>1 cGy
CT scan of abdomen or lumbar spine	3.5 cGy
CT pelvimetry	0.25 cGy

Adapted from American College of Obstetricians and Gynecologists. Committee Opinion. No. 299, September 2004. Guidelines for diagnostic imaging during pregnancy. Obstet Gynecol 2004;104: 647–51.

institutions decrease fetal exposure during fluoroscopy by limiting the number of views obtained. An example of these modifications is the limited or "single shot" IVP for the gravida who has pyelonephritis.

Ultrasonography

Ultrasonography involves the use of sound waves and is not a form of ionizing radiation [1]. There have been no reports of documented adverse maternal or fetal effects related to diagnostic ultrasound procedures [1]. With regards to infection in pregnancy, sonography is useful in the diagnosis of endocarditis, pyelonephritis, and some abdominal/pelvic abscesses.

MRI

MRI is capable of providing large field-of-view images of maternal abnormalities in any plane [4]. Images that are obtained with MRI do not expose the mother or fetus to ionizing radiation and often are diagnostic without the use of intravenous contrast [4]. Thus far, there are no reported harmful human effects from the use of MRI, including mutagenic effects [3]. Theoretic concerns include the effect of tissue heating on the fetus with certain magnetic resonance techniques and the unknown effect of gadolinium agents on fetal well-being [4]. Fetal compromise has never been documented with regard to either of these aspects of MRI.

MRI in the setting of pregnancy presents several unique challenges. Motion artifact is generated from maternal peristalsis and breathing as well as fetal movement [4]. Also, the patient's ability to suspend respiration for extended periods of times is limited in the third trimester [4]. To reduce maternal fatigue and discomfort, the left lateral decubitus position should be used and imaging times kept as brief as possible [4].

Contrast agents

A variety of oral and intravascular contrast agents are used with ionizing radiation and magnetic imaging procedures [1]. Iodinated contrast agents are used commonly with CT. These compounds contain iodine bound to a benzene ring [5]. The potential risk of iodine to the mother or fetus is negligible because the iodine remains bound to the benzene ring, and free iodine is not available for uptake [5]. Gadolinium agents used for MRI cross the placenta and may enter the fetal circulation [4]. The effects of gadolinium-based agents on fetal well-being are not understood fully; therefore, these compounds should be used only when compelling clinical indications exist [4].

Nuclear medicine

Nuclear medicine plays a limited role in the diagnosis of infection. Gallium has been used to evaluate for infection but more discriminating imaging, such as CT and MRI, are preferred in the setting of pregnancy. Nuclear medicine studies are not discussed in this article.

Central nervous system infections

Central nervous system infections in pregnancy are extremely rare. For example, epidural abscess complicating obstetric epidural analgesia occurs in only 1 to 2 cases per 10,000 admissions at major hospitals [6]. Prompt diagnosis is essential because reported mortality rates are nearly 25% [7]. MRI is the most common imaging technique that is used to diagnose spinal epidural abscesses, with a sensitivity approaching 100% [8]. MRI with gadolinium enhance-

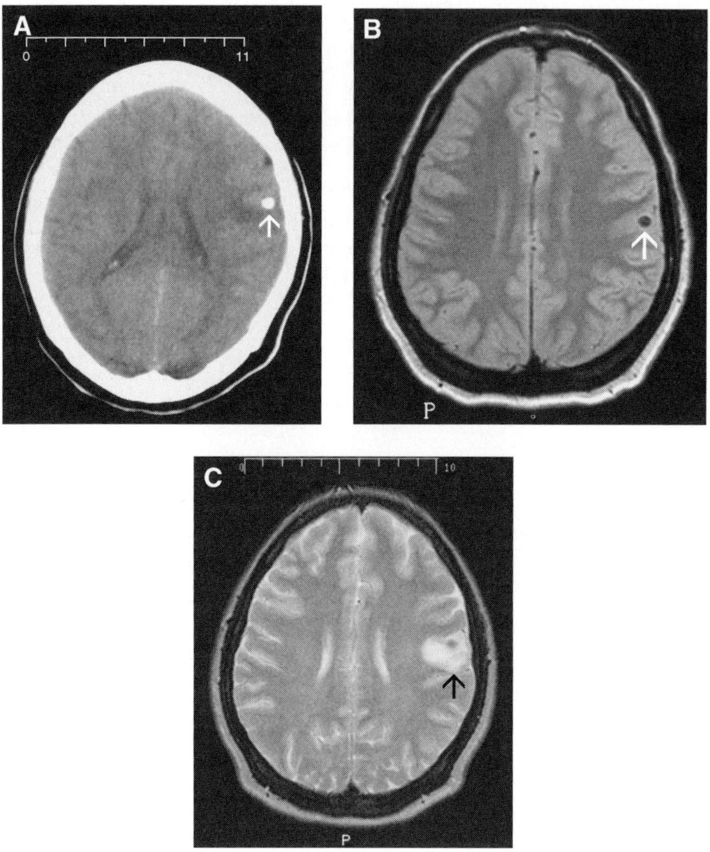

Fig. 1. Imaging of neurocysticercosis in a pregnant patient. (*A*) CT showing a small, rounded density in the brain (*arrow*). (*B*) T1-weighted MRI image displaying the same cystic-appearing lesion (*arrow*). (*C*) T2-weighted image highlights the lesion and surrounding edema (*arrow*).

ment surpasses CT myelography as the superior imaging technique with this condition because it better distinguishes hematoma, disc herniation, or tumors from purulent collections [6]. One 10-year retrospective study found equal sensitivity with CT-myelography and MRI in diagnosing epidural abscess but emphasized that a spinal tap was not required with the latter [6].

Few reports of brain abscesses or other intracranial infections affecting pregnancy exist in recent medical literature. These lesions usually result from complicated sinusitis, otitis media, meningitis, or systemic infections from a variety of microorganisms. MRI is the procedure of choice in evaluating suspected intracranial infections, primarily because of its inherent contrast resolution and multiplanar capability [9]. Brain lesions typically appear as rim-enhancing lesions with mass effect on MRI (Fig. 1) [10].

In summary, MRI is the optimal modality for diagnosis if physicians suspect CNS infection in pregnancy. Alternatively, patients who have extreme pain or who are unable to cooperate potentially should undergo CT scan because of motion artifact concerns [10].

Infections of the chest and thorax

Pneumonia complicates 0.04% to 1.0% of all pregnancies and represents a significant concern for the pregnant woman [11]. Clinicians rely upon plain chest film initially when evaluating pulmonary disease secondary to its wide availability and extremely low fetal exposure (Fig. 2). The absorbed radiation dose for the uterus and fetus is 100 times less than the estimated maternal dose

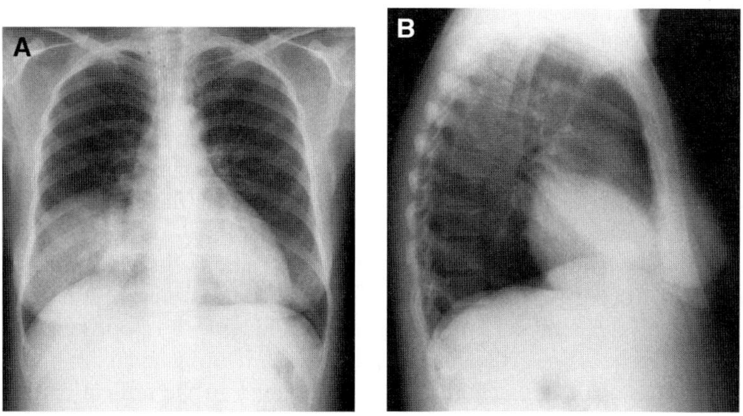

Fig. 2. Pneumococcal pneumonia in pregnancy. (*A*) Posteroanterior chest radiograph showing the right middle lobe infiltrate. (*B*) Lateral view in the same patient.

[12]. For complicated chest infections, such as empyema, CT serves as an excellent second-line study; however, few reports of pulmonary empyema complicating pregnancy exist in the current English medical literature. Obstetricians primarily should order posteroanterior and lateral chest radiographs for suspected pneumonia and reserve CT for more complicated infections.

The incidence of infective endocarditis during pregnancy has been reported to be 0.006% [13]. The maternal and fetal mortality rates can reach 33% and 29%, respectively [13]. Because endocarditis presents with protean manifestations, physicians usually establish the diagnosis with radiographic techniques. Chest plain films may show evidence of heart failure (enlarged cardiac silhouette, pulmonary venous congestion) or lung consolidation; however, M-mode and two-dimensional echocardiography endures as the study of choice in diagnosing infective endocarditis [14]. A transthoracic approach may show regurgitant flow, wall motion abnormalities, thrombi, or vegetations as small as 2 mm [14]. With inconclusive data on transthoracic echo, the more invasive transesophageal approach may elucidate the hallmark findings.

Acute viral pericarditis is the most frequent pericardial disease in pregnancy [15]. Echocardiographic findings include pericardial effusion and chamber enlargement [15]. Rarely, other infectious pericardial disease in pregnancy may result from tuberculosis, HIV, or other disseminated infections; two-dimensional echocardiography is the mainstay of diagnosis.

Hepatobiliary infections

Acute viral hepatitis is the most common cause of jaundice during pregnancy [16]. Reports on the imaging appearance of hepatic disorders in pregnancy are sparse [17]. Radiologists normally recommend ultrasound first when evaluating possible liver infection in pregnancy.

Sonography can distinguish between cystic and solid lesions, and distinguish a single mass from one with multiple satellite lesions [18]; however, even color-flow Doppler sonography cannot distinguish between solid liver masses and early abscess reliably [19]. MRI plays an important role in differentiating hepatic masses, and its safety in pregnancy makes it the better alternative study compared with CT [18]. If MRI is unavailable, CT has the ability to delineate potential liver infection.

Acute cholecystitis is the second most common surgical condition in pregnancy, and occurs in 1 in 1600 to 1 in 10,000 pregnancies [20]. This diagnosis carries a high incidence of maternal morbidity and a poor perinatal outcome [21]. Obstructive gallstones are the usual inciting agent in the gravid patient, whereas acalculous cholecystitis is common in the critical care setting. Clinicians should rely upon sonography as the initial, noninvasive modality if cholecystitis is suspected (Fig. 3). Ultrasound has a 95% sensitivity for detecting gallstones and also may show gallbladder wall thickening, pericholecys-

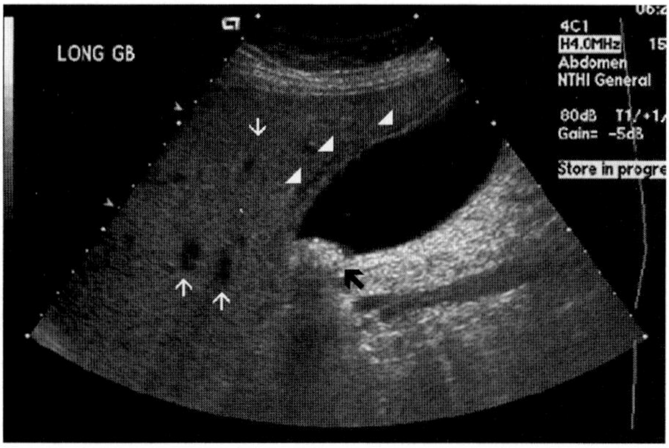

Fig. 3. Sonography in a gravid patient with cholecystitis showing a gallstone (*black arrow*), thickened gall bladder wall (*arrowheads*), and areas of biliary dilatation (*white arrows*).

tic fluid, bile duct dilatation, and sonographic Murphy's sign [21,22]. CT has been reported to be useful in the diagnosis of calculus cholecystitis but scanning an acutely ill patient may be difficult and the added time and expense rarely are justified [23].

Recent case series in the medical literature have demonstrated the effective use of radiological resources in the treatment of cholecystitis. Ultrasound-guided percutaneous cholecystotomy has been reported to be an effective means of treating cholecystitis in pregnancy with optimal maternal and fetal outcomes [24]. Endoscopic retrograde cholangiopancreatography procedure without fluoroscopic examination for pregnant patients was described in two recent case series with excellent outcomes [25,26].

Appendicitis

Appendicitis is the most common acute abdominal condition that requires surgery during pregnancy [27]. In recent years, the maternal mortality rate associated with appendicitis has declined to approximately 0.5% [27]. More concerning, the fetal loss rate has been reported as high as 4.8% with ruptured appendicitis [28]. Graded-compression sonography has been of value in the diagnosis of acute appendicitis in pregnancy [29]. One study that included 42 patients who had confirmed appendicitis reported a sensitivity and specificity of 100% and 96%, respectively [29]. Several studies have noted difficulty with sonography in diagnosing appendicitis, especially in the late second and third trimesters. Sonography is highly operator-dependent and the presence of bowel gas or obesity can impair image interrogation [30]. In addition, the large size of the gravid uterus and upward displacement of the abdominal contents does not allow adequate compression [29,30].

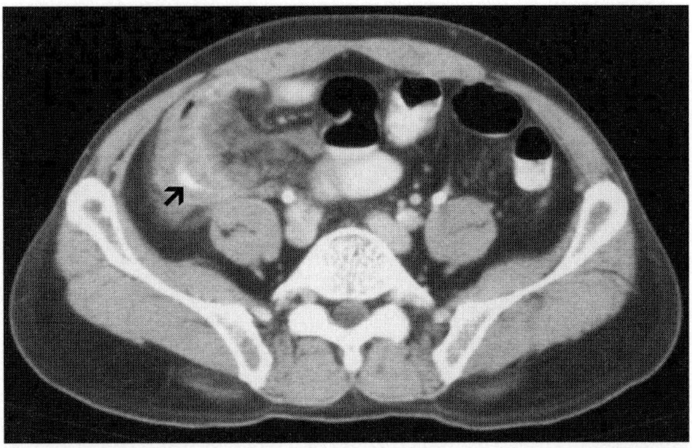

Fig. 4. CT displaying contrast in the appendix, a thickened wall (*arrow*), and periappendiceal inflammation of acute appendicitis in this woman whose pregnancy was in the first trimester.

Helical CT is highly sensitive and specific for the diagnosis of acute appendicitis in the nonobstetric population with sensitivity, specificity, and diagnostic accuracy of 98% each [31]. Although ionizing radiation and contrast medium are required, CT is able to overcome many of the shortcomings of ultrasound. Moreover, standard examination times are minimal and CT is widely available (Fig. 4).

MRI was investigated recently as an alternative to CT in diagnosing acute appendicitis. In a small study with 12 patients, MRI seemed to be a valuable and safe technique for the evaluation of pregnant patients who were suspected clinically of having acute appendicitis [30]. The ability of MRI to visualize the appendix in the third trimester was encouraging [30]. Because of the lack of experience with MRI in appendicitis, CT probably should be the second-line imaging modality ordered if doctors suspect the diagnosis.

Acute pancreatitis

The incidence of acute pancreatitis in pregnancy is approximately 1 in 2000 to 3000 pregnancies [20,32]. Rapid diagnosis is essential because the associated maternal and fetal morbidity and mortality rates are high, particularly with necrotizing pancreatitis. Most cases of pancreatitis in pregnant women are associated with choledocholithiasis [32]. Most radiologists depend upon sonography as a first-line test with pancreatitis in pregnancy. Besides the findings associated with obstructive stones, one may see ascites or diffuse pancreatic enlargement on sonography [33].

After sonography, CT with intravenous contrast medium injection is accepted as the imaging procedure of choice: to document the extent of pancreatic and extrapancreatic acute fluid collections and to detect pancreatic necrosis [34].

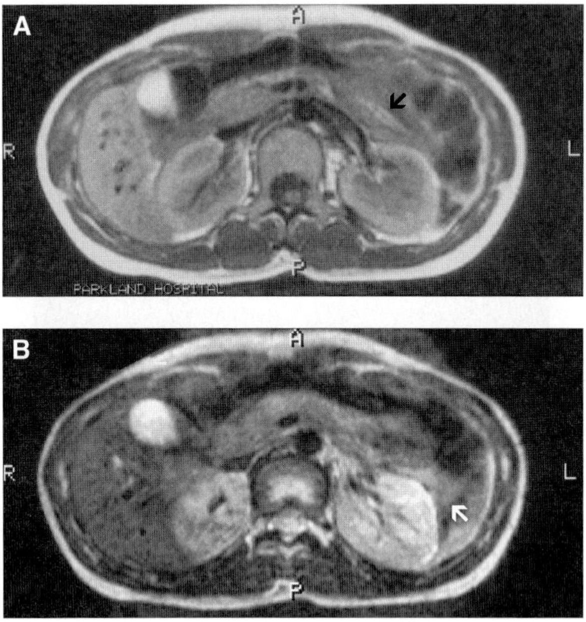

Fig. 5. MRI of pancreatitis in a pregnant patient. (*A*) Fluid in the dilated distal pancreatic duct (*arrow*). (*B*) inflammation of the tail (*arrow*).

For the pregnant woman, MRI has emerged as an alternative imaging technique for the diagnosis and management of complicated pancreatitis (Fig. 5). A recent study showed that MRI detected severe acute pancreatitis with 83% sensitivity and 91% specificity versus 78% and 86%, respectively, for CT [34]. Pregnant patients probably should undergo MRI instead of CT to evaluate severe, necrotizing pancreatitis, especially if multiple studies are required.

Abdominal and pelvic abscess

Cases of pelvic or abdominal abscesses complicating pregnancy are rare. Although etiologies of this unusual complication of pregnancy include nongynecologic conditions, such as ruptured diverticulitis or appendicitis, tuboovarian abscesses of unknown origin also have been reported [35]. Pelvic abscesses in the postpartum period are more common and usually are associated with complicated endometritis or wound infections (Fig. 6) [3]. Enhanced imaging modalities, including ultrasonography, CT, and MRI, have increased the likelihood of earlier diagnosis [35].

Because pelvic abscesses occur infrequently in pregnancy, the optimal imaging algorithms have not been studied well. Some reports describe ultrasound

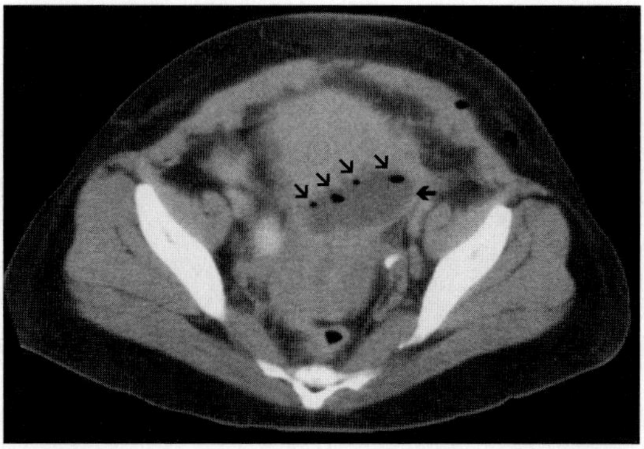

Fig. 6. Pelvic computed tomography of post partum endometritis showing dehiscence of the uterus with air in the uterine incision site (*small arrows*) and a large bladder flap abscess (*large arrow*).

followed by MRI as the best method to localize these fluid collections in pregnant patients [36]. Percutaneous imaging-guided (ultrasound or CT) transcatheter drainage of these abscesses has avoided exploratory laparotomy and surgical drainage in some patients [35]. The use of these drainage procedures in pregnant patients is sparse in current medical literature but good outcomes have been described [35]. Clinicians should rely on ultrasound primarily to be followed by MRI or CT to diagnose and treat abdominal/pelvic abscesses in pregnancy.

Urinary tract infections

Urinary tract infection is one of the most frequently seen medical complications in pregnancy [37]. Of these infections, acute pyelonephritis carries a high perinatal morbidity if left unchecked, is one of the most common indications for antepartum hospitalization, and complicates 1% to 2% of all pregnancies [38]. If clinicians suspect pyelonephritis, ultrasound should be ordered first and may demonstrate hydronephrosis, hydroureter, perinephric fluid collections, or urinary calculi (Fig. 7) [39,40]; however, the sensitivity and specificity of abdominal ultrasound in detecting renal stones in one study was approximately 34% and 86%, respectively [40]. If findings are inconclusive or indirect evidence of obstruction is visualized, limited IVP should be performed.

To limit the use of ionizing radiation, one group recommends a three-film IVP, including a scout view, a 30-second film, and a 20-minute film (they found that if the 20-minute film did not reveal a calculus, later films did not provide any additional information) [40]. Using an abdominal shield over the contralateral, unaffected side and obtaining a prone film helps to limit further fetal radiation exposure [40]. Thus, a limited IVP is an excellent second-line imaging modality after ultrasound.

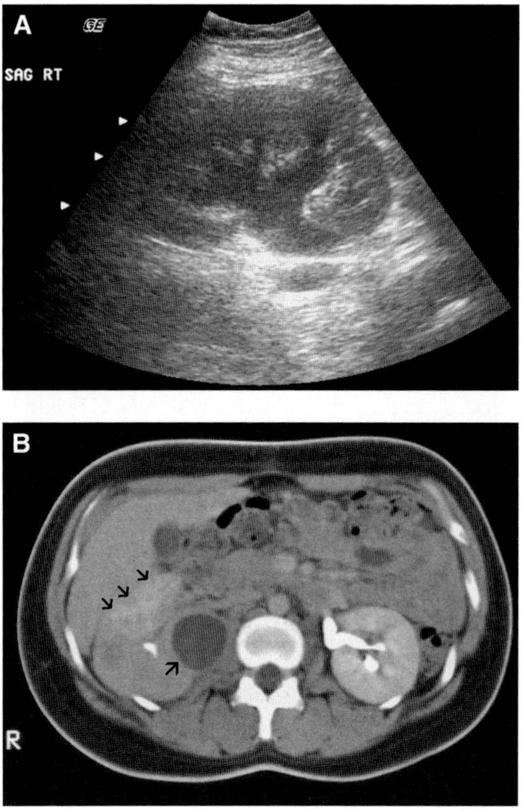

Fig. 7. Imaging of pyelonephritis in pregnancy. (*A*) Renal sonography showing hydronephrosis. (*B*) Computed tomography displaying a large renal abscess (*large arrow*) and areas of inflammation in the right kidney (*small arrows*).

CT may be used to evaluate obstruction in the context of pyelonephritis but it exposes the fetus to more radiation. One report described a low-dose CT technique using only four slices 5 mm apart to guide percutaneous drainage of a perinephric abscess [41]. MRI use in pregnancy for evaluation of pyelonephritis has not been reported and it is known not to visualize calculi well [41]. Ultrasound or CT-guided procedures to treat urinary tract obstruction or abscess in pregnancy are described in the literature with promising results [41].

Musculoskeletal infections

A paucity of literature exists to describe musculoskeletal infections in pregnancy. Psoas abscesses in pregnancy have been reported with MRI as the most effective means to diagnose these infections [42,43]. As in the non-pregnant patient, MRI is the most effective means to evaluate any musculo-skeletal pathology.

Puerperal septic thrombophlebitis

The incidence of septic thrombophlebitis is 1 in 3000 deliveries [44]. Obstetricians often struggle to make this diagnosis clinically; therefore, they rely upon pelvic CT or MRI [3]. One prospective comparison of MRI, CT, and sonography found that MRI and CT were the studies of choice in evaluation of ovarian vein thrombosis (Fig. 8) [45]. Specifically, MRI had 92% sensitivity and 100% specificity for detecting thrombosis, whereas CT had 100% sensitivity and 99% specificity [45]. One case series recently described the use of transvaginal sonography to identify pelvic venous plexus thrombosis in patients early in pregnancy, and concluded that this modality holds promise as a noninvasive diagnostic technique [46].

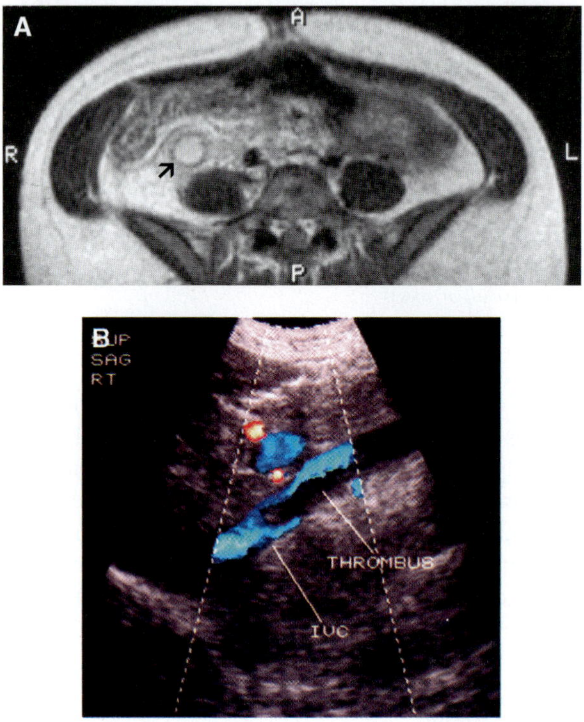

Fig. 8. Septic thrombophlebitis in a postpartum patient. (*A*) MRI showing a thrombosis in the right ovarian vein (*arrow*). (*B*) Sonography displaying a large thrombus in the inferior vena cava (IVC) originating from the ovarian vein.

Summary

The usefulness of sonography, plain film, CT, and MRI in diagnosing infections in pregnancy was discussed. Imaging modality choices for specific clinical indications in pregnancy were reviewed. The overall safety of most techniques in pregnancy was emphasized.

References

[1] American College of Obstetricians and Gynecologists. Committee Opinion. Number 299, September 2004. Guidelines for diagnostic imaging during pregnancy. Obstet Gynecol 2004;104:647–51.
[2] El-Khoury GY, Madsen MT, Blake ME, et al. A new pregnancy policy for a new area. AJR Am J Roentgenol 2003;181:335–40.
[3] Cunningham FG, Gant NF, Leveno KJ, et al. Williams obstetrics. 21st edition. New York: McGraw-Hill; 2001.
[4] Leyendecker JR, Gorengaut V, Brown JJ. MR imaging of maternal diseases of the abdomen and pelvis during pregnancy and the immediate postpartum period. Radiographics 2004;24(5): 1301–16.
[5] Gilstrap III LC, Little BB. Drugs and pregnancy. 2nd edition. New York: Chapman & Hall; 1998.
[6] Borum SE, McLeskey CH, Williamson JB, et al. Epidural abscess after obstetric epidural analgesia. Anesthesiology 1995;82(6):1523–6.
[7] Hlavin ML, Kaminski HJ, Ross JS, et al. Spinal epidural abscess: a ten-year perspective. Neurosurgery 1990;27(2):177–84.
[8] Schroeder TH, Krueger WA, Neeser E, et al. Spinal epidural abscess–a rare complication after epidural analgesia for labour and delivery. Br J Anaesth 2004;92(6):896–8.
[9] Falcone S, Post MJ. Encephalitis, cerebritis, and brain abscess: pathophysiology and imaging findings. Neuroimaging Clin N Am 2000;10(2):333–53.
[10] Wax JR, Pinette MG, Blackstone J, et al. Brain abscess complicating pregnancy. Obstet Gynecol Surv 2004;59(3):207–13.
[11] Ramsey PS, Ramin KD. Pneumonia in pregnancy. Obstet Gynecol Clin North Am 2001; 28(3):553–69.
[12] Lim WS, Macfarlane JT, Colthorpe CL. Pneumonia and pregnancy. Thorax 2001;56(5): 398–405.
[13] Montoya ME, Karnath BM, Ahmad M. Endocarditis during pregnancy. South Med J 2003; 96(11):1156–7.
[14] Cox SM, Hankins GD, Leveno KJ, et al. Bacterial endocarditis. A serious pregnancy complication. J Reprod Med 1988;33(7):671–4.
[15] Ristic AD, Seferovic PM, Ljubic A, et al. Pericardial disease in pregnancy. Herz 2003;28(3): 209–15.
[16] Doshi S, Zucker SD. Liver emergencies during pregnancy. Gastroenterol Clin North Am 2003;32(4):1213–27.
[17] Mortele KJ, Barish MA, Yucel KE. Fulminant herpes hepatitis in an immunocompetent pregnant woman: CT imaging features. Abdom Imaging 2004;29(6):682–4.
[18] Cobey FC, Salem RR. A review of liver masses in pregnancy and a proposed algorithm for their diagnosis and management. Am J Surg 2004;187(2):181–91.
[19] Read KM, Kennedy-Andrews S, Gordon DL. Amoebic liver abscess in pregnancy. Aust N Z J Obstet Gynaecol 2001;41(2):236–7.
[20] Dildy GA, Belfort MA, Saade GR, et al. Critical care obstetrics. 4th ed. Malden (MA): Blackwell Science; 2004.

[21] Elamin Ali M, Yahia Al-Shehri S, Abu-Eshy M, et al. Is surgical intervention in acute cholecystitis in pregnancy justified? J Obstet Gynaecol 1997;17(5):435–8.
[22] Laurila J, Syrjala H, Laurila PA, et al. Acute acalculous cholecystitis in critically ill patients. Acta Anaesthesiol Scand 2004;48(8):986–91.
[23] Yusoff IF, Barkun JS, Barkun AN. Diagnosis and management of cholecystitis and cholangitis. Gastroenterol Clin North Am 2003;32(4):1145–68.
[24] Allmendinger N, Hallisey MJ, Ohki SK, et al. Percutaneous cholecystostomy treatment of acute cholecystitis in pregnancy. Obstet Gynecol 1995;86(4 Pt 2):653–4.
[25] Simmons DC, Tarnasky PR, Rivera-Alsina ME, et al. Endoscopic retrograde cholangiopancreatography (ERCP) in pregnancy without the use of radiation. Am J Obstet Gynecol 2004; 190(5):1467–9.
[26] Bagci S, Tuzun A, Erdil A, et al. Treatment of choledocholithiasis in pregnancy: a case report. Arch Gynecol Obstet 2003;267(4):239–41.
[27] Andersen B, Nielsen TF. Appendicitis in pregnancy: diagnosis, management and complications. Acta Obstet Gynecol Scand 1999;78(9):758–62.
[28] Ueberrueck T, Koch A, Meyer L, et al. Ninety-four appendectomies for suspected acute appendicitis during pregnancy. World J Surg 2004;28(5):508–11.
[29] Lim HK, Bae SH, Seo GS. Diagnosis of acute appendicitis in pregnant women: value of sonography. Am J Roentgenol 1992;159:539–42.
[30] Cobben LP, Groot I, Haans L, et al. MRI for clinically suspected appendicitis during pregnancy. Am J Roentgenol 2004;183(3):671–5.
[31] Ames Castro M, Shipp TD, Castro EE, et al. The use of helical computed tomography in pregnancy for the diagnosis of acute appendicitis. Am J Obstet Gynecol 2001;184(5):954–7.
[32] Ramin KD, Ramin SM, Richey SD, et al. Acute pancreatitis in pregnancy. Am J Obstet Gynecol 1995;173(1):187–91.
[33] Gosnell JE, O'Neill BB, Harris HW. Necrotizing pancreatitis during pregnancy: a rare cause and review of the literature. J Gastrointest Surg 2001;5(4):371–6.
[34] Arvanitakis M, Delhaye M, De Maertelaere V, et al. Computed tomography and magnetic resonance imaging in the assessment of acute pancreatitis. Gastroenterology 2004;126(3):715–23.
[35] Sherer DM, Schwartz BM, Abulafia O. Management of pelvic abscess during pregnancy: a case and review of the literature. Obstet Gynecol Surv 1999;54(10):655–62.
[36] Matsunaga Y, Fukushima K, Nozaki M, et al. A case of pregnancy complicated by the development of a tubo-ovarian abscess following in vitro fertilization and embryo transfer. Am J Perinatol 2003;20(6):277–82.
[37] MacLean AB. Urinary tract infection in pregnancy. Int J Antimicrob Agents 2001;17:273–7.
[38] Wing DA. Pyelonephritis in pregnancy: treatment options for optimal outcomes. Drugs 2001; 61(14):2087–96.
[39] Johansen TE. The role of imaging in urinary tract infections. World J Urol 2004;22(5):392–8.
[40] McAleer SJ, Loughlin KR. Nephrolithiasis and pregnancy. Curr Opin Urol 2004;14(2):123–7.
[41] Athanasopoulos A, Petsas T, Fokaefs E, et al. Paranephric abscess during pregnancy: a case for a low-dose interventional CT. Urol Int 2004;73:185–7.
[42] Saylam K, Anaf V, Kirkpatrick C. Successful medical management of multifocal psoas abscess following cesarean section: report of a case and review of the literature. Eur J Obstet Gynecol Reprod Biol 2002;102(2):211–4.
[43] Kawamura K, Sekiguchi K, Shibata S, et al. Primary psoas abscess during pregnancy. Acta Obstet Gynecol Scand 2000;79(2):151–2.
[44] Brown CE, Stettler RW, Twickler D, et al. Puerperal septic pelvic thrombophlebitis: incidence and response to heparin therapy. Am J Obstet Gynecol 1999;181(1):143–8.
[45] Twickler DM, Setiawan AT, Evans RS, et al. Imaging of puerperal septic thrombophlebitis: prospective comparison of MR imaging, CT, and sonography. Am J Roentgenol 1997;169: 1039–43.
[46] Leibovitz Z, Degani S, Shapiro I, et al. Diagnosis of pregnancy-associated uterine venous plexus thrombosis on the basis of transvaginal sonography. J Ultrasound Med 2003;22(3):287–93.

ELSEVIER
SAUNDERS

Clin Perinatol 32 (2005) 803–814

CLINICS IN
PERINATOLOGY

Postpartum Endometritis

Sebastian Faro, MD, PhD

Department of Obstetrics, Gynecology, and Reproductive Sciences, The University of Texas Houston Health Sciences Center, 7400 Fannin, Suite 840, Houston, TX 77054, USA

Postpartum endometritis is a term that applies to a spectrum of infections: infection of the endometrial lining, the myometrium, and the parametrium. In the late 1970s and the early 1980s the term was used to imply the severity of infection. Postpartum endometritis defined a mild stage of infection involving the endometrium or inner lining of the uterine cavity and the superficial myometrium. Endomyometritis was a moderate stage of infection that involved the inner lining of the uterus and penetrated the full thickness of the myometrium. Endomyoparametritis, a severe infection, implied that the infection progressed from the inner lining of the uterus through the myometrium and extended into the parametrium (ie, the broad ligaments) [1]. The latter infection could also involve the mesosalpinx and fallopian tubes, and typically exosalpingitis occurs, not endosalpingitis, thereby avoiding any residual damage to the internal structure of the fallopian tubes. It is rare that a patient who suffers from endomyoparametritis develops any degree of infertility. Although these terms were used to denote the seriousness of postpartum endometritis, all uterine infections should be considered serious. Infection caused by either *Streptococcus pyogenes* (group A streptococcus [GAS]) or *Streptococcus agalactiae* (group B streptococcus [GBS]) are associated with significant morbidity and mortality, especially the former bacterium [2–5].

It is not infrequent that a patient developing postpartum endometritis coincidentally develops an abdominal incision infection (surgical site infection [SSI]). It is important to recognize the development of concomitant endometritis and SSI because the patient may develop an uterocutaneous fistula. The presence of an uterocutaneous fistula may indicate that the patient has developed necrotizing myositis of the uterus. This is an infection that does not respond to antibiotic therapy and requires surgery. The microbiology of SSI is usually derived from the patient's own skin microflora (eg, *Staphylococcus aureus*),

doi:10.1016/j.clp.2005.04.005 *perinatology.theclinics.com*

including community-acquired, methicillin-resistant strains (MRSA) and the patient's own endogenous vaginal microflora. The infection can be caused solely by skin microorganisms, solely by organisms derived from the endogenous microflora, or both. SSI can occur independently of endometritis, may accompany endometritis, or may be related to and communicate with endometritis. It is important when evaluating a patient who has an SSI, postpartum endometritis, or both that the physician considers the origin of the bacteria most likely to cause the infection. The best defense in dealing with postoperative infection, whether the patient is undergoing obstetric or gynecologic surgery, is to take measures to reduce her risk of developing a postoperative infection as well as to recognize the subtle signs of a developing infection. Every patient undergoing pelvic surgery should be considered at risk for developing a postoperative pelvic infection or SSI. The degree of risk can be related to several factors: (1) the body mass index (BMI), (2) the state of her vaginal microflora at the time of the operative procedure, (3) previous recent exposure to antibiotic therapy, (4) the presence of underlying chronic illness, and (5) the use of immunosuppressive medication [6–8].

Epidemiology

Approximately 10% of patients delivering by cesarean section and approximately 5% delivering vaginally develop postpartum endometritis [9]. The patients most likely to develop postpartum endometritis are those who either have chorioamnionitis or have a prolonged labor. Labor, especially in the presence of ruptured amniotic membranes, allows for bacteria from the vagina to ascend to the cervix, thus allowing bacteria to gain access to the uterine cavity. Risk factors associated with the development of postpartum endometritis or surgical site infections are listed below:

- Prolonged labor with ruptured amniotic membranes
- Lack of prenatal care
- Delivery by cesarean section following prolonged labor with ruptured membranes
- Cesarean delivery in a patient who has a BMI >25
- Use of intrauterine monitoring
- Multiple vaginal examinations
- Altered vaginal microflora (eg, bacterial vaginosis, heavy vaginal colonization by *S agalactiae* or *Escherichia coli*)
- Nasal carriage of *Staphylococcus aureus*

Microbial pathophysiology

Postpartum endometritis originates during labor as bacteria from the lower genital tract ascend into the cervix (these bacteria are listed in Box 1). Once colonization of the cervix has occurred, bacteria can ascend to the lower seg-

Box 1. Bacteria that constitute endogenous vaginal microflora

Lactobacillus crispatus, L casei, L jansei
Corynebacterium
Diphtheroids
Alpha hemolytic streptococci
Nondescript streptococci
Staphylococcus epidermidis
E coli
Enterobacter agglomerans, E cloacae, E aerogenes
Klebsiella pneumoniae
Morganella morgagnii
Fusobacterium necrophorum
Eubacterium
Prevotella bivia, P melaninogenicus
Mycoplasma genitalia, M hominis
Ureaplasma urealyticum

ment of the uterus, colonizing the decidua and gaining entrance to the amniotic fluid. In fact, membranes do not present a barrier to infection of the amniotic fluid once the bacteria have traversed the endocervical canal. Colonization of the amniotic fluid can be achieved by bacteria colonizing the amniotic membranes, then migrating across the intact membranes or causing the membranes to rupture. Bacteria can both colonize the amniotic membranes and grow on them. Through the production of collagenases and proteases, the amniotic membranes are weakened and eventually rupture. Artificial or spontaneous rupture of membranes can occur in the absence of bacterial colonization, but this will allow bacteria to colonize the decidua and amniotic fluid. If the bacteria fail to colonize the decidua, an amnionitis can develop in the absence of a deciduitis, and the uterus may not become infected, even though the patient has chorioamnionitis; however, deciduitis can lead to infection of the myometrium and this infection may initially go unnoticed. Following delivery, if these patients received appropriate antibiotic therapy, they are unlikely to develop postpartum endometritis.

If conditions favor bacterial growth, during labor the bacteria that have colonized the decidua will invade the myometrium and reproduce. This process can continue during labor, even though the patient is asymptomatic.

Once bacteria gain entrance to the amniotic fluid, they reproduce and significantly increase in number. The aerobic and facultative anaerobic bacteria increase from 10^2 to 10^6 bacteria/ml of amniotic fluid or more, and obligate anaerobic bacteria increase from 10^2 to 10^4 bacteria/ml of amniotic fluid or more over a 12-hour period [10].

This infection, postpartum endometritis, can be mild, moderate, or severe, and can develop into a necrotizing myometritis of the uterus or necrotizing fasciitis of the abdominal wall. Though infrequently, these latter infections do tend to occur with *S pyogenes* (GAS) and *S agalactiae* (GBS). These infections can also be polymicrobial and can involve the endogenous bacteria of the lower genital tract. Although the gram-positive bacteria produce a variety of endotoxins, the gram-negative bacteria produce exotoxins that cause a spectrum of clinical abnormalities.

The endogenous bacteria of the lower genital tract comprise a variety of gram-positive and gram-negative bacteria (see Box 1, above). Other bacteria such as *S agalactiae* and *Bacteroides fragilis*, as well as other members of the *B fragilis* group, can be found in the vagina.

A healthy endogenous vaginal microflora is characterized by the dominant bacterium of *Lactobacillus crispatus*, *L casei*, or *L jensenii*. Lactobacilli are present in a concentration of 10^6 bacteria/ml of vaginal fluid or more. The other bacteria are present in a concentration of less than 10^3 bacteria/ml of vaginal fluid. The ratio of lactobacilli to other bacteria is important because it is highly probable that when lactobacilli dominate, the risk of infection is small. *Lactobacillus* maintains dominance through the production of: (1) organic acids, mainly lactic acid, thus maintaining the vaginal pH between more than 3.8 and less than 4.5; (2) hydrogen peroxide, which is converted in the powerful oxidizing agents destructive to bacterial DNA that do not produce catalase; and (3) bacteriocin, a low–molecular weight protein that inhibits the growth of bacteria. Anything that upsets the pH balance, causing it to rise, or a decrease in the hydrogen ion concentration will result in the growth of bacteria other than the lactobacilli, and the suppression of lactobacilli. This change in the vaginal ecosystem can result in any number of bacteria becoming dominant, thus resulting in bacterial vaginosis (BV), GBS overgrowth, or *E coli* dominance [11,12]. Once the endogenous vaginal microflora undergoes a shift (eg, BV or GBS), the bacteria reach such high numbers that the inoculum is sufficient to initiate infection.

The gram-negative bacteria represent a group of virulent bacteria that can potentially cause severe infection resulting in septic shock and death. The gram-positive bacteria (eg, *S agalactiae*, *S pyogenes*, and *S aureus*, can cause severe infection resulting in septic shock and death. These bacteria can act in concert with gram-negative facultative and obligate anaerobic bacteria to cause infection. *S agalactiae* and *S pyogenes* can induce thrombosis of the myometrial vasculature thereby preventing antibiotics, oxygen, and nutrients from perfusing the myometrium. Hypoxia of myometrial cells results in apoptosis, eventually causing necrosis of the myometrium (ie, necrotizing myositis).

Clinical presentation and diagnosis

Postpartum endometritis can occur immediately following delivery or several days later. The time postpartum endometritis develops depends upon: (1) when the process actually started, (2) the duration of labor in the presence of ruptured membranes, (3) the status of the endogenous microflora at the time of labor, and (4) the actual bacterium or bacteria causing the infection. Patients entering active labor with an altered vaginal microflora or bacterial vaginosis are at significant risk for the development of postpartum endometritis. Bacteria such as *S agalactiae* (GBS), *S pyogenes* (GAS), and *E coli*, as well as other gram-negative facultative anaerobic bacteria, definitely place the laboring patient, especially one requiring cesarean delivery, at significant risk for the development of postpartum endometritis [4,8,13].

There is no doubt that the patient who labors with ruptured membranes for a prolonged period will have her decidua colonized by bacteria from the vagina. These bacteria have the ability to invade the myometrium and cause infection before delivery, even if the patient is asymptomatic. Clinical clues that infection may be developing are a rise in body temperature and a simultaneous rise in the maternal pulse rate. Patients who experience a difficult labor do not undergo progressive cervical change and descent of the present fetal part. A white blood cell (WBC) count that continues to rise and an associated increase in immature polymorpholeukocytes should alert the physician that the patient is developing chorioamnionitis. After recognition of these subtle signs, even though the patient may not have developed a fever (ie, an oral body temperature of 101°F or higher), the physician should initiate oral antibiotics, especially if the patient is delivered by cesarean section. Clinical signs of postpartum endometritis include the following:

- Oral body temperature ≥101°F at any time, or a temperature of 100.4°F measured on two separate occasions at least 6 hours apart
- A tachycardia that parallels the temperature
- Uterine tenderness
- A purulent vaginal discharge
- Associated findings with advanced endometritis (dynamic ileus, elvic peritonitis, pelvic abscess, bowel obstruction, necrosis of the lower uterine segment)

Postoperatively, patients who have an oral temperature of 101°F and a simultaneous tachycardia should be considered infected until proven otherwise. Delay in further evaluation and initiation of antibiotic therapy only worsens the infection and increases morbidity and the risk of death. Patients whose temperature is between 99.9°F and 101°F should have their temperature taken hourly until a directional trend is established. Individuals who have a temperature that is trending downward and normal vital signs do not need to be evaluated at that time; however, those whose temperature is trending upward should be evaluated as follows:

A complete review of current medications. Determine the possibility of drug fever.

A complete physical examination. Determine if there is a physical finding of infection (eg, pneumonia, pyelonephritis, endometritis, surgical site infection).

A complete white blood cell count with differential. An increase in both indicates infection.

Obtain serum electrolytes, blood urea nitrogen, creatinine, and glucose. A normal glucose indicates that WBC can phagocytize bacteria, and hypoglycemia indicates that sepsis may be present and phagocytosis is impaired.

Urine should be obtained via a catheterized specimen to avoid contamination from the vaginal lochia.

Imaging studies (ie, pelvic and abdominal ultrasonography or CT scan) should be obtained if indicated.

Pelvic examination should include obtaining specimens of the decidua for isolation, cultivation, identification and antibiotic sensitivities.

Patients who have tachycapnia or shortness of breath should have their oxygen saturation determined. Individuals who have abnormal oxygen saturation should have a chest radiograph and arterial blood gases to determine if there is atelectasis, pneumonia, or pulmonary embolus

Blood cultures should be obtained from individuals who experience shaking chills or rigors. Ideally, venous blood should be obtained at the time the temperature spike occurs or when the patient is experiencing rigors. Two sets of blood cultures should be obtained approximately 20 to 30 minutes apart. The blood culture bottles should be checked daily, preferably every 12 hours, to determine if there is growth in the media. If growth is detected, a Gram's stain should be performed and the physician notified of the characteristics of the bacteria growing in the blood culture bottles. The number of bottles exhibiting growth should also be reported. Growth in one bottle may represent a contamination; whereas growth in two or more bottles of the same bacterium should be interpreted as the patient being bacteremic.

Surgical site infection, abdominal incision or episiotomy site, is usually indicated by one or more of the following characteristics:

Advancing erythema (indicates cellulitis)

Induration (indicates that the infection involves the dermis and subcutaneous tissue)

Skin changes (ie, a sheen, edema, orange skin [pau d'orange]) or tense appearance

Drainage that can be serous, cloudy serous, dark brown or tea-like, serosanguinous, purulent, or bloody

Pain, which may be extreme

Areas of blackened discoloration

Response to gentle palpation

A suspicious surgical site infection should be evaluated as follows:

Ultrasonography or CT scan of the surgical site should be performed to determine if there is a fluid collection.

Aspiration of the fluid with a sterile needle and syringe

Gram's stain the fluid, and culture for aerobic, facultative, and obligate anaerobic bacteria

Gram's stain characteristics of the fluid can be extremely helpful in the management of a surgical site infection:

Fluid is serous and there are no white blood cells or bacteria = seroma
Fluid is cloudy, serous, and white cells are present but no bacteria are seen = probable *Mycoplasma* or *Ureaplasma* infection
Fluid is purulent, white cells are present and gram-positive cocci in chains are seen = *S agalactiae*, *S pyogenes*. or other *Streptococcus* sp
Same as item 3 above, but gram-positive cocci in clusters=*S aureus* (assume MRSA) or other *Staphylococcus* sp
Same as item 3 above, but gram-negative rods = facultative anaerobe
Same as item 3 above, with a foul odor and gram-positive cocci, rods or both = polymicrobial anaerobic infection
Same as item 3 above, but gram-positive cocci and gram-negative rods, no odor = polymicrobial infection

If the CT scan of the pelvis and abdomen reveals the presence of gas at the surgical site, aspiration should be performed and then the patient should immediately be taken to the operating room. Once anesthesia has been administered and the patient prepped and draped, the patient's incision should be completely opened. All necrotic tissue should be debrided and the surgical site thoroughly irrigated with saline or antibiotic solution (eg, bacitracin, 50,000 units plus kanamycin, 1 g in a liter of normal saline). The incision should be packed with moistened gauze, (eg, 0.25% acetic acid), and the packing should be changed three to four times daily. Dressing changes should be continued until a complete layer of granulation tissue forms over the surface of the surgical site. After this occurs, the incision can be closed or allowed to close by secondary intention.

During the initial surgical site examination, the wound and surrounding area should be palpated. If the patient responds that there is significant pain, and the pain is extremely severe to gentle palpation radiating out a significant distance (eg, 2 to 3 cm), consider the possibility of necrotizing fasciitis. Progression to advanced necrotizing fasciitis of the surgical incision is characterized by advancing cellulitis, necrosis as areas of blackened skin appear, and liquification of the underlying tissue. The patient becomes septic and develops the hallmarks of septic shock. The patient's WBC count also may be extremely high (eg, high 20,000 to low 30,000) with hypotension, rapid respiratory rate, oliguria, and cold clammy skin. Continuation of the septic process results in organ failure and eventually death [14].

Antibiotic management

Early postpartum endometritis

This is typically a unimicrobial infection with uterine tenderness, failure of the uterus to involute, and the cervix remains dilated. Antibiotic choices are:

- Piperacillin/tazobactam, 3.375 g IV every 6 hours; this antibiotic provides good coverage against gram-positive and gram-negative facultative anaerobes, as well as gram-positive and gram-negative obligate anaerobes
- Ampicillin/sulbactam, 3.1 g every 6 hours, plus gentamicin, 5 mg/kg of body weight every 24 hours
- Clindamycin 900 mg IV every 8 hours, which is active against 80% of GBS, *S aureus* including MRSA, and obligate anaerobes, plus gentamicin, 5 mg/kg of body weight every 24 hours, which provides excellent coverage against gram-negative facultative anaerobes and provides activity against MRSA
- Metronidazole, 500 mg every 8 hours, provides good activity against gram-negative facultative anaerobes, plus gentamicin, 5 mg/kg of body weight every 24 hours

Late postpartum metritis

This is typically a polymicrobial infection that involves both facultative and obligate anaerobes. Antibiotic choices are:

- Piperacillin/tazobactam, 3.375 g IV every 6 hours plus gentamicin, 5 mg/kg of body weight every 24 hours; this combination provides enhanced gram-negative facultative coverage, and the two antibiotics act synergistically against GBS and enterococci
- Clindamycin, 900 mg IV every 8 hours plus gentamicin, 5 mg/kg of body weight every 24 hours plus ampicillin, 2 g IV every 6 hours; the last two antibiotics act synergistically to provide activity against *Enterococci* and GBS
- Metronidazole, 500 mg IV every 8 hours plus gentamicin plus ampicillin

Evaluating the patient failing to respond to antibiotic therapy

Antibiotic therapy administered early in the infection will usually produce a positive response within 48 hours of its initiation [1,15,16]. Patients not demonstrating a positive response or whose condition is deteriorating should be re-evaluated for their failure to respond to therapy. Differential diagnosis for patients failing antibiotic therapy includes the following:

- The emergence of a resistant bacterium
- Development of a pelvic or surgical site abscess
- Inappropriate dosing of antibiotic therapy
- Antibiotic therapy started late
- Wrong diagnosis
- Septic pelvic vein thrombosis
- Thrombosis of the microvasculature of the myometrium
- Necrosis of the myometrium
- Drug fever

Because most patients delivered by cesarean section receive antibiotic prophylaxis, there is the potential for selection of a resistant bacterium. Studies have demonstrated that with the administration of a single dose of a cephalosporin there is a sixfold increase in enterococcal colonization of the lower genital tract [17,18]. There is also potential for the selection of resistant gram-negative facultative anaerobes toward the cephalosporins.

If a culture of the endometrium was obtained at the initial evaluation, the culture plates incubated in an aerobic atmosphere should reveal growth by 48 hours, if aerobic or facultative anaerobic bacteria are involved in the infection. Bacteria that are present on the agar plates can then be Gram's stained and additions to the present antibiotic therapy can be made. These are outlined in Box 2.

If adjustments to the initial antibiotic therapy were made and the physical examination was unrewarding (no mass was detected), but the patient did exhibit pain in the pelvic region, consider imaging studies. CT scan or ultrasonogram of the pelvis will assist in determining if a fluid collection is present. If a mass is present and is located in the cul-de-sac, it may be conducive to draining through a colpotomy incision. A fluid collection (ie, abscess or infected hematoma) may be drained percutaneously. If the physical examination is unremarkable, the imaging studies do not reveal any fluid collection, and there is no evidence of surgical site inflammation; the patient may have drug fever.

Drug fever can be diagnosed by noting the absence of any physical findings, and a pulse rate that does not vary significantly and does not parallel the patient's temperature. A WBC count may demonstrate an eosinophilia, but a rise in eosinophils occurs only in a small number of patients who have drug fever. In the case of drug fever, all nonessential medications, including antibiotics, should be discontinued. The fever should resolve within 24 to 96 hours of discontinuing all medications. If the patient exhibits a spike in temperature, however, then an entire evaluation should be performed. If an infection is suspected, antibiotic therapy should be reinstituted. This time it would be preferable not to use the same class of antibiotics that was previously administered.

Box 2. Adjustment to empirically administered antibiotic therapy

Initial antibiotic therapy

Piperacillin/tazobactam or ampicillin/sulbactam

- Gram's stain reveals gram-positive cocci, mostly *Enterococcus* or *Staphylococcus*—add gentamicin
- Gram's stain reveals presence gram-negative bacilli, most likely facultative anaerobe (eg, *E coli*)—add gentamicin

Piperacillin/tazobactam + gentamicin

- Gram's stain reveals gram-negative bacilli, most likely a resistant facultative anaerobe—change gentamicin to amikacin

Clindamycin + gentamicin

- Gram's stain reveals gram-positive cocci—add ampicillin
- Gram's stain reveals gram-negative bacilli—change gentamicin to amikacin

Metronidazole + gentamicin

- Gram's stain reveals gram-positive cocci—add ampicillin
- Gram's stain reveals gram-negative bacilli—change gentamicin to amikacin

Venous blood should be obtained to inoculate liquid medium (blood culture bottles) any time there is a suspicion of bacteremia, if the patient has rigors, or if she has failed antibiotic therapy. There are no specific signs or clinical findings on examination that indicate a patient has bacteremia, so the physician should check with the laboratory daily to determine if there is growth in the blood culture bottles.

Summary

Postpartum endometritis or a surgical site infection should be suspected if the patient develops an elevated oral temperature, of 100.4°F or higher with an associated tachycardia at any time following the procedure. A tachycardia that parallels the temperature is strongly indicative of infection. A thorough physical and pelvic examination should be performed. A complete blood count with WBC differential, serum electrolytes, blood urea nitrogen, creatinine, glucose, urine analysis, urine culture, and sensitivity also should be obtained. Patients failing to respond to initial antibiotic therapy in a positive manner should be thoroughly evaluated for the possible emergence of a resistant bacterium or the development of an abscess or septic pelvic thrombosis. Antibiotic therapy should be continued until the patient is afebrile for 24 to 48 hours, the WBC count returns to normal for that particular patient, and the patient is tolerating oral liquids and solids, and ambulating without difficulty.

When considering if a patient is ready for discharge, it is crucial to ensure that:

- her body temperature has been between 97.6°F and 99.6°F for the preceding 24 to 48 hours;
- her pulse rate has been within the normal range for the preceding 24 to 48 hours;
- she is tolerating oral liquids and solids;
- she is ambulating without difficulty;
- she is passing flatus and has active bowel sounds;
- she is micturating without difficulty; and
- the incision is without erythema, induration, edema, drainage, or significant pain.

References

[1] Faro S, Phillips LE, Baker JL, et al. Comparative efficacy and safety of mezlocillin, cefoxitin, and clindamycin plus gentamicin in postpartum endometritis. Obstet Gynecol 1987;69:760–6.

[2] Udagawa H, Oshio Y, Shimizu Y. Serious group A streptococcal infection around delivery. Obstet Gynecol 1999;94:153–7.

[3] Silver RM, Heddleston LN, McGregor JA, et al. Life-threatening puerperal infection due to group A streptococci. Obstet Gynecol 1992;79:894–6.

[4] Faro S. Group B streptococcus and puerperal sepsis. Am J Obstet Gynecol 1980;138:1219–20.

[5] Faro S. Group B beta-hemolytic streptococci and puerperal infections. Am J Obstet Gynecol 1981;139:686–9.

[6] Myles TD, Gooch J, Santolaya J. Obesity as an independent risk factor for infectious morbidity in patients who undergo cesarean delivery. Obstet Gynecol 2002;100:959–64.

[7] Tran TS, Jamulitrat S, Chongsuvivatwong V, et al. Risk factors for postcesarean surgical site infection. Obstet Gynecol 2000;95:367–71.

[8] Martens MG, Kolrud BL, Faro S, et al. Development of wound infection or separation after cesarean delivery. Prospective evaluation of 2431 cases. J Reprod Med 1995;40(3):171–5.

[9] Duff P. Pathophysiology and management of postcesarean endomyometritis. Obstet Gynecol 1986;67:269–76.

[10] Pinell P, Faro S, Roberts S, et al. Intrauterine pressure catheter in labor: associated microbiology. Infect Dis Obstet Gynecol 1993;1:60–4.

[11] Faro S, Phillips LE, Martens MG. Perspectives on the bacteriology of postoperative obstetric-gynecologic infections. Am J Obstet Gynecol 1988;158:694–700.

[12] Hillier SL, Kiviat NB, Hawes SE, et al. Role of bacterial vaginosis associated microorganisms in endometritis. Am J Obstet Gynecol 1996;175:435–41.

[13] Stefonek KR, Maerz LL, Nielsen MP, et al. Group A streptococcal puerperal sepsis preceded by positive surveillance cultures. Obstet Gynecol 2001;98:846–8.

[14] Faro S. Sepsis in obstetric and gynecologic patients. In: Remington JS, Swartz MN, editors. Current clinical topics in infectious diseases. Cambridge (MA): Blackwell Science; 1999. p. 60–82.

[15] Martens MG, Faro S, Hammill HA, et al. Metronidazole/gentamicin vs. Sulbactam/ampicillin

in the treatment of post-cesarean section endometritis. Diagn Microbiol Infect Dis 1989;12: 189s–94s.

[16] Sweet RL, Roy S, Faro S, et al. Piperacillin and tazobactam versus clindamycin and gentamicin in the treatment of hospitalized women with pelvic infection. The Piperacillin/tazobactam Study Group. Obstet Gynecol 1994;83:280–6.

[17] Faro S, Martens MG, Hammill HA, et al. Antibiotic prophylaxis: is there a difference? Am J Obstet Gynecol 1990;162:900–7.

[18] Faro S, Cox SM, Phillips LE, et al. Influence of antibiotic prophylaxis on vaginal microflora. Am J Obstet Gynecol 1986;6(Suppl):4s–8s.

ELSEVIER
SAUNDERS

Clin Perinatol 32 (2005) 815–824

CLINICS IN
PERINATOLOGY

Index

Note: Page numbers of article titles are in **boldface** type.

doi:10.1016/S0095-5108(05)00078-3

Q

R

S

ETHICAL REASONING IN ACCOUNTING AND AUDITING

by
Lawrence A. Ponemon
and
David R. L. Gabhart

CGA-Canada
Research Foundation

La Fondation de recherche
de CGA-Canada

Research Monograph Number 21

Canadian Cataloguing in Publication Data

Ponemon, Lawrence A.
Ethical reasoning in accounting and auditing

(Research monograph ; no. 21)
Includes bibliographical references.
ISBN 0-919521-45-2

1. Accountants—Professional ethics—Canada. 2. Accountants—Professional ethics—United States. 3. Auditors—Professional ethics—Canada. 4. Auditors—Professional ethics—United States. **I.** Gabhart, David R. L. **II.** CGA-Canada Research Foundation. **III.** Title. **IV.** Series: Research monograph (CGA-Canada Research Foundation) ; no. 21.
HF5616.C2P65 1993 174'.9657'0971 C93-091368-X

Ordering information is available from:
CGA-Canada Research Foundation
700-1188 West Georgia Street
Vancouver, BC Canada V6E 4A2
Telephone: (604) 669-3555
Facsimile: (604) 689-5845

ISBN 0-919521-45-2